Choices and Conflict

Explorations in
Health Care Ethics

Emily Friedman, Editor

AHA books are published by American Hospital Publishing, Inc., an American Hospital Association company.

The views expressed in this publication are strictly those of the authors and do not necessarily represent official positions of the American Hospital Association.

Library of Congress Cataloging-in-Publication Data

Choices and conflict : explorations in health care ethics / Emily Friedman, editor.
       p.   cm.
    Includes bibliographical references.
    ISBN 1-55648-082-2 (paperback)
    1. Medical ethics. I. Friedman, Emily.
  R724.C485   1992
  174'.2—dc20   92-8416
                                                                     CIP

Catalog no. 025105

©1992 by American Hospital Publishing, Inc.,
an American Hospital Association company

Printed in the USA

AHA is a service mark of the American Hospital Association used under license by American Hospital Publishing, Inc.

Text set in Garamond
4M/92—0318

Audrey Kaufman, Project Editor
Nancy Charpentier, Editorial Assistant
Marcia Bottoms, Managing Editor
Peggy DuMais, Production Coordinator
Luke Smith, Designer
Brian Schenk, Books Division Director

To the memory of David M. Kinzer, 1920–1990

Judgment is facts passed through values.
—Ray Brown

Contents

About the Editor

Emily Friedman is a health policy analyst, writer, and lecturer with a longstanding interest in bioethics and the social ethics of health care. She is contributing editor of *Hospitals and Healthcare Forum Journal* (for which she writes a bimonthly ethics column), and she is a contributing writer to the *Journal of the American Medical Association, Health Business, Health Management Quarterly,* and *Health Progress,* among other periodicals. She is a member of the editorial boards of *Health Management Quarterly* and the *Journal of Rural Health.* Ms. Friedman was Rockefeller Fellow in Ethics at Dartmouth College in 1987–1988 and currently is an adjunct assistant professor at the Boston University School of Public Health, where she teaches a course in health care rationing. Ms. Friedman was the editor of the previous volume in this series, *Making Choices: Ethics Issues for Health Care Professionals* (American Hospital Publishing, 1986). She is based in Chicago.

Foreword

The 1990s is the decade of ethics, ethics, ethics.

For example, what is a human life worth? Does the worth of a human life depend upon:

- What country, state, or city a person lives in?
- The color of a person's skin?
- The person's age?
- Gender?
- Sexual preference?
- Whether the person:
  - Has an IQ of 200 or 50?
  - Is a heart surgeon or a jaundiced newborn?
  - Is a violinist or has Alzheimer's disease?
  - Is a baseball pitcher or a quadriplegic?
  - Is a billionaire or an unemployed victim of AIDS?
  - Is a mother of five young children or a convicted felon?
  - Is a social worker or a street heroin addict?
  - Is an ethicist or a functional illiterate?
  - Is primarily productive or primarily consumptive?

Whether covertly or overtly, these questions are being asked and choices made daily. In virtually all societies, rank has its privileges. Is life itself one of these privileges in our society?[1]

In the 1990s we have so much science that is applicable to health and medicine. Some people even say we have too much technology. All members of our expanding population will get sick and all will die, but, on average, they will do so at a substantially older age than just a few years ago. We are using vast resources to prevent disease and treat illness—perhaps $800 billion in our country alone in 1992. We have created, by virtue of all of our successes and resources, an enormous opportunity to succeed, to fail, or just to muddle along.

To whom do we in health care report? Who keeps score? What distinguishes right from wrong? Who decides what we should expend resources for? These are the kinds of choices that challenge the field of medical ethics.

I believe that human beings behave on three fundamental ethical levels:

1. *Personal morality:* Morality is defined as "a quality or fact of conforming to or deriving from right ideas of human conduct; goodness and uprightness of behavior."[2]
2. *Societal ethics:* Ethics are "principles of conduct governing an individual or profession; the ideals of character manifested by a people."[3]
3. *Public law:* Law is "a rule or mode of conduct or action that is formally recognized as binding by a supreme controlling authority and is made obligatory by a sanction."[4]

I believe that these three controllers of human behavior represent a hierarchy, at the top of which is personal morality. If personal morality and/or societal ethics were widespread and powerful enough, there would be no need for public laws. The mere existence of public law in a given sphere represents the failure of both personal morality and societal ethics as controllers in that area.

Unfortunately, we have innumerable real and potential laws in the field of medicine and health. These would be unnecessary if morality and ethics were performing well as the best controllers of human behavior.[5]

A major effort, sponsored in part by the Agency for Health Care Policy and Research of the Department of Health and Human Services and sponsored by the American Medical Association and numerous specialty societies, is now under way to develop, evaluate, approve, and implement practice guidelines/standards/parameters/policies and to assess their effects on clinical outcomes. Outcomes research offers great hope that we will be able to document value gained for money spent in medical/health care.

Traditional crude outcome measures have included expected lifespan from birth and neonatal mortality rates. Starfield has recently utilized the following additional indicators of health in evaluating systems across geographic boundaries:[6] postneonatal mortality, total infant mortality, age-adjusted death rate, average life expectancy for males and females separately at 1, 20, and 65 years of age, years of potential life lost, and percentage of birth weights below 2,500 grams.

The Medical Outcomes Study measures the following characteristics[7]:

- Functioning
  - Physical capacity
  - Usual daily activities in role
  - Usual social activities
- Well-being
  - Mental health/mood–affect
  - Rating of current health
  - Bodily pains

I suggest that in addition to these outcomes, we consider measuring personal productivity, satisfaction of specific needs, welfare of the patient's family, the financial well-being of the patient and the family, and complications of diagnostic and therapeutic interventions. Of course, any intervention should be in comparison with *no* intervention.

I know of no one better qualified then Emily Friedman to bring to you a choice selection of reprinted and original articles for this book, *Choices and Conflict: Explorations in Health Care Ethics.* Its predecessor, published by American Hospital Publishing in 1986, was extremely well received. It offered a similar but earlier collection of articles of great value to those innumerable people in our society, both inside and outside medicine, who are interested in these vexing questions.

Reader, consider and be challenged.

References

1. Lundberg, G. D. Rationing human life [editorial]. *JAMA* 249(16):2223–24, Apr. 22–29, 1983.
2. *Webster's New Collegiate Dictionary.* Springfield, MA: G. & C. Merriam Co., 1975.
3. *Webster's New Collegiate Dictionary,* 1975.
4. *Webster's New Collegiate Dictionary,* 1975.
5. Lundberg, G. D. A decade of ethics. *ASCP News,* Aug. 1990, p. 2.
6. Starfield, B. Primary care and health: a cross-national comparison. *JAMA* 266:2268–71, 1991.
7. Tarlov, A. R., Ware, J. E., Greenfield, S., et al. The medical outcomes study. *JAMA* 262(7):925–30, Aug. 18, 1989.

George D. Lundberg, M.D.
Editor, *JAMA*

Preface

In 1986, when the previous volume in this series, *Making Choices: Ethics Issues for Health Care Professionals*, was published, the role of ethics in the provision of health care was still being defined. Relatively few Americans had signed living wills or other advance directives, and many states still had no legislation authorizing the use of such documents. Five years later, on December 1, 1991, the federal law known as the Patient Self-Determination Act went into effect, requiring hospitals and other health care providers to inform patients about state law regarding advance directives and to offer patients the chance to execute such directives.

Six years ago, there was no link between the debate over availability of abortion services and legal cases involving termination of treatment or life support for patients in persistent vegetative states. Today, after abortion rights opponents tried to intervene in the case of Nancy Cruzan, a comatose patient whose parents sought to terminate life support, two volatile, emotional ethics issues have become intertwined.

Back in 1986, most bioethics discussions, publications, and education focused on issues involving the individual patient—termination of treatment, the right to refuse care, the use of surrogates for making health care decisions. Today, social ethics issues such as whether access to health care is a right, what to do about the 35 to 40 million Americans who are uninsured, and especially the prospect (or the reality) of health care rationing are receiving equal attention.

In the mid-1980s, ethics and public policy seemed worlds apart. The stereotypes were of ivory-tower academic ethicists debating how many patients could dance on the head of a pin, and isolated, callous politicians who cared not a whit about human dilemmas. Never, it was said, would the twain meet. Indeed, there were those who wondered whether the policy-oriented 1983 recommendations of the President's Commission for the Study of Ethical Problems in Medicine and Biomedical and Behavioral Research might compromise the pristine purity of the bioethics endeavor.

These days, politicians write about rationing schemes in ethics journals, ethicists address gatherings of state legislators, Congress passes laws regarding advance directives, ethics analysts routinely comment on public policy and health, and ethicists hold positions in government. Times have indeed changed.

On many fronts, the situation has improved. More than 10 percent of the population have executed advance directives, and the often murky legal situation involving termination of treatment has been clarified somewhat—although at any moment the scales could tip back the other way. Ethics advisory committees are commonplace in hospitals and are a growing presence in other health care organizations. Ethics education and discussion in health care professions other than medicine is growing, and community-based ethics education and policy development efforts are ongoing in many states. Bioethical discourse has found its place in the health care sun.

However, I am reminded of a warning issued several years ago by William Campbell, M.D., a physician in St. Louis. Addressing the enormous improvements in health status wrought by the introduction of better public health measures, immunization, antibiotics, and "wonder drug" pharmaceuticals, he observed, "Most of the cheap and easy diseases have been taken care of." What confront us now, clinically, he said, are more intractable scourges, such as Alzheimer's disease, acquired immune deficiency syndrome (AIDS), and cocaine addiction.

And what confront us now, ethically, are the moral equivalents of expensive and difficult illnesses: conflicts between equal claims of rights, increasingly cloudy lines between life and death, the American love–hate–fear relationship with high technology in health care, and allocation of the admittedly huge, but also admittedly (and necessarily) limited health care pie.

Retired pathologist Jack Kevorkian facilitates the suicides of sick women; while the government indicts him for murder and noted ethicist Arthur Caplan calls him "a serial mercy killer," millions of Americans voice support for him. We spend more and more on health care, yet more people lack access to the system, and our health status indicators are slipping. Although we are living longer, agonizing questions are being asked about whether simple quantity of life is sufficient—and half of American Black men still do not live to see the age of 65.

Questions breed more questions, and the answers seem more elusive. The stakes seem higher. We may have more and better lights, but the darkness seems darker.

These changes in the environment of bioethics are reflected in this book. Its contents do not focus primarily on the hospital, as was true of the previous volume. Issues of ethics and public policy receive more scrutiny, as do the provider's role in rationing, ethics issues involving non-physician professionals, the changing patient–provider relationship, and the state of bioethics itself. These essays, in some ways, probe deeper. But that is appropriate, for bioethics itself has now burrowed beneath the surface of health care and is raising questions about the very structure and purposes of the system of care we have chosen.

Thanks are, of course, in order. As in any project of this nature, contributions were made by many individuals, some of whom do not appear in the book as authors. First and foremost among the latter is Audrey Young Kaufman, my editor at American Hospital Publishing, who has been a source of patience, discipline, and problem solving as both real and imagined obstacles clouded my way.

Paul Hofmann and William Minogue, M.D., made helpful suggestions regarding content. Several health care executives—Ron Anderson, M.D., of Parkland Memorial Hospital in Dallas; Ruth Rothstein of Mount Sinai Hospital Medical Center and now of Cook County Hospital in Chicago; Robert Sillen of Santa Clara Valley Medical Center in San Jose, California; Austin Ross of Virginia Mason Medical Center in Seattle; and Neilson Buchanan of El Camino Hospital in Mountain View, California—provided me with powerful reminders that an administrator who is committed to doing what's right can be as strong a force for moral change as the most silver-tongued ethicist who ever lived.

Corinne Bayley, Robert Keller, M.D., John Lewin, M.D., Sister Marie Madeleine, Max Michael, M.D., Charlene Rydell, Alan Sager, Ph.D., John Sbarbaro, M.D., James Tallon, Bruce Vladeck, Ph.D., and others furthered my own education in ethics, morality, and justice. And when I was in despair over the cruelty of this world, Stephen Lewis, former Canadian ambassador to the United Nations and a consultant to UNICEF, provided me with inspiration and collegial support.

Among those whose work does appear here, I wish especially to thank George J. Annas, J.D., Kate Brown, Ph.D., Renée Fox, Ph.D., Andrew Jameton, Ph.D., William Nelson, Ph.D., and Judith Swazey, Ph.D., for friendship and ethical discourse, and George Lundberg, M.D., for having the courage of his convictions in public.

Finally, the deaths of several friends—Elizabeth Bonnett, David Kinzer, Peter Bellamy, and Gamble Rogers among them—taught me anew about the fragility of human life and the need for a good death. In connection with that, heartfelt personal thanks to Margaret, Louis, Judy, Don, Betty, Herb, Ariel, Sharon, Katy, Diane, Kate, Don, Walt, Jim, Roger, and other friends who helped me through all the miserable things that happened while I was putting this book together. And thanks to N.S.B. for caring.

Emily Friedman
January 1992

Part I

Rationing: Issues and Reasons

In a nation that spent $740 billion on health care in 1991, it seems absurd to even suggest that health services are rationed in the United States. On the other hand, in a nation where 35 to 40 million people lack any form of health insurance and face severely compromised access to care, how can it be suggested that health services are not rationed? The debate rages on as to whether, how, and to whom health care can or should be limited or denied. The answers to these questions, at least at the moment, appear to be that health care does now or will in the future need to be rationed; that we all want someone else's care rationed, rather than our own; and that we do not have much sense of how to go about it.

In this section, lessons from the past and proposals for the future are provided. Henry Beecher, M.D., tells how health care resources were allocated historically and applies what was learned to contemporary dilemmas. Daniel Callahan, Ph.D., suggests that advanced age could serve as a criterion for termination of care. John Kilner counters by pointing out that the traditional healers of the Akamba people of Africa use age as a standard in precisely the opposite way, favoring the aged over the young. And Albert Jonsen, Ph.D., offers the "rule of rescue": his belief that human beings are unable to resist the urge to save those at imminent risk of death, no matter how inappropriate or futile that urge. His message is that rationing as a conscious, predetermined act may be an impossibility in human society.

Chapter 1

Scarce Resources and Medical Advancement

Henry K. Beecher, M.D.

Scarce Resources and Medical Advancement reprinted by permission of *Daedalus,* Journal of the American Academy of Arts and Sciences, from the issue entitled, Ethical Aspects of Experimentation with Human Subjects, Spring 1969, Vol. 98/2.

Before his death, Henry K. Beecher, M.D., was Dorr professor of research in anesthesiology at Harvard University. He was a pioneer in examining ethical issues in medical research with human beings. Henry Beecher's classic analysis of rationing and resource allocation was originally published in 1969. Although much of the essay is as relevant today as it ever was—indeed, much of it is more relevant—certain sections concerning the clinical details of hormone therapy, the legal implications of research involving children, and the state of the art in organ transplantation are now outdated and have been omitted. Some of his information concerning kidney dialysis is also dated; however, it was included here so that the reader may better understand the issues Beecher raises in connection with what was then an emerging technology.—Editor

---

There is profit in most fields of human endeavor in taking an appraising look at past and present practices. Such comparison can tell much about the direction we are traveling, whether up or down. In medicine, there are a number of routes that can lead to useful insights. Present concern with human experimentation is a case in point. Within this field one can find various levers useful for prying loose significant information. The attitudes of the past and the present toward scarce resources in medical research are revealing. It is our purpose to examine them in some detail.

Among the recurring problems in the history of medicine, from ancient times to the present, is that of the sound allocation of scarce resources. A fairly comprehensive history of medicine could be written on the subject. But our immediate interest is an attempt to identify and to face up to several grave problems created by existing knowledge and limited resources. Nearly all advances in medicine involve experimentation and, usually, experimentation is hampered by scarce resources in its early period.

Scarce resources in the advancement of medicine are attributable to a variety of causes—some are deliberate, man-made, and some are owing to "natural" scarcities that obtain when a rare and newly discovered drug is found to have great effectiveness, where facilities for its adequate production have to be developed despite almost overwhelming difficulties. Sometimes the difficulty is a costly technique, where the problems are monetary cost and shortages of competent manpower. Sometimes moral and ethical considerations determine shortages. There is reason to believe that these may in some cases be based on outmoded views: The use of children is fraught with many problems and, in England at least, with legal difficulties; this area needs and is getting study. Another area where customs and moral, ethical, and legal problems abound is the definition of brain death with surviving heart beat. Clearly, the first problem is definition, but not to be neglected is the secondary fact that many tissues and organs not now adequately available for transplantation would be were the proposed new definition of irreversible coma accepted. *To do nothing in this area is far more radical than to act as proposed.*

I believe that the understanding of scarce resources and recognition of their causes can do much to alert us to such blocks and to their avoidance or correction in future growth. In the preparation of this manuscript, any early thoughts that the two aspects—availability and allocation—could be neatly divided had to be abandoned; the two are usually inextricably interwoven.

Once availability was assured, even though of limited extent, it was often surprisingly difficult or impossible to discover the *principles* that determined allocation of the new substance or technique to one man while it was withheld from another. Many of those who could have answered questions as to underlying principles of allocation are dead; but firsthand experience with the living does not lead to optimism as to what the dead might have divulged. Some of those who could still give information have failed to reply to requests. Some have said it was "too dangerous" to spell out the principles involved. One is led to the conclusion that in many cases no very extensive, thought-out policies were involved. A first-come-first-served basis seems to have been employed. There are notable exceptions to this. Some have evidently enjoyed the power of allocation and exercised it in a personal but nevertheless usually responsible way. And some—such as Professors Charles H. Best, William Castle, and George Thorn—have been completely helpful in discussing their pioneer work.

Our present concern is for the ethical use of scarce resources in medical experimentation in man. Passing references have been made above to areas where shortages and other difficulties have been encountered. It may be helpful for the purposes of orientation to spell them out a little more fully.

I. A Few Historical Examples from the Last Three Hundred Years

The Chamberlen Forceps

A member of the Chamberlen family (probably Peter, Sr.) developed an obstetrical forceps in the seventeenth century.[1] A similar instrument had been suggested by Pierre Franco in 1561. Nonetheless the Chamberlen family kept the secret of their instrument secure for many years.[2] At any rate, no outsider saw it until Hugh Chamberlen decided to sell it, for a high price, first in Paris to François Mauriçeau, the leading obstetrician of his time. That sale was lost owing to the demonstration's fatal outcome. Eventually Hugh sold the secret in Holland to Roger Roonhuysen and others. There was limitation on the use of a discovery for private gain.

Ignorance and the Scurvy

Sometimes ignorance is responsible for the scarcity of essential material. The importance of lemon and orange juice for seafarers had been known by the Dutch and others at least from 1564.[3] Lind published his "Treatise of the Scurvy" in 1753; but it was not until 1796, more than forty years later, that the Admiralty added lime juice to the naval ration, and the dread scurvy vanished from the fleets. The British sailors were referred to contemptuously by the Yankees as limeys. The Yankees took no stock in lemon juice, with the result that our Navy and merchant sailors suffered from scurvy for a century longer than the British, until steam shortened voyages to a safe duration.[4]

Anesthesia

During the first public demonstration of anesthesia at the Massachusetts General Hospital on October 16, 1846, William Thomas Green Morton was permitted to keep secret the nature of his "Letheon" and to obscure the fact that the active agent was diethyl ether. But a few days later, despite the resounding success of the first public demonstration, Morton was informed that the "surgeons of the hospital thought it their duty to decline the use of the preparation until informed what it was."[5] Under this pressure, Morton capitulated and revealed the nature of his agent.

He was attacked; some held his attempt at secrecy to be monstrous. Others defended him on the basis that he was not a physician, but a dentist. It was then customary for dentists to patent their devices, and no one thought the worse of them for it. Morton had worked hard, and a great discovery had come from his labors. He claimed that the reason for keeping his preparation secret was that he wished to perfect the method of its use and not come before the world until he was certain of the efficiency of his discovery. The surgeons of the Massachusetts General Hospital believed in Morton's sincerity and maintained their confidence in him.

Whatever Morton's true motivations were, selfish or not, he attempted to maintain his epoch-making material as a scarce resource. He was prevented from doing so by the surgeons of the Massachusetts General Hospital; the pressure of society removed his substance from the limited category and made it available to anyone who could learn to use it.

The Thyroid Hormone and Myxoedema

Until the latter part of the nineteenth century, myxoedema was considered to be an incurable disease. Observations in man and experimentation in animals led to the suggestion by Victor Horsley that a sheep's thyroid be transplanted into a patient suffering from myxoedema. This was done in Portugal with immediate improvement of the patient, improvement that was evident the day after operation, far too soon to have been the result of the graft "taking." The reasonable conclusion was made that the benefit came from absorption of the "juice of the healthy thyroid." With this information in mind, G. R. Murray cut up a sheep's thyroid and placed it in a little glycerine and 0.5 per cent solution of carbolic acid.[6] After standing for twenty-four hours, the juice was filtered off and injected into a woman suffering from myxoedema, twice weekly at first and later at two- or three-week intervals. Over three months' time, two and a half sheep's thyroid glands were used. The recovery of the patient was spectacular. The tedious and other unsatisfactory aspects of this procedure led to the isolation by Kendall of thyroxine from the thyroid gland. Its chemical structure was established, and finally it was prepared synthetically. Thus the remedy that had been so successful for one patient became easily available, through physiological and chemical studies, to all who need it.

Insulin

Ever since von Mehring and Minkowski had produced diabetes by excision of the pancreas in dogs in 1889, a number of attempts had been made to isolate the pancreatic substance that controlled carbohydrate metabolism. Finally this was accomplished by F. G. Banting and Charles H. Best in 1920 (published in 1922). They isolated the secretion of the islands of Langerhans and called it insulin.

Professor Best has recently had this to say:

The general principle involved in the early days of the clinical use of insulin was that only severe cases, who were desperately in need of some better treatment, would receive insulin. Furthermore it was felt that these cases should have had a very careful and thorough study so that any changes ascribed to the new therapy would be, in fact, due to it and not be within the variations encountered in diabetics.

In 1922, six distinguished physicians from the United States were invited to Toronto and fully briefed on the available information concerning insulin, and a revolution in medical care was launched. One of these six was Dr. E. P. Joslin of Boston. Dr. Priscilla White, his junior colleague in those early days, has described how Dr. Joslin's first concern was for those who were beginning to fail, especially children where the mortality was 100 per cent. They got first priority. Other considerations in the use of the scarce insulin were psychological stamina and "people who could take the routine and not break."

Penicillin

Investigations of the therapeutic usefulness of penicillin and measures to increase its supply were carried out by the Committee on Medical Research of the Office of Scientific Research and Development, by the Division of Medical Sciences of the National Research Council, and by certain commercial companies. These studies were initiated and continued as a phase of the war effort, *primarily for the benefit of the Armed Forces.*[7]

Although discovered by Fleming in London in 1929, penicillin's unique capabilities were revealed only in 1940–41 by Florey, Chain, and their collaborators at Oxford. Stimulated by Florey's visit to this country in the summer of 1941, some sixteen companies soon (by 1943) became engaged in the production of penicillin.

The first clinical tests of penicillin in this country were reported in 1941. In June of 1942, the Committee on Chemotherapeutic and Other Agents of the National Research Council, under the chairmanship of Dr. Chester S. Keefer, was invited to organize and to supervise clinical investigations in selected hospitals, the records to be coordinated by Dr. Keefer and his Committee.

In April 1943, the Surgeon General of the Army arranged for clinical tests to be made at the Bushnell General Hospital in Utah. There were many soldiers in that hospital who had returned from the Pacific area with unhealed compound fractures, osteomyelitis, and wounds containing long-established infections. The results of treatment with penicillin were so encouraging that within a matter of weeks similar studies were planned in ten General Army Hospitals and venereal studies in six. Plans were made for the Navy to carry on comparable but less extensive studies.

By the time Dr. Richards' report was made (May 22, 1943), more than three hundred patients were being treated with penicillin despite the great production problems. The earlier Oxford studies were confirmed. At the time of his report, Dr. Richards foresaw that the supply for civilian medical needs would be extremely limited.

On August 28, 1943, Dr. Keefer and his Committee reported on five hundred cases of infection treated with penicillin. Twenty-two groups of investigators were involved. Penicillin was then a scarce resource, and the situation urgent. In order to conserve material and time, the use of penicillin was restricted to a limited number of infectious states. After penicillin had been established as effective in treating staphylococcus and streptococcus infections, its use was soon extended to pneumonia and pneumococcal infections. Then it was shown to have an almost miraculous effect on gonorrhea and later a similar effect on syphilis, and a considerable number of other infections.[8] First came the concept, then the availability of the agent. As the material became plentiful, the breadth of its usefulness widened. The Committee saw it as their responsibility to direct "study toward those infections that are most likely to occur in our armed forces and to those that are resistant to the sulfonamides." A few cases (seventeen at the time of Keefer's 1943 report) of subacute bacterial endocarditis, however, were studied with disappointing results. Owing to the scarcity of penicillin and the lack of extensive experience, inadequate doses were used in those early days. Later, penicillin was found to be very effective in treating subacute bacterial endocarditis. This is an indication of the types of erroneous conclusion one may encounter while materials are scarce and experience limited.

Allocation of penicillin within the Military was not without its troubles: When the first sizable shipment arrived at the North African Theatre of Operations, U.S.A., in 1943, decision had to be made between using it for "sulfa fast" gonorrhea or for infected war wounds. Colonel Edward D. Churchill, Chief Surgical Consultant for that Theatre, opted for use in those wounded in battle. The Theatre Surgeon made the decision to use the available penicillin for those "wounded" in brothels. Before indignation takes over, one must recall the military manpower shortage of those days. In a week or less, those overcrowding the military hospitals with venereal disease could be restored to health and returned to the battle line. Moreover, no one is going to catch osteomyelitis from an associate; venereal disease was a widely disseminated and serious hazard to the individual and to the war effort.

When penicillin became available for civilians, the aim was to widen its spectrum of usefulness and to determine the doses needed for effectiveness. To do this, Chester Keefer, who was in charge of the program, carried out a model project, notwithstanding extreme pressures to accede to the importunities of friends, strangers, even the White House, indirectly.

II. The Present

Intermittent Hemodialysis

Intermittent hemodialysis is of very limited availability. It does not, of course, involve the transplantation of tissues or organs, but it is often a means of maintaining life while awaiting the availability of a suitable kidney for transplantation.

Hemodialysis is an example of a limited experimental-practical procedure that is enveloped in problems both mundane and ethical. H. E. de Wardener has discussed the ethical and economic problems of keeping people alive with hemodialysis.[9] The main function here, of course, is the adjustment of the electrolyte and water content of the body so that they are kept within constant limits and certain wastes derived from protein metabolism are eliminated. If the kidneys cannot do this, the subject will die; life can be maintained even in the absence of kidney function, however, by circulating the blood through an artificial kidney. This process is called hemodialysis. It requires that the patient be placed on the artificial kidney some twelve to fourteen hours twice weekly. It is customary to carry this out at night in order to interfere as little as possible with normal activities. The patient's liberty is severely curtailed; the site of the arterial

and venous connections must be kept absolutely clean and cannot be put into a bath; nor can the subject swim. Vigorous exercise is unwise. The site must be protected from injury. Strict dietary limitations are necessary. In most cases, the procedure much [must] be carried out, at the present time at least, in a hospital.

Correctly carried out the mortality is low. For example, J. P. Pendras and R. V. Erickson at Seattle have treated twenty-three patients for over forty patient-years with three deaths.[10] De Wardener reports that he at Charing Cross and Shaldon at the Royal Free Hospital have treated thirty-five patients for a period of forty-three patient-years with one death owing to a technical accident.[11] Eight of Shaldon's patients are on home dialysis. Combining the data from the three centers gives a total of fifty-eight patients treated for eighty-three patient-years with four deaths.

With these elementary considerations in mind, one can turn to the ethical questions that must be faced, and in this it will be helpful to follow de Wardener's thoughtful comments.

Have we the right to prolong life in this way? Despite the limitations imposed, life can still be pleasant and productive; the answer is an unqualified yes to the general question.

Granted that the procedure is justified, who shall be treated? It has been the practice of the initial center to broaden responsibility by committee action, as at Seattle, where the committee includes both lay and medical members.

De Wardener doubts that the results of spreading responsibility are any better than decisions made by one or two individuals. G. E. Schreiner also argues against committee decision as to which candidate will be placed on dialysis, for a committee decision that involves laymen requires in the end organization and presentation of medical data to the lay group and in this the physicians' biases can be expressed.[12] But many aspects of society must be considered in the decision of who will and who will not be accepted in a dialysis program, aspects where the physician is as incompetent to make decisions as the layman is to decide on medical issues. Pendras seems to be on firm ground. His group considers two bases for selecting patients: the medical-psychological aspect and the social-moral, rehabilitation one. In essence, the Seattle screening is done by two committees in which laymen as well as physicians function.[13] In choosing candidates, they consider "worth to the community." For example, a thirty-two-year-old man with a stable history of employment and responsibility, with a family of six to support, was chosen over a forty-five-year-old widow whose children were grown up and had left home. Pendras is a strong advocate of the group decision.

In de Wardener's program, decision has to be made only when a place becomes available; the first obligation is toward those patients who are already being treated.[14] A new patient is not accepted until the last one has been well launched, for experience has shown that most difficulties occur in the early weeks of treatment. Moreover, a new patient is not accepted when any staff shortages are present. To be chosen, the subject must be showing signs of deterioration notwithstanding a low-protein diet. Since hemodialysis facilities are in short supply, a choice must be made among needy candidates. Usually such a choice is made among those between puberty (below this age, they will not mature if on dialysis) and menopause, subjects who are clear mentally and cooperative, and not suffering from some other disease that dialysis will not control. Often patients who have young children are chosen.

A definition of suitability for dialysis depends on a number of factors, some arbitrary, some empirical. For instance, the subject chosen should have the possibility of a prolonged survival. It seems reasonable during the period of establishment of a new technique to choose in the early years those subjects who will probably do best.

What are the financial consequences? The initial cost of the equipment is $4,200 (1966) per bed in England. When dialysis is carried out for three patients six nights a week, the capital cost per patient, thus, is $1,400. (This does not include the cost of housing.) Maintenance cost, nursing staff, technicians, and disposable items come to $84 per patient per week. De Wardener estimates that 2,230 patients in England in 1962 would have been acceptable and would have profited from dialysis. Aside from initial capital expenditure, the cost of treating this number in a hospital would be $9,800,000 for one year. He also estimates the British need to be ultimately the care of eleven thousand patients where the annual cost would be equivalent to the cost of two 800-bed district hospitals; clearly, dilemmas persist. He provides other interesting estimates of cost over a period of years.

In America, Pendras at Seattle estimates the cost at $5,000 to $10,000 per patient per year.[15] He believes that present facilities can accommodate only about 10 per cent of those in need. He estimates that with a cumulative patient load, after five years, 75 to 250 million dollars would be required for therapy for some fifteen to twenty-five thousand patients. At present, hemodialysis can be offered only on a limited basis owing to the scarcity of dialysis centers and the great cost.

Who ought to pay? Few individuals can afford the cost of dialysis. In some countries, only those who can pay are accepted for hemodialysis; in other countries, the State pays; in still other countries, no hemodialysis is available to anyone.

The cost is such that few can pay for the procedure without reducing their standard of living and without jeopardizing their children's future. Such a patient has to choose between family problems and dying. Some call this a form of suicide, a charge hotly denied by others. The sad fact is that a patient may feel obliged to make such a choice when his judgment may be clouded by disease. Once the treatment has begun, a drastic step is required by the sick man to stop the treatment and spare the family further financial distress. He can do this, for example, by a dietary indiscretion, such as choosing a high potassium diet, or by tearing out the tubes allowing himself to bleed to death. It is unquestionably true that financial hardship preys on the minds of many confronted with these problems.

In the face of such tragic decisions, it is good to know that the United States is financing programs from both government and charitable funds. These are still in short supply, but the trend is hopeful. In Britain, if the Health Service is to be truly comprehensive, it is the responsibility of the Ministry of Health to provide for intermittent hemodialysis. The Minister of Health accepted this responsibility in 1965.

Is it right for the large sums involved to be directed to the purposes of hemodialysis? The size of the financial commitment has discouraged some. De Wardener takes the creditable view that this is nothing new because, as Lord Platt has pointed out, in earlier years vast sums were spent on tuberculosis patients without questioning the cost. De Wardener has recently found that the cost per week of sanatorium care of a patient with tuberculosis is the same as maintaining a patient on intermittent hemodialysis in a hospital. Few tuberculosis patients confined to a sanatorium can lead productive lives, whereas those on intermittent hemodialysis can. This is a sound argument in favor of extending the availability of hemodialysis. Others can argue, if they choose, that the placement of the tuberculosis patient in a sanatorium removes a threat to the health of those who might otherwise come into contact with him; that the man with renal failure will not infect those about him, and therefore there is less urgency in treating him—a specious argument.

De Wardener presents interesting comparisons of the cost of treating or housing those with mental disease and those with renal failure. If those with mental disease are not treated or confined, they will roam the streets and prod our conscience. In contrast, those with failing kidney function will die and leave us in peace. The treatment of those with hemodialysis is not so radical an economic venture in the treatment of disease as some have supposed.

A further ethical question to be considered is whether the considerable number of skilled individuals involved in hemodialysis should be utilized in this way, taking into account, for example, the shortage of nurses. Wards in some hospitals are closed because of this shortage. De Wardener estimates that if the present nurse-to-patient ratios in Britain hold ten years hence, some four thousand nurses will be engaged in this activity. Automation as well as the employment of less skilled personnel may help with the staffing problems. But legal problems can arise when care of patients is delegated to "unqualified" staff. The numbers of doctors involved is less important than the number of nurses; but, even so, too few nephrologists are willing to take on the time-consuming demands involved in maintaining a hemodialysis program.

Schreiner has raised the question as to whether the physician might possibly be better occupied with trying to discover how the streptococcus produces glomerular nephritis than with treating the consequences of this infection. This question is really not relevant: Many physicians are quite competent to supervise a dialysis program, but few are competent by native research ability to get at the cause of the kidney failure. Schreiner says it is the old problem of research versus patient care. A more basic problem is the availability of the necessary kinds of talent.

III. Ethical Problems Arising in Transplantation of Tissues and Organs

Some General Comments

Whenever the transplantation of tissues or organs is concerned, the material needed is in short supply now and will continue to be so into the foreseeable future. It is evident that the transplantation of tissues or organs is not purely a medical problem. Perplexing questions abound; some are medical or partly medical, and some are not. The Ciba Foundation symposium was primarily interested in transplantation, but it considered subjects pertinent that are as diverse as how and when can a potential donor be considered to be free of undue influence? How long should "life" be maintained in a patient with irrevocable brain damage? When does death occur in an unconscious patient maintained only on artificial aids to the circulation and the respiration? Are there ever circumstances when death may be mercifully advanced? Can a parent rightly refuse necessary treatment of his child? How can minors, the ignorant, prisoners, be protected in the transplant situation? When may pregnancy be terminated? Is it legal to mutilate a donor for the sake of another person? What protection from society do medical men need in the development of new life-saving techniques? What is the community's financial responsibility in developing and maintaining life-supporting measures? Clearly, problems arising in transplantation are wide ranging.

Nearly all cases of transplantation where homografts are concerned involve experimentation for the benefit of the ailing subject, and thus the ethical problems encountered are usually relatively straightforward. The donor, with reasonable explanatory effort on the part of the physician, cannot help knowing that he is participating in a therapeutic experiment. There are instances of trans-

plantation, however, where the above situations are not present, where transplantation has been carried out in an experiment not for the benefit of the subject. The author has discussed elsewhere a study in which skin homografts were carried out in children who had been subjected to thymectomy in order to see if thymectomy provided a better "take"; it did not.[16]

J. E. Murray believes that the lung is a likely organ to be transplanted and that, of the non-paired organs, the liver is the most promising. Remarkable progress has already been made in liver transplantation. Transplantation of the endocrine organs is being studied.[17] But it is impossible to discuss usefully the ethical problems arising in the rejection phenomenon until it is better understood—beyond acknowledging that its existence must act as a cautionary deterrent in the field. On the other hand, it is difficult to get around the possibility that some organs may be less subject to deleterious action by this phenomenon than others. It seems reasonable to proceed therefore, especially when the only alternative is death.

An especially difficult problem with single organ transplants, such as the heart or liver, is that this is a once-and-only procedure, whereas with the kidney as many as three transplants in a single patient have been carried out. Then, too, in the case of renal disease the fact must be weighed that the man with no kidney function can often be kept alive and functioning for years with intermittent hemodialysis. There are, clearly, basic differences in the problems surrounding the several organs.

If there were no legal or logistical problems, there would be available each year, it is estimated, over 10,600 cadaver kidneys in the United States, for approximately 7,600 kidney recipients, and 6,000 livers for 4,000 potential liver recipients.[18] These data are based on "neurological" deaths when the tissues to be transplanted would be satisfactory.

Some generalizations can be supplied as useful guides in the transplantation field.[19] These have been emphasized for years by responsible investigators in the area. It may be helpful to summarize them: Before transplantation is undertaken there must be a reasonable chance of clinical success. An acceptable therapeutic goal must be present. Adrenal or pancreatic transplants violate this "rule" since acceptable replacement secretions can be obtained. The risks and uncertainties must be presented to the families of the donor and the recipient as well as to the two principals. The protocol for each transplantation must be devised so as to gain and preserve the maximum information. There must be probing evaluation of the results by independent observers. Careful, accurate, conservative information is to be disseminated through legitimate channels, both medical and lay, in order that cruel hopes will not needlessly be raised. The field of transplantation carries great hope for the future; this should not be discredited by unscientific practices or proclamations.

Blood Transfusion

In 1668, an eighty-page pamphlet on blood transfusion was published at Bologna. It is fair to call this the first text book on this subject.[20] Thus for three centuries the possibility of the transfusion of blood had been in men's minds, although its widespread practice really dates from about the time of World War II. Between 1668 and World War II, the scene was fraught with animal as well as human experimentation, some of it wild. Blood transfusion has interest and relevance to the present consideration: It represents the greatest and most successful transplantation of tissue. The considerable seventeenth-century interest in blood transfusion was followed by little interest in the eighteenth century, a sequence one often finds in the history of science: Men turn away from insoluble problems, only to return to them when some event or discovery gives renewed hope that they can be solved. In the nineteenth century, several books on the subject published in Europe stimulated an ever expanding interest that has continued to the present.

From the earliest times, blood has been considered to have an almost mystic importance, doubtless because of the plain fact that much loss of blood promptly leads to loss of life. It was believed that the weak could be made strong by drinking the blood of the latter, so the blood of bulls or of gladiators became a popular beverage. Keynes describes the attempt, near the end of the fifteenth century, to rejuvenate the aged Pope Innocent VIII by giving him a drink prepared from the blood of three young boys who thus died in vain.

The history of blood transfusion follows a common pattern of science. First there was the *concept* of introducing various materials into the circulation of an animal, then this was *extended* to blood. *Animal experiments* were carried out. Finally, these were *applied to man*.

Very often before the eruption of a great new advance in science, a *climate* appears wherein many men have similar ideas, and it becomes impossible to be sure who had the new concept first. It is certain, however, that Dr. Wren (later Sir Christopher) must get the credit for first experiments, in 1657, of intravenous injection of foreign substances into animals' veins. Then toward the end of February 1666, Richard Lower first demonstrated to a distinguished company at Oxford that a bled-out dog could be revived at once by the blood from a donor dog. The bled-out recipient "promptly jumped down from the table, and, apparently oblivious of its hurts, soon began to fondle its master, and to roll in the grass to clean itself of blood." This was the first public demonstration of a successful dog-to-dog transfusion. Lower's priority was challenged by one Jean Denys of France, who managed to get *his* claim translated into English and even published

in the *Transactions* of the Royal Society for June 22, 1667, without the knowledge of the Secretary, Henry Oldenburg, who unfortunately at the moment was confined in the Tower. He got out just in time to have Denys's letter suppressed, although some copies still exist.[21]

In experiments in 1667, Denys succeeded for the first time in transfusing animal blood into men, first into a sick boy who was made miraculously well by a lamb's blood and then in an experiment in a *well* man, without ill effects. Similar experiments were carried out in England, until inevitably, disaster struck in 1668 in France: A patient died and the widow sued Denys. Denys lost, with the injunction that no further transfusions were to be made unless approved by a member of the Faculty of Medicine at Paris. Opposition there led to discontinuance of the procedure.

Samuel Pepys recorded in his *Diary* on November 14, 1666, comments on an animal-to-animal transfusion and, nimble-witted man that he was, suggested it would be interesting to inject the blood of a Quaker into an Archbishop. On November 21 of the next year, Pepys wrote of a "poor and debauched man, that the College have hired for 20s. to have some of the blood of sheep let into his body." There were no apparent ill effects, although considerable uncertainty as to the outcome had been expressed before the fact. This "poor and debauched" man may have been the first *paid* experimental subject, at least in England. (There is some evidence that the French had preceded the English in this.)

In 1794, Erasmus Darwin proposed the *hiring* of a donor so that frequent transfusions could be made into a sick man. The potential recipient "now found himself near the house of death"; he felt it useless to proceed with the experiment, and it was not carried out. The use of a subject paid to participate in an experiment three hundred years ago and Darwin's suggestion that a donor be hired indicate that some of our modern practices have ancient origins.

The world had to wait until December 22, 1818, for Blundell's account of the first successful man-to-man transfusion. In 1907, Jansky identified four blood groups, and transfusion was well on its way to acceptance as a standardized technique.

O. H. Robertson made use of stored blood in World War I, a practice widely followed in World War II first by the British and then by the United States forces after a tragic error made in Washington was overcome.[22] The American Forces entered North Africa essentially without adequate blood transfusing equipment. Here was human experimentation of a negative sort, but on a massive scale. This incredible mistake came as a result of believing that the newly developed blood plasma, wet or dried, would suffice. It soon became apparent that the infusion of plasma would indeed restore the blood pressure to a level where bleeding would be resumed in those already nearly exsanguinated and much of the remaining essential hemoglobin washed out.[23] (This is not the place to attribute blame. Edward D. Churchill, Consulting Surgeon for the Mediterranean Theatre, is writing the history of this titanic error.) The first blood bank for civilians was established as part of a military effort in Barcelona in 1936. The following year Fantus in Chicago founded the first completely civilian blood bank. Blood substitutes ranging from milk to modified fluid gelatine have been disappointing. Fractionating blood into its components has made it possible to satisfy a patient's needs more accurately than formerly.

G. E. W. Wolstenholme has taken a look at those who give and those who receive blood. He estimates that some seven million transfusion units are presently administered in the United States each year.[24] The donors are usually eighteen to sixty-five years of age, from whom 500 ml. are drawn without ill effect. The use of cadaver blood was suggested by G. Rubin in 1914,[25] and had considerable vogue in Russia during the 1930's. Such a practice is limited by infection developing after death and by the difficulties in obtaining an adequate history to rule out infectious hepatitis, malaria, and syphilis in its early stage. Sometimes blood is taken over a period of weeks, stored for re-infusion into the donor at the time of operation.

Even when infection-free and compatible blood is available, it is not always welcomed. Wolstenholme tells of a press report during World War II of a fanatical Nazi soldier captured at Tobruk who killed himself as soon as he realized he was being given British blood. Some British held a similar aversion. In North Africa, a British general ordered the destruction of one hundred blood transfusion units derived from German prisoners of war rather than have any of it used to save the lives of British wounded. One learns with relief that as soon as the general's back was turned the order was ignored. Arkansas has introduced legislation to control or to prevent the administration of "racially different" blood.[26]

Aside from these bizarre cases, the Jehovah's Witnesses provide a greater and more serious difficulty, one that bristles with ethical problems. One eminent chief of service at a Harvard hospital decided, on the advice of counsel and with Trustee support, to overrule the wishes of an adult "Witness." She was transfused. If one can ignore—overcome—such blood prejudice, can one also force a kidney transplant? What are the limits of coercive therapy? What is to be the end of this complex decision? The rather large group of Jehovah's Witnesses would prefer to lose their life than go against what they believe to be God's instruction (Leviticus XVII, 13, 14): "You shall eat the blood of no manner of flesh for the life of all flesh is the blood thereof." It is customary to accede to such prejudice, but not always. A great ethical problem arises in the case of the children of Jehovah's Witnesses or in the case of a Witness too ill to make a rational decision. If the emergency is not great, legal advice can be sought; if the situation is desperate, some physicians have desisted, some have not. The law is not yet helpful in this area.

It is unquestionably true that blood transfusion is too often too lightly undertaken. One distinguished authority in the field has argued vehemently in the past that blood transfusion should not be carried out during surgery under general anesthesia lest a previously undetected incompatibility or a frank error in matching go unnoticed. To accept as decisive this remote possibility against the undoubted life-saving power of blood transfusion during surgery is sadly unrealistic. When contemplating over-use, one must always remember the possibilities and hazards of sensitization. Wolstenholme estimates the over-all mortality rate for transfusion to be "not higher than three in 10,000."[27]

In extra pay for those who engage in hazardous pursuits, society has accepted the view that risk is reimbursable. One wonders if the question of whether the sale of major organs with the risk this entails will eventually find the same acceptance as the sale of blood for transfusion. When the immunological problem is solved, this question could become a pressing one. Legislation now pending in Italy would make illegal any payment for an organ.

Corneal Transplantation

In reviewing the history of corneal transplantation, Rycroft has concluded that credit must go to Pellier de Quengsy for attempting in 1789 to stitch a glass disc into the cornea after removing a scarred patch of that tissue; he does not record the outcome.[28] A few years later (1796) Erasmus Darwin, in London, wondered if a "small piece of cornea" could not be trephined out. Such ideas led to the first graft of corneal tissue on a human cornea by Reisinger in 1817. He got the idea from watching Astley Cooper place a skin graft on the stump of an amputated limb at Guy's Hospital. The first successful human corneal graft was achieved by Zirm in 1905. The donor in this case was a small boy who had to have his eye removed because of an intraocular foreign body. Later the Russian Filatov demonstrated that donor material from cadavers could be used, after storage at low temperatures.

Unlike other material where grafting has been attempted, corneal grafts involve avascular tissue, and this undoubtedly accounts for the early and continued success. Since the material can be obtained from cadavers or surgical sources and stored, most of the harassing ethical problems surrounding other tissues or organs are not present here. Prior to World War II, donor material was difficult to find and came mainly from eyes containing tumors. After World War II, when the demand for donor material greatly increased, surgeons turned to cadaver material. Once again the Anatomy Act of 1832 hindered this approach in Britain, and one had to depend on the occasional permission of relatives of the deceased. This situation was improved by the 1952 Corneal Grafting Act, which was later incorporated in the Human Tissue Act of 1961.

The Queen Victoria Hospital's Eye Bank at East Grinstead received in 1965, about fifteen years after its founding, over four hundred eyes. International donor services are now provided. These widespread activities have been made possible by public education through lectures, the press, radio, and television. Such success can doubtless be extended to more complicated transplantation problems by similar educational efforts.

The law concerning what can and cannot be removed from a body and under what circumstances varies with the country or state involved. Much of it is unclear or ambiguous.

Kidney Transplantation

The general, although not unanimous, view is that an individual with two healthy kidneys can ethically give one, providing the gift is truly voluntary and is given with the full knowledge of the risks, including the information that his sacrifice may turn out to be useless. Still, family pressures are often so great that it is difficult to impossible to determine if the donor is truly a volunteer. Attempts to ensure voluntariness have sometimes led to standardized psychological examination where the examiner attempts to determine if the potential donor is "stable, well-balanced and rationally motivated." Such an examination can also uncover possible pressure from the family. The donor is told that if he does not want to give a kidney, no one will know, for the physician will state that the donor is unsuitable. In these circumstances, about three out of five are found to be genuine volunteers. A major purpose is to prevent external pressure on the prospective donor. There is the recurrent question as to whether one is justified on ethical grounds in refusing to transplant a kidney from a relative who would feel that he had in the refusal failed to save the life of a loved one. One can ask whether it is really ever possible to exercise truly free choice in a situation where the inherent pressures are so strong as they are in family situations. Family pressures can lead to choice of a donor on the basis of his presumed expendability. Family pressure is, however, "consonant with the dignity and responsibility of free life."[29] There are also subtle and strong internal pressures within each possible donor. These pressures are rooted in common religious and social attitudes concerning the propriety of self-sacrifice. It is difficult to see how anyone or any panel of experts could be absolutely certain that free and uninhibited consent exists when the prospective donor is aware that he is making a life or death decision, and that the decision is under scrutiny. The potential anguish of such a situation could be most acute for the identical twin who is a unique donor. But in view of the

excellent results after other intrafamilial transplantations, the situation is not limited to twin cases.[30] Excepting identical twins or other close relative donors, the whole issue is clouded by the brief prognosis, in most cases one or two years, at present.[31] It has been estimated that, excluding fraternal twins, there are probably no more than fifteen patients in the world who have survived kidney transplantation for more than three years.[32] It is, thus, not now possible to know the value of the procedure in terms of a five- or ten-year prognosis. Even if the benefit proves to be limited to a few years, this gain is significant for the individual who fills a useful place in society. Starzl asks searching questions as to who is equipped to determine the "usefulness" or "value" of a given individual: "A system of selection based upon such materialistic criteria is founded on the dangerous assumption that a few people are qualified and have the right to adjudicate the value of someone else's years."[33]

Under some circumstances, it is not ethical, or perhaps even legal, for a patient to accept an organ. For example, if the patient knows that the donor's spouse strongly disapproves of the donation, it may be unethical for him to accept. If he knows that a prisoner or a lunatic is giving the organ, it might be not only unethical, but illegal to accept it. A "person under restraint cannot be presumed to consent."[34]

M. F. A. Woodruff finds it curious that so much emotional concern is voiced over a kidney donation, yet during the Battle of Britain no one saw any moral problem in allowing a man to become a fighter pilot.[35] Most would rather give a kidney than become such a pilot. Bentley objects to such an analogy, for moral theologians make a distinction between direct and indirect effects. For the fighter pilot, the possible maiming is never the means of achieving what he wants to do. The maiming, if it occurs, is an indirect effect, foreseen as possible; but in transplantation, the maiming—the loss of a kidney—is the direct means to the end desired. Thus, a moral difference is present.

One can speculate on the consequences of a breach in the present immunological barrier: The transplantation of skin could be life-saving in the severely burned. In another area, with the present population of the United States at 200 million, one can estimate ten thousand kidney transplants each year.[36]

A difficult early period in any specific experimental work is likely to be the time when success is rare. Lord Platt believes the ethical position of removing a kidney from a healthy person when the chance of it surviving as a transplant for a long time is 5 per cent is different from what it would be if the success rate were 90 per cent.[37] "Rarity of success" is a real and complicating factor not usually discussed. In such a situation, whether to continue or to call it quits is a troubling decision. If an acceptable success rate is to be achieved, experimentation must continue. This problem is not limited to organ transplantation; it is common in the development of most complex diagnostic and therapeutic procedures.

Lord Platt takes the view that in certain rare and dangerous developmental procedures, not yet ready for general use, but nevertheless *for the patient's welfare:* "There is a slight danger here, in that one is selecting patients for such procedures partly because they may benefit other people in the future and not wholly because of possible benefit to the present patient."[38] As long as the purpose of the procedure is truly diagnostic or therapeutic for the given individual, there can be little ground for complaint, if at the same time it adds to knowledge or benefit to others. It seems likely that the only questionable situation would grow out of deception of the subject or one's self when there was no true expectation of helping the patient.

Lord Platt is of the opinion that too little thought is given to whether the proposed experiment is really a *sound* experiment.[39] The writer has emphasized for years that the improperly designed experiment, one that cannot give useful data, is an unethical experiment, regardless of whether it is "harmless" or not. There is the requirement in all human experimentation that the ends sought not be trivial.

The next few years may show that kidney transplantation has a better chance of success than has resection of the esophagus for cancer: 15 per cent five-year cures for the lower third; 5 per cent for the middle third; no five-year cures for the upper third.[40] Esophageal surgery would not ordinarily be called experimental, yet kidney transplantation is usually so designated. One may not fairly equate experimental procedures with procedures that have a low success rate. It must be borne in mind that for some diseases—as, for example, cancer of the esophagus—there is no real alternative to surgery, whereas there is an alternative to kidney transplantation: intermittent hemodialysis.

Murray has made the point that an operation on the donor is not a medical procedure at all; it is not making a sick person well, but a well person sick.[41] Any maiming of a patient should be for his benefit. The principle of totality covers this: A part of the body may be sacrificed for the good of the whole. The donor loses a kidney, but has spiritual gain in his sacrifice.

Questions involve both donor and recipient: whether a kidney transplant, for example, will do any good and, if so, to whom. If the transplant lives, the recipient is obviously benefited. Whether the transplant lives or dies, the donor can be benefited psychologically and spiritually. This was affirmed by the Supreme Judicial Court of Massachusetts in the case of the first identical twin transplant.

G. B. Giertz has proposed that a considerable number of persons might agree when healthy, when fully conscious, that a kidney might be taken if certain conditions ensue later in life,[42] or a second solution might stem from a re-evaluation of widely accepted moral principles with alteration of legislation.

Heart Transplantation

Transplantation of the heart represents a desperate effort to save a desperate situation. It is a therapeutic effort that will be widely practiced, once the rejection phenomenon is overcome. Just as attention to various unethical procedures has focused our thought on the necessity to straighten out our practices, so also in an opposite sense Barnard's first heart transplant focused attention on a great need. The resultant excitement and the educational effect will in all probability lead to the acquisition of funds and the stimulation of investigators so that the transplant problems—not only of hearts but of other organs as well—will be solved sooner than would otherwise have been the case. While granting a pre-eminent place for the individual's rights, it would be wrong to overlook the fact that society has rights too, especially relevant to the possibilities of successful transplantation.

A considerable debate is at present under way concerning whether or not further heart transplants should be attempted until the rejection phenomenon in general is better understood and better controlled. Another imponderable in the heart transplant situation is that it is impossible to judge with accuracy the prognosis in survival time of the prospective recipient without transplantation. Certainly a heart transplant would not be contemplated if widespread and crippling atherosclerosis were present.

While a great deal has been learned about transplantation in general from work with the kidneys, transplantation of the heart presents certain crucial differences. In the case of the kidney, the donor can survive following the loss of a kidney; the donor of a heart cannot survive. If the transplantation of a kidney is not successful, the subject can be placed on hemodialysis, and two or three attempts can be made at transplantation. No such possibility exists with cardiac transplantation; it is a once and only possibility. The restrictions on this scarce resource are thus more severe with the heart than with paired organs.

A further restriction pointed out by the Board on Medicine of the National Academy of Sciences is that a greater number of surgeons have the knowledge and skill to perform the actual transplantation of the heart "than have available the full capability to conduct the total study in terms of all relevant scientific observations."[43] The Board would restrict cardiac transplantation to those institutions in which there are present not only surgical expertise, but also a thorough understanding of the biological processes that lead to rejection and its control. In this hazardous field it is especially important that careful planning be established prior to the event, that systematic observations be recorded, and that all findings, good and bad, be communicated to the few others engaged in such activity. Rigid safeguards must be established to cover the choices of donor and recipient.

Legal Problems in the Field of Transplantation

A considerable dilemma is encountered in this area. The rights of donors, alive or cadaver, insofar as the latter can be said to have "rights," as well as the rights of recipients have not been spelled out in law; at the same time experience indicates that it is often undesirable to bring legal decision into a situation that is in a state of rapid change, as this one is.

The use of live donors who have been properly informed, who understand the risks involved and the uncertainty of success, who have agreed in writing, has not led to serious legal problems.

For those who, like G. P. J. Alexandre, believe that the removal of organs is proper in patients after the brain is dead, but whose heart still beats, the philosophy is simpler than for others who do not agree.[44] There is a difference, of course, when one of paired organs is removed and the removal of single organs, like the liver or the heart. Such a situation falls into the category of "statistical morality," for all major surgical procedures have their own mortality rates. When enough operations are carried out, even the removal of one of a pair will lead to death.

Cadaver donors are a special problem. In the first place, true emergency planning is involved so that the kidneys or other organs can be removed and perfused in an hour or less. In such a case, good hope for success is justified. Since the cadaver transplant must be effected in minutes, not hours, what legal procedure can be prepared ahead of time? Eventually, as Giertz has suggested, it may be possible to get enough individuals to agree, when healthy, to organ removal if brain death later occurs.[45] This procedure could, if extensive enough, make a real impact on the situation. Or legislation might be arrived at whereby tissues might be taken legally after death without further ado, unless the individual or his family explicitly objected or his religion was opposed to such a practice. The situation might also be handled by legal authorization for a previously designated person to give consent to tissue or organ removal after death. Under present legal restrictions, a living person has limited powers to dispose of his body or its parts after death, although some states permit such disposal by will, as in California and recently in Massachusetts.

When Woodruff set about organizing a skin bank in Scotland, he discovered that, under the Anatomy Act of 1832, it was illegal to proceed. The Act had been passed as a consequence of the activities of the Edinburgh murderers, Burke and Hare. The need for a skin bank was appreciated and the situation set to right by the passage in 1961 of the Human Tissue Act. The unethical act

(murder) led to restrictive legislation (the Anatomy Act of 1832), a sequence one can often observe when less final ethical violations occur than murder. One can take some comfort from the fact that when need for revision was demonstrated, correction of the law followed.

Another example of the restraining power of the courts was demonstrated in the 1932 case of the rich man who bought a testicle from a young Neapolitan. A surgeon transplanted it with the result that article 5 of the Italian common code of civil rights was promulgated in 1940. This forbade the donation of organs or other parts of the body that could produce a *permanent* deficiency in the donor. Blood transfusion or skin grafts were thus not made illegal.[46] A more enlightened bill is currently before the Italian Parliament for final approval. In the United States, the law has not kept pace with science, but, as suggested above, this may be a good thing until many situations and problems are better clarified than is presently the case.[47]

IV. General Comment

It was a considerable disappointment to the writer, after the examination of more than a dozen areas where scarce resources were involved, to find statements of only the most rudimentary principles of procedure. (One must face the fact that this, too, is a kind of principle.)

The guiding factors encountered (rather than principles in most cases) can be summarized: *Avarice* is exemplified in the secrecy surrounding the Chamberlen forceps. Although lemon and orange juice were in short supply, their effectiveness in treating the scurvy was a matter of record; yet decades passed before the general *ignorance* was overcome. *Self-interest* or dedication to high principle is not clear in the case of anesthesia.

This is not to say that in early times only avarice, ignorance, or self-interest determined the allocation of scarce resources; but it seems evident that these factors were determinants then more often than is now the case.

Continuing with our arbitrary list of examples, the next one, chronologically, is the thyroid hormone. With this, a new and much higher realm of procedure was entered; it could be called a prototype for present action: Myxoedema was recognized as an incurable disease of the thyroid; animals, presumably, had normal thyroids. Seventy-seven years ago the difficulties lying in wait for the transplanter were not known; "transplant" of a sheep's thyroid was carried out. The curative properties of the procedure were evident in a matter of hours, far too soon for grafting to explain the success. It was assumed and later proved true that the infusion of the thyroid "juice" accounted for the good effect. The active element was found to be thyroxine, which was synthesized. The early scarcity of the material and the tedious procedure gave way to the ready availability of the crucial substance as desired for anyone in need. This is a beautiful example of the selfless and effective work of many men, typified also in the triumphs of insulin, penicillin, and the adrenocorticotrophic hormone and cortisone.

There are at the present time plentiful reasons for despairing of mankind, but not in the standards evident in the progress of medicine. In the Western world, at least, the pre-eminence of the welfare of the individual is recognized as an indispensable component in the welfare of society. (It is inconceivable that a healthy society could be based upon exploitation of individuals, a sick use of individuals.) There is a considerable and growing recognition that science is not necessarily the highest value, that it must be placed in a hierarchy of values.

Some may consider these statements rather too grand. Yet what other conclusion can one come to with such visible evidence for them? Consider some major current concerns of today. May children be used in experimental procedures not for their direct benefit? (The answer seems to be "yes" in certain well-defined children's areas, "no" in others.) Relevant to our present interests is the fact that concern for "yes" or "no" *is* present.

It is now recognized that intermittent hemodialysis, as costly and inadequately available as it is at present, can be given to all who need it, at no greater cost than once was required by tuberculosis, even at less cost than mental disease now exacts. These latter unfortunates can add little to the world; hemodialysis can and does add years of productivity to those with otherwise fatal kidney disease.

Moreover, those who were once a grave and growing burden, the hopelessly comatose, can now be the means of extending life for desperately ill, but still salvageable individuals through a new understanding that the brain can die while other parts of the body remain sound and useful. It is also recognized that to *fail* to utilize this material is far more radical than not to use it.

The current requirements of an ethical approach to the transplantation of tissues and organs are a credit to our present standards of morality. All of these concerns, when contrasted with earlier years, offer heartening evidence of the growth of conscience, the advance in philosophical awareness, the gain in spiritual values, the sound growth of medicine.[48]

References

1. F. H. Garrison (*An Introduction to the History of Medicine* [Philadelphia, 1914], p. 208) says 1670; A. Castiglione (*A History of Medicine* [New York, 1941], p. 554) says 1647.
2. The usually accurate Garrison says two hundred years. Castiglione says more likely fifty years. *Ibid.*
3. F. H. Garrison, *An Introduction to the History of Medicine* (fourth ed.; Philadelphia, 1929), p. 363.
4. W. Dock, "How the Investigative Scot Foiled the Continental Conqueror," *The Pharos* (April, 1967), pp. 56–58.
5. F. R. Packard, *History of Medicine in the United States,* Vol. 2 (New York, 1931), p. 1096.
6. G. R. Murray, "Note on the Treatment of Myxoedema by Hypodermic Injections of an Extract of the Thyroid Gland of the Sheep," *British Medical Journal,* Vol. 2 (1891), p. 796.
7. A. N. Richards, "Penicillin" (Statement by the Chairman of the Committee on Medical Research), *Journal of the American Medical Association,* Vol. 122 (1943), p. 235.
8. A. Fleming (ed.), *Penicillin, Its Practical Application* (Philadelphia, 1946).
9. H. E. de Wardener, "Some Ethical and Economic Problems Associated with Intermittent Hemodialysis," *Ethics in Medical Progress: CIBA Foundation Symposium* (Boston, 1966), pp. 104–125.
10. J. P. Pendras and R. V. Erickson, "Hemodialysis: A Successful Therapy for Chronic Uremia," *Annals of Internal Medicine,* Vol. 64 (1966), pp. 293–311.
11. De Wardener, "Some Ethical and Economic Problems Associated with Intermittent Hemodialysis."
12. G. E. Schreiner, in *Ethics in Medical Progress: CIBA Foundation Symposium,* pp. 100, 118.
13. The Medical Advisory Committee is made up of eighteen physicians. The Admissions Advisory Committee is made up of seven individuals from all walks of life: two physicians, a lawyer, a housewife, a businessman, a labor leader, and a minister. Thus the community participates.
14. De Wardener, "Some Ethical and Economic Problems Associated with Intermittent Hemodialysis." Subsequent allusions to de Wardener in the text are to this article.
15. J. P. Pendras, "Experience with Patient Selection," unpublished data (1967).
16. H. K. Beecher, "Ethics and Clinical Research," *New England Journal of Medicine,* Vol. 274 (1966), pp. 1354–60.
17. J. E. Murray, "Organ Transplantation: The Practical Possibilities," *Ethics in Medical Progress: CIBA Foundation Symposium,* pp. 54–77.
18. N. P. Couch, "Supply and Demand in Kidney and Liver Transplantation: A Statistical Study," *Transplantation,* Vol. 4 (1966).
19. E. D. Robin, "Rapid Scientific Advances Bring New Ethical Questions," *Journal of the American Medical Association,* Vol 189 (August 24, 1964), pp. 624–25.
20. Sir G. Keynes, *Blood Transfusion* (London, 1949).
21. *Ibid.*
22. O. H. Robertson, "Transfusion with Preserved Red Blood Cells," *British Medical Journal,* Vol. 1 (1918), pp. 691–95.
23. See H. K. Beecher, "Preparation of Battle Casualties for Surgery," *Annals of Surgery,* Vol. 121 (1945), pp. 769–92; E. D. Churchill, Personal Communication by Letter (June 28, 1968).
24. G. E. W. Wolstenholme, "An Old-established Procedure: The Development of Blood Transfusion," *Ethics in Medical Progress: CIBA Foundation Symposium,* pp. 24–42.
25. G. Rubin, "Placental Blood for Transfusion," *New York Medical Journal,* Vol. 100 (1914), p. 421.
26. Arkansas Statutes 1947 Annotated, 1960 Replacement, Vol. 7A, Chapter 16, "Blood Transfusions":

"82-1601. Blood labeled as to race.—All human blood used or proposed to be used in the State of Arkansas for transfusions of blood, except such units of blood which will have been transported across the State line into Arkansas, shall be labeled with word 'Caucasian,' 'Negroid,' 'Mongoloid,' or some suitable designation so as to clearly indicate the race of the donor of such blood. No human blood not labeled in accordance with the provisions of this act [82-1601—2-1605] shall be used for transfusions in the State of Arkansas." [Acts 1959, No. 482, 2, p. 1923.]

"82-1602. Notice when blood of different race to be used in transfusion.—Any person about to receive a blood transfusion or a parent of said person, or the next of kin of said person shall be informed of the race of the donor of the blood proposed to be used if blood from a person of a different racial classification is to be used." [Acts 1959, No. 482, 2, p. 1923.] Certain emergency provisions are also spelled out.

27. Wolstenholme, "An Old-established Procedure: The Development of Blood Transfusion."

28. P. V. Rycroft, "A Recently Established Procedure: Corneal Transplantation," *ibid., pp.* 43–53.

29. D. Daube, "Transplantation: Acceptability of Procedures and the Required Legal Sanctions," *Ethics in Medical Progress: CIBA Foundation Symposium,* pp. 188–201.

30. T. E. Starzl, "In Discussion: 'Organ Transplantation: The Practical Possibilities,' by J. E. Murray," *ibid.,* p. 98.

31. W. E. Goodwin, "In Discussion: 'Transplantation: The Clinical Problem,' M. G. A. Woodruff," *ibid.,* p. 17.

32. Starzl, "In Discussion," *ibid.*

33. *Ibid.*

34. Daube, "Transplantation: Acceptability of Procedures and the Required Legal Sanction," *ibid.*

35. M. F. A. Woodruff, "Transplantation: The Clinical Problem," *ibid.,* pp. 6–23.

36. Murray, "Organ Transplantation: The Practical Possibilities," *ibid.*

37. Lord Platt, "Ethical Problems in Medical Procedures," *ibid.,* pp. 149–70.

38. *Ibid.*

39. *Ibid.*

40. E. W. Wilkins, Personal Communication, 1967.

41. Murray, "Organ Transplantation: The Practical Possibilities," *Ethics in Medical Progress: CIBA Foundation Symposium.*

42. G. B. Giertz, "Ethical Problems in Medical Procedures in Sweden," *ibid.,* pp. 139–48.

43. Statement Prepared by the Board on Medicine of the National Academy of Sciences, "Cardiac Transplantation in Man," *Journal of the American Medical Association,* Vol. 204, No. 9 (1968), pp. 147–48.

44. G. P. J. Alexandre, "In Discussion: 'Organ Transplantation: The Practical Possibilities,' by J. E. Murray," *Ethics in*

Medical Progress: CIBA Foundation Symposium, pp. 68–71. Compare also in this connection Report of an *Ad Hoc* Committee at Harvard Medical School to Examine the Definition of Brain Death.

45. Giertz, "Ethical Problems in Medical Procedures in Sweden," *ibid.*

46. R. Cortesini, "Outlines of a Legislation on Transplantation," *ibid.,* pp. 171–87; "In Discussion, 'Transplantation: The Clinical Problem,'" *ibid.,* p. 16.

47. C. E. Wasmuth and B. H. Stewart, "Medical and Legal Aspects of Human Organ Transplantation," *Cleveland-Marshall Law Review,* Vol. 14 (1965), pp. 442–71; also, C. E. Wasmuth, "Law for the Physician: Legal Aspects of Renal Transplantation," *Anesthesia Annals,* Vol. 46 (January–February, 1967), pp. 25–27.

48. In preparing this article, the author also had occasion to use the following sources not directly cited: Charles H. Best, Personal Communication by Letter (June 28, 1968); E. D. Churchill, "Wound Shock and Blood Transfusion" (in preparation); Editorial, "Ethics in Research," *Hospital Medicine,* Vol. 2 (April, 1968), p. 759; C. S. Keefer, Chairman, F. G. Blake, E. K. Marshall, Jr., J. S. Lockwood, and W. B. Wood, Jr., "Penicillin in the Treatment of Infections. A Report of 500 Cases"; Statement by the Committee on Chemotherapeutic and Other Agents, Division of Medical Sciences, National Research Council, *Journal of the American Medical Association,* Vol. 122, No. 18 (1943), pp. 1217–24; S. Krugman, J. P. Giles, and J. Hammond, "Infectious Hepatitis," *Journal of the American Medical Association,* Vol. 200, No. 5 (May, 1967), p. 365–73; P. Lieberman, *Medico-legal Monograph,* Law Department, American Medical Association (1966); F. Mauriceau, "Des Maladies des Femmes Grosses et Accouchées" (Paris, 1968; also English edition: "The Diseases of Women with Child and in Child-bed," trans. Hugh Chamberlen [London, 1672], see translator's note concerning the Chamberlen secret); J. R. Mote, Personal Communication by Letter (June 26, 1968); *Report of the Medical Research Council for 1962–63* (Cmnd. 2382), "Responsibility in Investigations on Human Subjects," pp. 21–25; D. H. Russell, "Law, Medicine and Minors—Part I," *New England Journal of Medicine,* Vol. 278, No. 1 (1968), pp. 35–36; D. H. Russell, "Law, Medicine and Minors—Part II," *New England Journal of Medicine,* Vol. 278, No. 5 (1968), pp. 265–66; D. H. Russell, "Law, Medicine and Minors—Part III," *New England Journal of Medicine,* Vol. 278, No. 14 (1968), pp. 779–80; P. White, Personal Communication (1968); R. M. Zollinger, Jr., M. D. Lindem, Jr., R. M. Filler, J. M. Corson, and R. E. Wilson, "Effect of Thymectomy on Skin-homograft Survival in Children," *New England Journal of Medicine,* Vol. 270 (April 2, 1964), pp. 707–710.

Chapter 2

Terminating Treatment: Age as a Standard

Daniel Callahan, Ph.D.

This article [also published in: *Hastings Center Report*, October–November, 1987, pp. 21–25] is an excerpt from *Setting Limits: Medical Goals in an Aging Society* by Daniel Callahan. Copyright ©1987 by Daniel Callahan. Reprinted by permission of Simon & Schuster, Inc.

Daniel Callahan, Ph.D., is director of The Hastings Center, Briarcliff Manor, New York.

Death, we are told, is no longer a hidden subject. That is at best a half-truth. The aged constitute the majority of those who die, some 70 percent, but a specific discussion of their dying is remarkably scant in legal, ethical, and medical writings. That omission is probably not accidental. The modernization of aging induces a sharp separation between aging and death. The latter is often treated as if it had little to do with the former, a kind of accidental conjunction. In medicine, the long-standing tradition of treating patients regardless of their age works against an open discussion, even though many physicians admit it is a consideration in their actual practice. The courts appear to follow a similar tradition. Despite the large number of decisions in recent years bearing on cases of elderly patients, that fact is typically not mentioned, though it is an obvious feature of the cases.

These inhibitions against explicit discussion of the elderly dying doubtless serve a valuable function. They reflect a sensible fear that the aged might be singled out for unfairly discriminatory treatment. They are a way of acknowledging the difficulty of sharply differentiating the medical conditions of the aged from those of other patients. Yet the pervasiveness of backstage debate about the care of the elderly dying among physicians and nurses, jurists and legislators, and the elderly themselves makes it imperative now to deal explicitly with the issue. There are also other reasons for having such a discussion. What is the proper goal of medicine for those who have already lived out a natural life span, by which I mean a full biographical, not a maximum biological life? That goal is, I believe, the relief of suffering rather than the extension of life. What are the practical implications of that position for the care of the critically ill, or elderly dying? If the goals of the aging ought to be service to the young and coming generations, what follows for their way of thinking about death? How does the ready availability of technology sway the making of decisions about the dying? I want to start with that last question.

Medical Technology: A House Divided

One of the hardy illusions of the past few decades has been the belief that with a few changes in law and attitudes, the dying can be spared excessive medical treatment and be allowed to die a "death with dignity." Yet the termination of treatment seems to remain almost as hard, if not harder, in practice now than in earlier times. That is true with the old as much as with the young. Despite the public debate and soothing words, both the public and physicians remain profoundly ambivalent about stopping the use of life-sustaining medical technologies. It is often and accurately said that the elderly do not want excessive and useless treatment. They greatly fear a death marked by technological oppressiveness, wrapped in a cocoon of tubes and machines. Yet they have also no less come—as we all have—to expect medicine whenever possible to extend their lives as well as alleviate or cure their diseases. These are not logically incompatible impulses, but they can be psychologically at odds.

Two fears seem to compete with each other among the elderly: on the one hand, that they will be abandoned or neglected if they become critically ill or begin to die and that few will care about their fate; or, on the other hand, that they will be excessively treated and their lives painfully extended. Death after a long, lingering illness marked by dementia and isolation in the back room of a nursing home similarly competes as a vision of horror with that of death in an intensive care unit, a dying constantly interrupted by painful and unwanted interventions. There is reason for such fears. Medicine steadily extends to the elderly the use of drugs, surgery, rehabilitation, and other procedures once thought suitable only for younger patients. Ever-more-aggressive technological means are used to extend the life of the elderly. On the whole, the elderly welcome that development—even as they fear some of its consequences. They want, somehow, that most elusive of all goals: a steadily improving medical technology that will relieve their pain and illness while not leading to overtreatment and to a harmful extension of life.

The difficulty of making accurate prognoses is part of the problem. In all too many cases, technology is used because it is not known that a patient is dying or in irreversible decline. The prognosis of a terminal illness is always difficult to achieve. The problem is even greater, a recent Office of Technology Assessment (OTA) study concluded, when immediate decisions must be made about initiating treatment. Only for patients who have been fully diagnosed can estimates of survival probability be made. Even then, the probabilities are very likely to be insufficient for guiding decisionmaking about withholding or withdrawing treatment for an individual patient.[1]

The ordinary, almost instinctive, tendency of physicians faced with that uncertainty is then to use technology, to treat with vigor. For his or her part, the patient—who will ordinarily want to live, but may also be fearful of useless overtreatment—will be faced with a no less highly uncertain situation. How sick am I? What are my chances? Both patients and families are likely to have the same inclination as the physician, to treat. Given a normal desire to preserve life and to use available technologies, those impulses of both patients and physicians are understandable. The hard question, therefore, is not why technology is used so much by physicians, or why patients want it no less than doctors. We have to ask instead why it is so hard to *stop* using it, even when patient welfare and plain common sense appear to demand just that.

We should not see the question of terminating treatment as a sharply focused "yes" or "no" decision to treat vigorously or allow to die, a kind of binary "1" or "0" gate-

way to life or death. It is more realistically viewed as a continuum in which the odds of effective intervention slowly decline. At age sixty-five, a person (call him Mr. Smith) in otherwise good health who suffers a heart attack will be treated, and the available technology makes the odds of saving him good.[2] Then imagine Mr. Smith being diagnosed for an operable cancer of the colon at age seventy-five, with a 50 percent chance of full recovery. If he is still mentally alert and eager to live, both doctor and patient will most likely choose to go forward with the operation. Imagine still another phase: at eighty, he again suffers a heart attack of moderate severity, with the odds of complete recovery if vigorously treated at about 20 percent and partial recovery at about 60 percent. He will probably be treated. Then, at eighty-two, he suffers a moderately severe stroke, one from which his life can most likely be saved but which will almost certainly leave him semiparalyzed and probably only semicompetent thereafter (but amenable to rehabilitation efforts). Thereafter, he gradually declines and suffers a series of other strokes in his mid to late eighties, spending his last years debilitated and demented in a nursing home before dying at eighty-eight.

When, in that continuum, was he dying? There is no straightforward answer to that question, for he was—but for the technology—dying at many points. Each crisis presented the need to make a choice for or against initiating treatment. A familiar story then unfolded: since physicians generally aim to save life, and since patients ordinarily prefer to live rather than to die, and since at each point there was some realistic hope, treatment was undertaken. The good fight was fought.

Mr. Smith lived on because we expect medicine to continue to devise ever-more-ingenious ways to save our lives. That is why the annual budget of the National Institutes of Health (NIH) has always risen, budget crises or not. Few congressmen can resist the plea to appropriate funds to save lives through medical research. Why should anyone be astonished, much less indignant, that the other message many are trying to deliver—the need to stop treatment—has such a hard time getting through? Unrelenting "wars" against disease are being pursued by thousands of dedicated medical researchers and physicians at the same time that "natural death" legislation is being passed. The former campaigns are much more dedicated and powerful than the latter. We have been told endlessly—and truthfully, with the support of hard data—that more effective emergency care and the improvement of intensive-care units will save additional lives, and that better geriatric rehabilitation services (for which Mr. Smith was an ideal candidate at many points) will help restore the functioning of the lives thus saved. In the meantime, of course, physicians are being exhorted to stop trying so hard to perform technological miracles with those destined—assuming we can know that—to die.

The double message is just about perfect, designed for maximum confusion. As a group the elderly dying are to be saved and those diseases which cause death eliminated. As individuals, however, the elderly dying should be allowed to die when it is right to do so and their diseases allowed to run their course.

Age as a Criterion

Could we not, however, turn to age as a criterion in order to know when to stop, when to say that no more should be done? I want to look first at one great source of confusion: the common failure to distinguish between age as a medical or technical criterion, pertinent to prognosis, and age as a person- or patient-centered criterion. By age as a medical criterion, I mean treating chronological age as if it were the equivalent of other physical characteristics of a patient—that is, as the equivalent of such typical medical indicators as weight, blood pressure, or white-cell count. Just as those characteristics would be reasonable considerations in treating a patient, so also would age if it could be treated as a reliable technical consideration. Age as a person-centered characteristic, by contrast, would be understood as the relevance of a person's history and biography, his situation not as a collection of organs but as a person, to be taken into account when that personal situation could legitimately be considered. I will argue that age as a medical standard should be rejected, while age as a person-centered (what I will call a "biographical") standard can be used.

Age as a medical standard. The principal use of age as a medical standard would be in prognosis of treatment outcome: how well will an elderly person respond to and benefit from a treatment? In that respect, the main problem in using age as a standard is twofold. It is difficult to disentangle age from a wide range of other conditions that may coexist with old age. Do kidneys fail because a person is old, or simply because of the ravages of a disease that anyone could have, whatever his age? It is no less difficult to distinguish between the general characteristics of the aged as a group and the unique characteristics of any given aged person. The OTA report on aging and life-extending technology medicine notes the difficulties in making the necessary distinctions (which I have reordered slightly to bring out the underlying logic):

(a) increasing age is associated with greater likelihood of physical decline, increased comorbidity, reduced physiological reserve, and cognitive impairment. Clinically, the probability of these decrements increases notably after age eighty-five; *but,*

(b) chronological age turns out to be a poor predictor of the efficacy of a number of life-sustaining technologies

(dialysis, nutritional support, resuscitation, mechanical ventilation, and antibiotics); *while,*

(c) efficacy may be lessened for older patients in general; *but,*

(d) improved medical assessment and care could improve that efficacy; *while,*

(e) in any case very little is currently known about differences in treatment outcome that are due to age *per se* and those that are due to increased prevalence or severity of diseases in older ages; *but,*

(f) in some classification systems (for the purposes of, say, admission to an ICU), chronological age functions as a proxy measure for age-associated factors that cannot be easily measured.[3]

I do not cite the OTA material with any intent to amuse. It is a careful set of distinctions based on the best empirical evidence available and makes perfectly clear why age alone is not a good predictor of medical outcome. It also nicely helps explain why physicians can also say that, in practice, they do make decisions based on the age of patients—but rarely can give a wholly defensible scientific account of themselves if pressed to do so. The puzzle, I think, is partially explained by the difference between (1) perceiving a patient as a whole person, whose combination, or gestalt, of characteristics makes it evident that he is old rather than young, which makes a difference in his future; and (2) perceiving and medically treating the person part by part, organ by organ. If we look at a person only as a collection of organs, any given characteristic may well be identical with that found in younger persons (some of whom have wrinkled skin, or failing kidneys, or are bald, or have osteoarthritis, for example). Moreover, even if in some cases, with some conditions, we know age to be generally relevant, we may not know where, on a continuum of characteristics of the aged as a group, any particular old person falls in terms of likely medical outcome. For all these reasons, age as a medical criterion is unreliable.

Age as a biographical standard. If we know someone's age, but nothing else about him, what do we know of significance? If the person is old—say, in his seventies (and certainly by his eighties)—we would know that most of his chronological life is in his past rather than his future, would not expect to find him playing football or climbing trees for recreation, might not be surprised to find that most of his friends are older rather than younger people, and might expect him to have two or more physical impairments, minor or major. Certain "age-associated" traits would almost invariably be present.

What makes him the person he is, and not someone else, is the combination of his age-associated traits and other, more idiosyncratic personal and social traits. That he was very old, with a statistically short life expectancy, would hardly be irrelevant to him as he thought about his life and his future or to the rest of us for many (even if not all) purposes. As Malcolm Cowley has noted, "we start by growing old in other people's eyes. Then slowly we come to share their judgment."[4] We would not make long-range plans with an elderly person the way we might with a younger person, nor would we likely invite him to take charge of strenuous long-term projects, even if he were highly talented. For his part, he would not be likely to undertake a total change in his way of life, such as immigrating to a new country, or undertaking extensive training for a new career. While age alone would not tell us whether he was lively or dour, bright or dull, we would most likely be far more impressed with great physical vitality in someone that age than in a teenager.

His age would, in other words, surely be a part of our overall understanding of him—not the whole story, but hardly of no consequence either. While many "age-associated" traits will bear on the functioning of an elderly person, age as a biographical trait does not reduce to that. Age encompasses a relationship to time—less time statistically remains for an old person than a young person, and there is more personal history behind him as well. It encompasses a relationship to self-consciousness—life and its prospects will usually be thought about differently. And it encompasses a relationship to the passing of the generations—the old are next in line to pass as individuals. The old know they are old, and so does everyone else. Age is not an incidental trait of a person. Might the combination of age and other characteristics then be allowed to have a bearing on medical treatment, and particularly termination, decisions?

The morality of age as a standard. Before attempting to answer that last question, it is necessary to inquire whether it is moral to make the attempt. Some would say no: age as a criterion for the termination of treatment should be ruled out of bounds altogether. A central strand of medical ethics holds that patients should be treated only on the basis of their strict medical needs, and that age should no more influence the way they are treated than should their race, sex, or ethnic background. Mark Siegler has pointed to one source of the objection, noting that a failure to retain "need-specific criteria with respect to elderly patients . . . [would] undermine the traditions of clinical medicine, which are based upon medical need and patient preferences . . . and [would] undermine the traditions of our society, which are based upon moral virtues of charity and compassion."[5] The immediate force of such objections is evident. While there has been some toleration in the medical-ethics literature for the idea of rationing by imposing external policy constraints on physicians, there has been little if any toleration for the idea of physician rationing at the bedside. Doctors are enjoined by medical morality to be unstinting advocates for the welfare of their individual patients and no less enjoined to use medical criteria only—"medical need"—in making their decisions. Yet it is precisely that tradition which my approach to limitation of health care for the aged calls into doubt. The high cost of health care, unrelenting technological developments, and the good of the elderly themselves require that it be examined afresh.

"Medical need," in the context of constant technological innovation, is inherently elastic and open-ended; as a guide to what is actually good for patients or what physicians are obliged to give them, it is highly unreliable. Experienced and conscientious physicians do in fact take age into account in termination decisions, and always have. Why should we therefore assume that age is not, and should not be, part of a responsible moral judgment? The problem in responding to this question is in distinguishing between a medical and a moral judgment. That an elderly person should be given a different drug dosage than a younger patient is ordinarily considered a purely medical judgment. By that statement is meant that if the aim is proper physical care of the patient in both cases, then different dosages may be indicated to achieve identical outcomes. A judgment of that kind can be based on scientific evidence. But the use of age as a "medical" indication is ambiguous. If it means that because of a person's age, medical treatment will be futile, do no good whatever, then it may properly be called a medical and not a moral judgment. It is a judgment about medical efficacy only. Yet if a judgment is also being passed about the worth of the life—that the treatment is futile not because it will fail technically but because the life saved is not worth saving because of age—then it has passed into the moral realm. According to the tradition of medical ethics, judgments about the social worth of a patient's life are unacceptable as grounds for terminating care. That is a solid and necessary tradition; but it does not touch the question of whether age as a standard might be defensible.

There is also another possibility for ambiguity. What is medical "need"? If understood as the needs of a patient's organs, or other physiological systems, treatment may (by ordinary standards) be required; otherwise they will fail. But if "need" is understood to be the needs of the patient as a person, not merely as an assemblage of deficient organs, no clear answer about the requirement of "medical need" may be forthcoming. Then the physician may have to make a moral judgment: will meeting the needs of the patient's organs meet his needs as a whole person? They are not necessarily the same. It is not clear which need the tradition invoked by Siegler has in mind. More than that, the technological possibilities of medicine for organ sustenance, quite apart from overall patient welfare, mean that "medical need" can rarely if ever be kept free of moral evaluation and judgment. The good of organs is always subordinate to the good of the person.

Daniel Callahan, Ph.D.

There is no such thing as pure "medical need"; it always presupposes some value judgment about the desirability of treatment.

Will it necessarily be the case, as James Childress has suggested, that the use of an age standard would symbolize "abandonment and exclusion from communal care"?[6] That would be likely only if it were widely believed or perceived that an age standard for exclusion from care came into use as a manifestation of society's rejection, denigration, or devaluation of elderly people. It would be a different matter if, instead, it emerged from a prudent effort to find an appropriate balance between the needs of the aged and those of younger generations, and from a conscientious effort to determine, in the face of potentially unlimited technological innovation in care for the aged, where a reasonable limit on care could be set. The "symbolic significance" of an age standard depends not on the mere fact of using age but on the meaning attributed to that fact; context, perceived motive, and articulated rationale determine that symbolic meaning. Childress would most likely be right if age were used as a standard in the present situation; but that would not necessarily be the case if its use were transformed so as to be seen as part of an affirmation of old age and not its denigration.

Age as a biographical standard for terminating treatment. How can a combination of age and other characteristics be allowed to have a bearing on the termination of treatment? How, I respond, can it not any longer? If "medical need" is too indeterminate and elastic a concept to be used by itself, then some use of age will be *necessary* to make a judgment about terminating care of the elderly. Since age is an important aspect of the patient as a person, someone who is not just a collection of organs, it falsifies the reality that is part of a person in his fullness to set it aside as irrelevant. Moreover, in addition to being a necessary part of a full and proper medical-moral judgment, age is a valuable and illuminating part, telling us where the patient stands in relation to his own history. There are a large and growing number of elderly who are not imminently dying but who are feeble and declining, often chronically ill, for whom curative medicine has little to offer. That kind of medicine may still be able to do something for failing organs; it can keep them going a bit longer. But it cannot offer the patient as a person any hope of being restored to good health. A different treatment plan should be in order. That person's history has all but come to an end, and medical care needs to encompass that reality, not try to deny it.

For many people, beginning with the aged themselves, old age is a reason in itself to think about medical care in a different way, whether in forgoing its lifesaving powers when death is clearly imminent, or in forgoing its use even when death may be distant but life has become a blight rather than a blessing. The alternative is not, as some would have it, respect for life but an idolatrous enslavement to technology.

We should want to know not just what chronological age may tell us about the state of a person's body (as a technical criterion), but also what it morally and psychologically signifies for a person to have an old rather than a young body; or what it means for a person to be old rather than young when considering the prospect of painful treatment; or what it signifies to live life as an old person—or as a sick old person—who cannot expect to recapture the vitality of youth, or even of an earlier old age. When considered in those ways, age becomes a category of evaluation in its own right, something reasonable and proper to wonder and worry about. It bears not only on physical characteristics, but on a person's self-understanding, as something intrinsic (with varying degrees of intensity, to be sure) to a person's individuality and life story. The whole person—and it is that whole person who presents himself or herself for treatment—is a person of a certain chronological age: that determines many characteristics, and much of the coloring, of a person's life. That is the importance of the biographical point of view.

Principles for the Use of Age

How, from a biographical vantage point, should we formulate age as a criterion for the termination of treatment and make use of it in termination decisions? I will begin by proposing some general background principles for the termination of treatment of the aged, each meant to articulate themes developed earlier.

After a person has lived out a natural life span, medical care should no longer be oriented to resisting death. No precise chronological age can readily be set for determining when a natural life span has been achieved—biographies vary—but it would normally be expected by the late seventies or early eighties. While a person's history may not be complete—time is always open-ended—most of it will have been achieved by that stage of life. It will be a full biography, even if more details are still to be added. Death beyond that period is not now, nor should it be, typically considered premature or untimely. Any greater precision than my "late seventies or early eighties" does not at present seem possible, and extended public discussion would be needed to achieve even a rough consensus on the appropriate age range. That discussion would also have to consider whether, for policy purposes, it would be necessary to set an exact age or a range only, and that would pose a classic policy dilemma. Too vague a standard of a "natural life span" would open the way for too great a flexibility of application to be fair or workable, while too specific a standard—one indifferent to the unique features of individual biographies—would preclude prudence and appropriate room for discretion.

Problems of that kind, however difficult, should not be used as an excuse to evade the necessity of setting some kind of age standard, or to conclude that any age standard must necessarily mean denying the value of the elderly. The presumption against resisting death after a natural life span would not in any sense demean those who have lived that long or to suggest that their lives are less valuable than those of younger people. To come to the end of life in old age does not diminish the value of the life; that remains until the very end. This is not a principle, in short, for the comparison of lives. It reflects instead an acceptance of the inevitability of death in general and its acceptability for the individual after a natural life span in particular. Death will then take its proper place as a necessary link in the transition of generations.

Provision of medical care for those who have lived out a natural life span will be limited to the relief of suffering. Medicine is not in a position to bring meaning and significance to the lives of the old. That only they can do for themselves, with the help of the larger culture. Yet medicine can help promote the physical functioning, the mental alertness, and the emotional stability conducive to this pursuit. These remain valuable goals, even when a natural life span has been attained. The difference at that point is that death should no longer be treated by medicine as an enemy. It may well be, of course, that medical efforts to relieve suffering will frequently have the unintended but foreseeable consequence of extending life expectancy. That is to be expected. A sharp line between relieving suffering and extending life will be on occasion difficult to draw, and under no circumstance would it be acceptable to fail to relieve suffering because of the possibility of life extension. The bias of the principle should be to stop resisting death after a certain age, but not when the price of doing so is unrelievable suffering. At the same time—as the success of the hospice movement proves—it is perfectly possible to relieve suffering while not seeking to extend life.

The existence of medical technologies capable of extending the lives of the elderly who have lived out a natural life span creates no presumption whatever that the technologies must be used for that purpose. The uses of technology are always to be subordinated to the appropriate ends of medicine: that is, to the avoidance of premature death and to the relief of suffering. The alternative is slavery to the powers of technology—they, not we, will determine our end. Medicine should in particular resist the tendency to provide to the aged the life-extending capabilities of technologies developed primarily to help younger people avoid premature and untimely death. The use of those technologies should be subordinate to what is good for the elderly as individuals, good for them as members of society, good for them as a link in the passing of the generations, and good for the needs of other age groups.

The three principles detailed above are not so radical as they may first appear. They come close to actually articulating what many elderly express as their fears about aging and death. They indicate a wish that their life not be aggressively extended beyond a point at which they still possess a good degree of physical functioning and mental alertness, a life that has value and meaning for them; they are asking not for more years as such (though some would want just that), but for as many *good* years as possible; and that medical technology be limited in its use to those situations in which it will maintain or restore an adequate quality of life, not sustain and extend a deteriorating one.

References

1. U.S. Congress Office of Technology Assessment, Biological Applications Program, *Life Sustaining Technologies and the Elderly* (Washington, DC: OTA, July 1987), 1–22ff.
2. I have adapted this description from a similar one developed by Jerome L. Avorn, "Medicine, Health, and the Geriatric Transformation," *Daedalus* 115 (Winter 1986), 215–17.
3. OTA, *Life-Sustaining Technologies,* I-39-45.
4. Malcolm Cowley, *The View from Eighty* (New York: Penguin Books, 1982), 5. That line was quoted in G. C. Prado's remarkably interesting book *Rethinking How We Age* (Westport, CT: Greenwood Press, 1986), which analyzes psychological and social age, as distinguished from biological age.
5. Mark Siegler, "Should Age Be a Criterion in Health Care?" *Hastings Center Report* 14:5 (October 1984), 27.
6. James F. Childress, "Ensuring Care, Respect, and Fairness for the Elderly," *Hastings Center Report* 14:5 (October 1984), 29.

Chapter 3

Who Shall Be Saved? An African Answer

John F. Kilner

John F. Kilner is assistant professor of social ethics, Asbury Theological Seminary, Wilmore, Kentucky, and adjunct professor of medical ethics at the University of Kentucky, Lexington.

Daniel Ngwala and I drive our dusty, dented four-wheel-drive Subaru into a little market area where cars are not often seen. Getting out, Ngwala wanders over to where several older men are talking while younger faces eye me cautiously. Ngwala asks if there are any traditional healers in the area. With a casual gesture, someone tells him: a witchdoctor named Kavili Nduma lives "out that way," but why does he want to know? After due assurances that we are not government agents come to cause trouble, Ngwala returns to the car and we head "that way."

A mile or so down the rutted dirt road we stop to greet a woman with fifty pounds of firewood on her back, and we ask the whereabouts of Nduma. She says we have gone too far and must return to the second path on (she points) "that" side of the road. We do so, taking the car as far down the path as we can before thornbushes and rocks force us to stop.

We leave the car at a mud and grass hut nearby, but only after we have secured a pledge from an adult to keep the fascinated children from pulling the car apart. Now setting out on foot, we travel twenty minutes through meandering maize fields and up a rocky hill, finally reaching Nduma's home—and she is home, thank God! Ngwala explains the reason we have come, and Nduma calls others to bring us chairs. Though the chairs are rickety and lack upright backs, I quickly forget how uncomfortable they are during the two-and-a-half hour interview that follows.

Questioned about how best to cope with the frequent scarcity of medical resources, which may allow her to save only one of two dying people, Nduma says to save an old man rather than a young, a man without children rather than a father supporting five. She affirms these priorities even when it is revealed that in both cases those preferred arrived second rather than first for treatment. When she adds that it really would be better to try to save none rather than one, little doubt remains that I have encountered a perspective on scarce resource allocation very different from those generally found in the United States.

In fact, this was precisely the reason for the long journey to Africa. The trip was inspired by my conviction that an ethical analysis of alternative approaches to the microallocation of scarce lifesaving medical resources would be greatly enhanced by discussing the problem with people operating out of a different cultural framework. (Microallocation focuses on determining who gets how much of a particular lifesaving medical resource, once budgetary and other limitations have determined the total amount of the resource available.) With support and guidance both in the United States and Kenya, I decided to investigate in particular the views of the Akamba people of Machakos district, Kenya, by means of personal interviews. Special assistance was provided by Ngwala, one of the Akamba himself, lifelong resident of Machakos, and part-time farmer with a variety of skills.

The Akamba are traditionally subsistence farmers and herders. But their young men are increasingly seeking jobs in the district's towns or the nation's capital, Nairobi, as the rapidly growing population of 1.2 million fills the district's 14,183 square kilometers (5,475 sq. mi.). The land is largely semi-arid—a major exception being some very hilly areas—so life here is not easy. Moreover, droughts are not unusual; roads and infrastructure are not yet well developed, and government services are limited.

Health care in Machakos reflects the general scarcity of resources. While much development is taking place, the efforts of government and religion (mainly Christian) have so far produced only a few modest hospitals, health centers, and health subcenters (four or five each). Most public health care is provided at the more than fifty small dispensaries scattered throughout the district. But even the most basic critical drugs such as penicillin are frequently out of stock, especially in the dispensaries. Accordingly, many, if not a majority, of the people still depend upon traditional healing even though for the most part it has been forbidden by the government, which is promoting a more "modern" (Western) approach to health care.

Having decided to focus upon the Akamba people, I next had to identify those in the Akamba culture who are most knowledgeable about the ethical as well as medical issues involved in allocating scarce medical resources. I learned that those I was seeking are the "healers" of the culture, for Akamba healers have consistently been concerned with both physical and religious/moral health. Akamba healers are of two types: traditional healers (witchdoctors, herbalists, and midwives) and health workers (those who work in government or mission health care facilities). I randomly selected a sample population of 132 persons, with equal representation from both groups.[1]

Since the Akamba think in terms of stories,[2] it seemed appropriate to pose my questions as a series of stories (see box). The stories focused mainly on a healer named Mutua and two patients, Mbiti and Kioko. Resources are so scarce that only one of the two can be saved. In each situation, Mbiti arrives earlier, which, according to the Akamba, is a presumptive reason for treating him before Kioko. But different facts about the two people are also stated in successive questions—for example, Kioko is helping many people in his area whereas Mbiti is not—in order to see if the Akamba ever view such considerations as more important than order of arrival.

People were generally willing to talk at great length about these matters, with a few notable exceptions. One witchdoctor suddenly stopped in the middle of an answer, and said that she could tell me no more. When

asked why, she replied that not she but a spirit had been speaking up to that point and the spirit refused to continue today. Plead as we might, she insisted she had nothing more to say but we could return the next day for more. We did, and she finished the interview. Was she merely eccentric? Another witchdoctor told us she could not be a Christian because whenever she started going to church an evil spirit killed a member of her family after telling her the day the murder would happen. She had lost her husband and two children this way, a fact that others confirmed. If I had not accepted the reality of spiritual beings before going to Kenya, I might well have left a believer. Such spiritual involvement added a striking dimension to the tremendous friendliness, hospitality, and thoughtfulness of the Akamba people.

Two Dying Patients, One Dose of Herbs

Mutua was an herbalist in Ukambani, who treated people for many different illnesses. Some patients, such as those with kiathi [a severe bacterial infection], received a rare herb called kitawa. But sometimes Mutua's supply of kitawa would run out. Mutua had seen people die because there was no kitawa. One morning a person dying of kiathi was waiting when Mutua finished treating his first patient. The person's name was Mbiti. But before Mutua called Mbiti in to examine and treat him, another person came in and asked to speak to Mutua. He told Mutua that a man named Kioko was dying from kiathi and had just arrived. The person urged Mutua to see Kioko right away. Mutua knew that there was only enough kitawa left to cure one person.

Suppose that Kioko was involved in a number of projects of great benefit to the peoples in Mutua's area. Moreover, if he died the projects would probably soon fail. Should Mutua save the life of Kioko or that of Mbiti, who had arrived earlier? Why?

Suppose that Kioki was the father of five children, whereas Mbiti had no children. Should Mutua save the life of Kiolo or that of Mbiti, who had arrived earlier? Why?

Suppose that Mbiti was over sixty years old, whereas Kioko was twenty-five. Should Mutua save the life of Kioko or that of Mbiti, who had arrived earlier? Why?

—**Example of scenario with some follow-up questions.**

John F. Kilner

The Akamba View of Life

The answers to our questions proved well worth waiting for, especially where they reflected outlooks different from those commonly encountered in the United States. For instance, where only one person can be saved, many Akamba favor saving an old man before a young, even where the young man is first in line. Whereas in the United States we tend to value the young more highly than the old because they are more productive economically, these Akamba espouse a more relational view of life. Life, they insist, is more than atomistic sums of individual economic contributions; it is a social fabric of interpersonal relations. The older a person becomes, the more intricately interwoven that person becomes in the lives of others, and the greater the damage done if that person is removed. At the same time, the older person has wisdom—a perspective on life that comes only with age—which is considered to be a particularly important social resource.

Another Akamba priority documented by the study is: where only one person can be saved, save a man without children rather than one with five. Whereas in the United States many would favor the opposite choice for the children's sake, many Akamba counter that the man without children faces annihilation and must be allowed to live so that he can "raise up a name" for himself by having children. The self, for the Akamba, is not solely an individual, mortal life in the present; it is also a vital link in a chain that reaches through time. To drop a link before subsequent links have been fashioned is to destroy all future links (persons) as well as the perpetual life of the link in question.

A third surprising (by U.S. standards) priority acknowledged by numerous Akamba is the insistence that it is better to give a half-treatment to each of two dying patients—even where experience dictates that a half-treatment is insufficient to save either—than to provide one patient with a full treatment which would almost certainly be lifesaving. Under these circumstances many in the United States would abandon substantive equality (or equal treatment, which would here probably mean equal death) in favor of procedural equality (or equal access, which would here probably entail saving one person according to a first-come, first-served principle).

But many Akamba argue that the whole point of equality is what a person receives. They live according to the proverb, "No matter how many Akamba are gathered the mbilivili will be shared." (A mbilivili is the smallest bird known to the Akamba and one that provides very little food.) Their outlook is sustained by the conviction that God is prone to heal not only where medical personnel have faithfully applied all available scientific knowledge but also where they have been faithful to the moral law as they are capable of knowing it. As long as

healers remain faithful (that is, moral), they maintain, the responsibility for patients' lives remains God's.

These views bring into question some Western assumptions that dictate allocation decisions in the United States and elsewhere. Moreover, they remind us of the error in too quickly concluding, from the fact that people of different cultures support conflicting policies or actions, that morality is relative and that people's basic moral sensibilities may differ significantly. Often, as here, the difference is one of knowledge or beliefs (about what contributions benefit society most, or the nature of eternal life, or God's role in healing) rather than of moral judgment.

Cultural differences affect more than allocation decisions, however. They help shape the way that medical personnel view and treat patients. For instance, because the Akamba traditionally see God as active in healing and people as both spiritual and material beings, they are more likely than their Western counterparts to perceive a need for treatment that addresses health problems on a spiritual as well as a physical level. While Akamba healers do not generally distinguish a psychological component of illness, their emphasis on relationships (regarding their valuing of the elderly) disposes them, together with the entire community, to provide the care and support required to meet this dimension of illness.

The different approaches of Akamba health workers and Akamba traditional healers reflect similar considerations. Health workers, shaped as they are by Western education and medical training, are much more apt to see an illness in purely physical terms and to be skeptical about spiritual diagnoses, not to mention spiritual treatment. To be sure, of the three types of traditional healer, only the witchdoctors make use of spiritual powers (to help those who have been spiritually victimized by "witches" or "wizards"). Yet, even the more physically oriented herbalists and midwives display a level of caring and personal availability to patients that sets them apart from many of the more Western health workers.

Health workers concentrate more on efficient treatment, and are more apt to devote time to research. They are more likely to employ varied (and scientifically better) treatments, even if their quality of caring does not always equal that of traditional healers. Health workers also use Western-developed medicines rather than the traditional herbs, though the administering and even effectiveness of the two do at times appear to be similar.

Scoring Values

Though I was eager to understand the full range of Akamba perspectives on the allocation of scarce lifesaving medical resources, I was especially interested to learn what significance, if any, they attach to four basic values frequently invoked in the U.S. allocation debate. Informal preliminary research revealed that the Akamba appeal to these values in the following particular form:

- *Equality:* All people are fundamentally equal where life itself is at stake, so the first to arrive should be treated when only one life can be saved.
- *Usefulness:* The most important goal in deciding whom to treat is to achieve the greatest social benefit possible.
- *Need:* Whoever is in the greatest danger of dying right away should be saved.
- *Life:* The most important goal in deciding whom to treat is to save as many lives as possible.

To determine the significance that the Akamba attach to these values, we asked our participants twenty-four questions and assigned value-significance points to their answers according to the values they expressed. Participants could earn a point for equality on twenty-three of the questions. Six questions pertained to usefulness; three to need; three to life; and others to a variety of values such as choice. For example, if a healer maintained that Mbiti, who arrives first, is to be treated rather than the patient Kioko, who is involved in projects to benefit the community, then the healer received an equality point. However, to receive this point the healer had to justify her or his choice with some sort of reference to the notion that people equally warrant treatment where life-threatening health problems are concerned. The implicit idea expressed here is that treatment should do nothing but proceed according to the natural lottery: first-come, first-served. (As noted previously, a significant number of healers were so strongly egalitarian that they never chose one patient over another. These healers automatically received a high number of equality points.)

Where Kioko rather than Mbiti was chosen because of his greater social usefulness, then the healer received a usefulness point rather than an equality point. Other questions presented the possibility of receiving, say, a need or life point as against an equality point. In nearly all of the questions it was possible to accumulate either an equality point or a point of some other type—the three categories mentioned here being the major ones. That virtually every question involved a possible equality point does not mean that equality is in some sense more "important" than the other values but merely reflects the manner in which the moral choice typically arises for the Akamba healers. They must choose between their adopted norm of first-come, first-served and some competing moral claim arising from the particulars of the case before them.

Once assigned in this manner, points of each type were summed for each person. The resulting equality scores ranged from 3 to 23 (average 14.3), usefulness scores

from 0 to 6 (average 2.1), need scores from 0 to 3 (average 2.4), and life scores from 0 to 3 (average 2.3). (In each case the highest score reflects the number of questions pertaining to that category.)

As the averages suggest, most of those interviewed placed a high value on need and life. Perhaps this is to be expected since the Akamba working in health care settings are dedicated to the health of their people. Another finding was somewhat less predictable. While one-third of those questioned viewed usefulness as completely irrelevant in the context under consideration, the remaining two-thirds saw it as a legitimate consideration, at least sometimes, when deciding whose life to save. This latter outlook had a definite impact upon the significance accorded to equality. Nearly two-thirds of the Akamba scored less than 17 on the equality scale—17 being the score of one who would allow the claims of equality to be set aside only where need, life, or choice (not usefulness) is at stake.[3]

What accounts for a healer's particular set of value-significance scores? Whether a person is a health worker or traditional healer appears to matter, for equality, usefulness, and life scores. But what, more precisely, accounts for the difference between the two groups? In order to attempt a partial answer to this question, personal information was gathered at the start of each participant's interview. Specifically, we ascertained each person's sex, age, marital status, length of marriage, number of children, level of education, length of (medical) training, job responsibility, years worked, and religion. Doing so was not always easy. Age was particularly troublesome since many people did not know their age. Sometimes only through the ingenuity of Ngwala—who quizzed them about their knowledge of certain natural disasters and their estimated age at the time of those they could remember—was it possible to obtain this information. We examined potentially significant relationships between the ten personal factors and the value-significance scores.

With regard to nine of the ten items no consistent correlation emerged between the factors and the value-significance scores. (Perhaps surprisingly, religion was one of the nine. Probably this is because the only two religions our respondents acknowledged were the traditional Akamba religion and Christianity. Both, as the Akamba understand them, promote a fairly egalitarian outlook and place similar degrees of emphasis upon the three other basic values examined in this study.) Only education appeared to make a difference. In the table on the next page, the health workers were divided as evenly as possible into three groups according to the highest level of education completed. (Kenyans complete the "standard" grades and then the "forms" before becoming eligible to enter a college or university.) Because none of the traditional healers interviewed had more than a primary education, they were treated here as a separate group and served as a check upon the other results, as will be explained shortly.

Statistical analysis of the scores suggests that the importance health workers attach to equality, usefulness, and life (not need) is significantly influenced by their education. (In fact, all three correlations are statistically significant at well above a 99 percent confidence level.) The more education one has received, the lower her or his equality score. This drop corresponds to a rise in both usefulness and life scores. However, when the weight ascribed to equality is changing most rapidly—beyond the primary educational level—the rise in usefulness scores is the primary change associated with the drop in equality scores.

Two other findings would appear to substantiate these conclusions. First, since the educational level of the traditional healers as a whole is only a little above that of the least-educated group of health workers, one would expect their mean value-significance scores to fall between the mean scores of the two least-educated health worker groups, though closer to those of the least-educated group. The table confirms that such is the case for all four values.

Second, in order to obtain a fourth educational level and thereby ascertain whether or not the observed trends continue through university education, the only three Akamba "doctors" (in the Western, university-educated sense) of Machakos district were interviewed. None had previously been selected through the sampling procedure employed. All of the observed trends do in fact persist at this fourth level. To the average equality scores (see the table) of 15.5, 14.1, and 9.8 the doctors add a 7.0; to the average usefulness scores of 1.6, 2.1, and 3.8 they add a 5.3; and to the average life scores of 2.1, 2.7, and 2.9 they add a 3.0.

My language regarding correlations between education and value-significance scores has been purposely tentative. Any quantitative measurement of the significance that people attach to particular values can only be approximate. Furthermore, while the data lead me to think that a decreasing equality-oriented and increasingly usefulness-oriented outlook is traceable directly to the Kenyan educational system, I am aware that this contention has not been conclusively proven. For instance, those who go on

for more education may—at least theoretically—be those who already have a more usefulness-oriented outlook.

However, two considerations cast doubt on this alternate explanation. First, this explanation gives no account of what does prompt the values to change. Since the nine other items apparently do not account for the differences in values according to this study, the best explanation seems to be that education is affecting values rather than vice-versa. Second, it seems highly unlikely that the reason many people stay in school through secondary school and beyond is their preference for one particular moral value over another. However, this question could be studied empirically.

If in fact basic values are being altered by the educational process in Kenya, then the institution of education, even when "purged" of religious instruction, is not as "value-free" as some contend. The real issue may be *which* values education is going to instill—those that it teaches implicitly, or "better" (if different) values, which are explicitly taught and otherwise encouraged.

A Shared Experience

As we brought the interviewing to a close I did not know exactly what the results of the study would be, but I knew it would be long before I forgot the process by which the results were obtained. One of the greatest challenges came near the very end. We completed the interviews a week ahead of schedule, but the heavy rains came ten days early. Those last three days were quite muddy. I never did get the hang of walking down a steep mud-path in the rain—without the dubious pleasure of sitting down in it at least once. But what a privilege to be able to see the task of healing through very different eyes.

In exchange for sharing their perspective, the Akamba health workers and traditional healers were eager to learn my views on medical resource allocation as well as the views of other Akamba. The problem of allocating scarce lifesaving medical resources, particularly the resource of their own time, is tragically real and urgent. One worker described to me a more than weekly occurrence at the district hospital. In a typical scenario, she is providing "intensive care" for a child who will not survive the night

Table. Average Value-Significance Scores by Education

Type of Healer	Level of Education	Average Scores			
		Equality	Usefulness	Need	Life
Health Workers	None—Standard 7	15.5	1.6	2.3	2.1
	Standard 8—Form 2	14.1	2.1	2.4	2.7
	Form 3—Form 4	9.8	3.8	2.4	2.9
Traditional Healers	None—Standard 8	15.2	1.8	2.4	2.2

without her when another child who also requires her undivided attention in order to live through the night is unexpectedly brought into the hospital. She herself is the scarce resource, and the allocation decision is hers.

In response to the interest expressed by many of those I interviewed, I decided to write up a final report for the participants. The report was translated into Kikamba and hand-delivered even to the most remotely located participants by persons who could read the reports out loud to those who were not able to read for themselves. The participants were grateful, even as they had been gracious in sharing their outlooks. They also remain eager to learn what others think of their views.

The dusty journey across the plains and hills of central Kenya was more than a strenuous physical trek. It was a moral excursion of the most challenging kind. Confronted by strange, new perspectives on an old and familiar problem, I found that my capacity to wrestle with these perspectives depended upon my willingness to question and struggle anew with my own views and my fixed notions of the range of viable alternatives. While the study is done, the journey continues.

Acknowledgments

In addition to those who were interviewed, many others have made important contributions to this study. I am deeply grateful to Daniel Ngwala, my ever-present Akamba research assistant, as well as to others in Kenya who provided governmental, academic, and personal support and counsel. Francis Massakhalia, James Kagia, Dan Kaseje, Dennis Willms, and Joyce Scott stand out among many others. In the United States, the Danforth Foundation and Harvard University (Sheldon Fellowship) provided major funding for the study, while key planning assistance and critical evaluation were provided by Margot Gill, Ralph Potter, Preston Williams, and Sissela Bok. A special word of thanks belongs to Arthur Dyck who helped guide this project from start to finish.

References

1. For a detailed explanation of the methodology, including a description of the sampling technique and questionnaire pre-testing as well as a copy of the basic questionnaire, see John F. Kilner, "Who Shall Be Saved?: An Ethical Analysis of Major Approaches to the Allocation of Scarce Lifesaving Medical Resources" (Cambridge, MA: Ph.D. dissertation, Harvard University, 1983).

2. Cf. John S. Mbiti, *Akamba Stories* (Oxford: Oxford University Press, 1966).

3. The issue of choice arises once in the questionnaire, when the respondents are asked whether or not patients should be allowed to forego treatment voluntarily (e.g., when they discover that all of the waiting patients cannot be treated). For a normative defense of a United States allocation policy which would more or less allow equality (as expressed in random selection) to be over-ridden only where need, life, or choice is at stake, see John F. Kilner, "A Moral Allocation of Scarce Lifesaving Medical Resources," *Journal of Religious Ethics* 9 (Fall 1981), 245–85.

Chapter 4

Bentham in a Box: Technology Assessment and Health Care Allocation

Albert R. Jonsen, Ph.D.

Reprinted, with permission, from *Law, Medicine, and Health Care* 14(3–4):172–74, Fall–Winter, 1985.

Albert R. Jonsen is professor of ethics in medicine and chief of the Division of Medical Ethics at the School of Medicine, University of California at San Francisco.

Jeremy Bentham, the founding father of utilitarianism, would have been delighted by technology assessment. Contemporary health policy planners are, unwittingly, aping the great man's felicific calculus, as they attempt to discern the efficacy and safety of magnetic resonance imaging or cardiac bypass surgery or extracorporeal shockwave lithotripsy. They try to design methods to calculate the effects of these technologies on mortality and morbidity and to compare the costs of one to the costs of alternatives. In recent years, the methods of technology assessment have been refined, but they remain, in essence, a copy of Bentham's proposal to plan and effect a rational course of action and to create a rational world.

The great philosopher and social reformer is, of course, still with us in a desiccated form. He bequeathed his body to the fellows of University College, London, and to this day his mummified figure is encased in a glass box, sitting in his favorite chair, dressed in his own clothes, his waxen face peering out with a bemused smile. He is trundled out from time to time for sherry with the dons. Bentham in his box is, in my opinion, an apt symbol for the boxed-in felicific calculus that is modern technology assessment. It is constrained from drawing into its calcu-

lations certain crucial elements and thus, like the mummy of its founder, it is but the lifeless, impotent relic of a powerful and vital way of thinking about, and dealing with, the world.

I venture this bizarre and exaggerated image in order to make vivid my thesis about our current efforts to allocate health care resources and to ration medical technologies. We labor under a cribbed, cabined, and confined way of thinking about allocation of medical care; we are as constrained as the great man in his box and we cannot, any more than he can, exercise power and control over the distribution of health care. I shall explain my thesis in several steps: first, by saying something about the philosophers' endeavors to elucidate a theory of justice about health care; second, by relating my personal experience with technology assessment; and third, by stating the reason why I believe we have, and are possibly destined to have always, a boxed-in approach to the problems of health resource allocation.

First, a word about the philosophers' endeavors. During the last few years, the attention of philosophers has been drawn to the problem of justice in health care. A somewhat neglected problem, it moved up the agenda with the research generated by the President's Commission for the Study of Ethical Problems in Medicine and Biomedical Research for its report, *Securing Access to Health Care*. Many fine studies were prepared in the course of that research. At the same time, in the political and social world, the costs of care had caught the attention of policy-makers and the Reagan administration had begun its retreat from—or should we say, its attack on—the federal subvention of health care in the United States.

The conceptual problem and the practical difficulties combined to bring the issue of just and fair allocation of health care to the head of the agenda, just as it was at the top of the agenda of the Sydney '86 conference. A few years ago this topic was always the last session in bioethics conferences.

The philosophers rightly noted that a theory of justice was needed to resolve the practical problems of just and fair allocation. Several very interesting attempts have been made to supply this theoretical approach. All those efforts have their strengths and weaknesses, which I shall not detail here. I merely want to point to an issue little noted by the philosophers, because of the level of generalization at which they work. All efforts to sketch a theory of justice about health care refer to the utility of medical intervention. It is obvious that there is a problem of just distribution only if that which is to be distributed is a good. Thus, the philosophers presuppose that in some sense, and in some form, health care activities are beneficial.

The President's Commission report concludes that it is the duty of society to assure equitable access to an adequate level of care for all. It described that adequate level as "enough care to achieve sufficient welfare, opportunity, information and evidence of interpersonal concern to facilitate a reasonably full and satisfying life." As Norman Daniels notes, this description shares with his own "[a] certain abstractness, that sanctuary for philosophers and den of inequity for health policy planners."[1]

One way to descend from that abstractness is to inspect with great attention the various forms of health and medical care, in order to determine the extent to which they actually do effect, on the whole, the benefits desired.

Technology assessment is one way in which that work is carried on. This art is still quite undeveloped, but it is improving in sophistication and extent. In my exaggerated simile—technology assessment is like Bentham in his box—I alluded to the similarity between the modern methods and the felicific calculus. This was, of course, a somewhat facetious allusion. Modern health planners are not avid readers of Bentham, Mill, or Sidgewick; they are not utilitarians in theory. But they are, to some extent, utilitarians in practice; the question they ask is whether a particular technology can be shown, in some quantitative way, to effect more benefit than harm in relationship to alternatives. In the words of the President's Commission, "The level of care deemed adequate should reflect a reasoned judgment not only about the impact of the condition on the welfare of the individual, but also about the efficacy and costs of care itself in relation to other conditions and the efficacy and costs of care available for them."[2]

These words are the familiar vocabulary of the utilitarian language, even though they are spoken, like Australian (Strine), at some distance from the mother tongue. During the last decade, I have been involved in several major efforts at technology assessment. I served on two National Institutes of Health working groups to assess the artificial heart, on a Department of Health, Education and Welfare project to assess cardiac transplantation, on an NIH committee to assess amniocentesis, and on a State of California Task Force on liver transplantation. I am now a member of the Medical Advisory Committee of National Blue Cross–Blue Shield, which issues advisory opinions about the efficacy of old and new medical technologies—everything from autologous bone marrow transplantation to neonatal circumcision. Since I am an ethicist, not a health planner, it has usually been my assigned task to point out the ethical, moral, and social implications of these technologies, a task I have always found extremely difficult.

Still, despite the difficulty, I continue with these activities because I find them extremely revealing for the problem of allocation of health care. It is at this level, rather than that of ethical theory, that the allocation policy can be determined. If Bentham were with us in person rather than in relic, he might be involved in such activities, just as he was in prison reform, legislative reform, and sanitary reform, for he was much more of a social activist and planner than a social philosopher and theorist. And if he were the member of a working group on the artificial heart or on liver transplantation, he would, I think, notice the barrier to the complete assessment of social utility to which I have referred.

That barrier is our practical incompetence in dealing with life-saving or life-sustaining technologies. Many of the technologies under assessment relieve illness or pain or disability, but do not directly save life, do not rescue people from imminent death. Those technologies that do stave off death and sustain life pose a particularly daunting problem to the assessor; they interpose into the miniature felicific calculus a barrier difficult to climb, a chasm difficult to leap: namely, the imperative to rescue endangered life.

Major organ transplantation and implantation are the most striking examples of these technologies. Our working groups were able to calculate the extent of possible use, the potential efficacy, and the costs of these technologies. The artificial heart, for example, might annually bring four years of extended life to some 25,000 persons, at a cost of some $100,000 per life saved. Allowing these people to die without any treatment for cardiomyopathy would be much less costly, since the alternative for them is not a lifetime of expensive chronic care but death. Also, the burden of paying for these transplants might eventually pinch the nation's health resources budget, depriving many of less dramatic but nonetheless life-enhancing forms of care. Should we encourage the development of the artificial heart? Of course we must, it is said, because it rescues the doomed from certain death. And those doomed to death are certainly quite visible individuals — Dr. Barney Clark, William Schroeder, Baby Jamey Fisk, and Baby Jesse, my son, your wife, the nice man next door — rather than the invisible multitudes who may die of exposure to toxic chemicals, cigarette smoke, or radiation, or those deprived of immunization or adequate nutrition. We reach a conclusion contrary to the utilitarian principle: We benefit a few at cost to many.

This occurs only when technology assessment becomes specific and explicit. The barrier will not rise up if we let these life-and-death decisions slip by, politely unnoticed, in a general rationing or allocation policy (as the British National Health Service learned to do long ago). But if we work at explicit evaluations of single technologies, the barrier is bound to appear.

I call this barrier the rule of rescue. Our moral response to the imminence of death demands that we rescue the doomed. We throw a rope to the drowning, rush into burning buildings to snatch the entrapped, dispatch teams to search for the snowbound. This rescue morality spills over into medical care, where our ropes are artificial hearts, our rush is the mobile critical care unit, our teams the transplant services. The imperative to rescue is, undoubtedly, of great moral significance; but the imperative seems to grow into a compulsion, more instinctive than rational.

I am, of course, familiar with what the philosophers call deontological principles: principles that command or forbid absolutely, regardless of the consequences. I had read about them, and thought about them, but I had never come smack up against one until engaged in the assessment of a life-saving technology. The evidence appeared to be leading to the logical and reasonable conclusion that the technology was not cost-effective. Before that conclusion could be drawn, however, the rule of rescue threw up an impassable barrier. The logical conclusion of the assessment faltered and fell, and the technology — hedged around with cautions, to be sure — won the day. Renal dialysis was such a victor in the 1960s; major organ transplantation recently carried off a federal task force.

This then is Bentham in a box: the rational effort to evaluate the efficacy and costs, the burdens and benefits, of the panoply of medical technologies — an effort essential to just and fair allocation — encounters the straitened confines set by the rule of rescue. Even the soundest consequentialist arguments against that rule seem unable to break out of the box.

Appeals to quality of life or to the impact of a technology on society or culture carry little weight, probably because they lack the force of quantification that is the strength of utilitarian arguments. Thus, as we find ourselves becoming more and more skilled at sorting out the efficacious from the useless and the cost-efficient from the wasteful, we find ourselves, at the same time, unable to extend our felicific calculus to the very expensive technologies that will rescue the relatively few.

The rule of rescue is indeed a deontological imperative. Utilitarians are not fond of deontological imperatives. Bentham's progeny devised many ways to interpret them, diminish their power, or banish them from moral discourse. But I am speaking of practice and policy and planning, not of philosophical theory. Even the most evangelical utilitarian would find it difficult to expunge the rule of rescue from the psychological dynamics of technology assessors. As a law reformer, Bentham would have had to take account of this strong imperative that resists the rational authority of the utilitarian principle.

I am not repudiating the moral significance of the rule of rescue. I am not claiming that this impasse is either salutory or malign; I am not suggesting that we are better off living within this limit or breaking through it. I merely report my experience with serious, conscientious efforts to discern the utility of medical technology, and I will close by posing the questions that my experience has raised for me. Should the rule of rescue set a limit to rational calculation of the efficacy of technology? Should we force ourselves to expunge the rule of rescue from our collective moral conscience? How should law deal with this powerful moral imperative? Might a world with less cost-effective health care be a morally better place? Perhaps we should resuscitate the estimable and eccentric Bentham — provide him with artificial heart and brain — and free him from his box so that we may ask him that same question. I do not know what a revived Bentham might answer.

References

1. N. Daniels, *Just Health Care* (Cambridge University Press, 1985) at 82.
2. President's Commission for the Study of Ethical Problems in Medicine and Biomedical Research, Securing Access to Health Care (Washington, D.C., 1983) at 36.

Part II

Rationing: The Health Care Professional's Role

It is well and good, many health care practitioners say, for bioethicists to sit in their splendid isolation and expostulate on theories of rationing and resource allocation. After all, the further away one is from a dilemma, the clearer that dilemma appears. But for the hospital administrator facing a budget shortfall, the emergency physician confronted by a bleeding indigent patient, the nurse who is begged by a terminally ill patient for help in committing suicide, or the trustee wrestling with formulating a policy on use of resuscitation, the blacks and whites fade to gray in short order.

Nevertheless, it is practitioners who often must carry out the rationing of care. In this section, some rules of the road are proposed. Leslie Blackhall, M.D., discusses the irrational proliferation of cardiopulmonary resuscitation and raises the deeper question of why inappropriate or ineffective treatments are offered to patients in the first place. William Kirkley, M.D., asks whether saving extremely low-birthweight infants is done in the interest of the infant, the parents, or the neonatal intensive care unit staff—and provides an uncomfortable answer. Lawrence Schneiderman, M.D., and his colleagues offer a theory of medical futility that, if accepted, would allow physicians to restrict the availability of some forms of care without undue suffering on anyone's part.

Marcia Angell, M.D., suggests that moderate forebearance on the part of physicians in ordering tests and using marginal procedures would prevent the rationing of necessary care and would spare physicians the moral pain of denying help to patients. John Wennberg, M.D., suggests that patients should have a much stronger role in determining their own treatment, arguing that patients' and physicians' preferences are not always the same. And Norman Daniels, Ph.D., outlines a key problem of justice in rationing care: that a physician who says "no" to an inappropriate patient demand has no guarantee that the resources saved by his or her action will be used to fulfill unmet need.

Chapter 5

Must We Always Use CPR?

Leslie J. Blackhall, M.D.

Reprinted, with permission, from *The New England Journal of Medicine* 317(20):1281–85, Nov. 12, 1987.

Leslie J. Blackhall, M.D., is on the staff of the general medicine section of Los Angeles County Hospital.

Cardiopulmonary resuscitation (CPR) as we know it today came into being after the invention of closed-chest cardiac massage in 1960.[1] This technique was originally developed for victims of sudden cardiac or respiratory arrest. As the introduction to one monograph on CPR, written in 1965, says, "The techniques described in this monograph are designed to resuscitate the victim of acute insult, whether it be from drowning, electrical shock, untoward effect of drugs, anesthetic accident, heart block, acute MI [myocardial infarction] or surgery."[2] At present, however, it is standard practice to attempt CPR on any patient in the hospital who has a cardiac arrest, regardless of the underlying illness. The exceptions, of course, are patients who request not to receive such treatment. The rights of patients to refuse this intervention have been well delineated in the courts, yet despite 27 years of experience with CPR and approximately 10 years of experience with "do-not-resuscitate" (DNR) protocols, many questions concerning CPR remain, including who should be involved in decisions about DNR orders and under what circumstances such decisions should be made. Infrequently discussed (although perhaps not infrequently encountered) is the situation in which a patient wants CPR but the physician believes that it is contraindicated. In these cases, patients almost invariably remain "full code," and physi-

cians feel obligated to provide a treatment that they have reason to believe will not be beneficial and may actually be harmful. Are they so obligated?

I was recently involved in a case that illustrates this conflict. A 30-year-old woman with acute myelogenous leukemia who had relapsed from her second remission approximately one month earlier was started on an experimental chemotherapeutic regimen that left her with profound neutropenia and thrombocytopenia for almost four weeks. After four weeks, a bone marrow biopsy revealed regeneration with blasts, indicating failure of the chemotherapy. The patient also had pneumonia thought to be fungal, which was not responding to treatment with broad-spectrum antibiotics, including amphotericin. She (with her family) was asked, "If your heart or lungs stop working, do you want us to pump on your chest and put you on a breathing machine?" The patient and her family decided that she should receive a full CPR effort. The house staff and nursing staff were opposed to this decision, and much conflict ensued.

We use CPR in the way we do for a variety of medical, historical, and psychological reasons. Although CPR was initially used selectively on patients with acute illness—mainly because those trained in its use were cardiologists, anesthesiologists, and surgeons, whose patients tended to have the reversible causes of cardiac arrest described in the quotation above—the increased training of nurses and physicians in the technique and the development of "code teams" rapidly expanded the patient population undergoing CPR. The development of code protocols in hospitals, whereby CPR was promptly begun on any patient discovered to have no pulse, extended the indications for this technique to include all patients with cardiac arrest, regardless of the underlying illness. These changes were instituted to improve the chances of a response to CPR and to ensure good neurologic function in patients who did respond. They created a problem, however, because many physicians recognized that there were some patients for whom CPR was inadvisable because of terminal illness or poor quality of life. The dilemma was how to decide when not to do CPR. After many court cases and much discussion among physicians, DNR orders were developed to encourage open discussion of these issues and to allow patient participation in the decisions. Analysis of the legal and ethical aspects of such orders has focused on the issue of patient autonomy—the right of competent patients to refuse any procedure and of incompetent patients to refuse through a surrogate. Thus, although the DNR order is written by a physician, its legitimacy comes from the patient; the order signifies that the patient has refused a procedure. The development of DNR protocols has not solved all the problems associated with CPR, however. Since CPR is performed routinely in the absence of a DNR order and because physicians frequently do not offer their patients a choice between CPR and a DNR order,[3-7] the decision to perform CPR is usually made without the patient's involvement.

The case I described earlier, however, presents a different problem. In this case the patient and family were consulted. The problem was that their decision ran contrary to the physician's medical judgment. The conflict that then arose was difficult to resolve, but in such cases it seems insufficient for physicians to cite patient autonomy and wash their hands of further responsibility. When a patient's request for treatment is in conflict with a physician's responsibility to provide what he or she believes to be good medical care, the calculation is difficult. A recent paper concerning this type of conflict concluded that there is no ethical imperative requiring physicians to perform procedures in the absence of at least a "modicum of medical benefit."[8] A review of the literature on the medical aspects of CPR, therefore, may aid us in our analysis of the ethical aspects of this case.

Kouwenhoven et al., in a paper that first described closed-chest cardiac massage, reported a long-term survival rate of 70 percent (14 of 20 patients).[1] This impressive rate has never been duplicated. In 13 papers published since 1960, the rates for survival until hospital discharge ranged from 5 to 23 percent.[9-21] Most papers report a survival rate of less than 15 percent, and one of the three studies with rates higher than 15 percent excluded patients with cancer, repeated arrests, or chronic illness and total dependence—all conditions associated with poor outcome. It is clear that survival after CPR is related to the underlying illness that leads to the arrest and that patients with certain conditions very rarely survive. For example, Bedell et al., in a study of 294 consecutive patients who had cardiac arrest at the Beth Israel Hospital in Boston,

found that although 44 percent initially responded to CPR, only 14 percent survived until discharge. No patient with metastatic cancer survived until discharge, nor did any patient with an acute stroke, sepsis, or pneumonia. Only 2 percent of patients with severe cardiomyopathy and 2 percent of patients who had had hypotension for 24 hours survived. Only 3 percent of the patients with renal failure (defined as a blood urea nitrogen level >50 mg per deciliter) survived, and no patient who required dialysis or had oliguria for 24 hours before the cardiac arrest survived until discharge.[7]

These dismal results only confirmed what numerous other studies had shown before—that CPR is frequently ineffective, even in patients in whom it has the best chance of succeeding: those with acute myocardial infarctions or complications due to anesthesia. It is almost never successful in patients with chronic debilitating illnesses.

Peatfield et al. assessed the results of CPR in 1063 patients over a 10-year period. The initial response was 32.4 percent, but only 8.7 percent survived until discharge. All patients with cancer or gastrointestinal hemorrhage died. In contrast, 15 percent of patients with acute myocardial infarction who required CPR survived.[10] In a study by Hershy and Fisher, 14 percent of all patients undergoing CPR survived, but only 6 percent of patients on the general wards survived.[12] The authors attributed this to the fact that most patients with the acute, reversible causes of cardiac arrest were in critical care units or the emergency room, whereas the patients on the general wards had the types of chronic illnesses associated with a poor outcome. No patient with cancer or an acute stroke survived CPR in their study. Similarly, a study by Johnson et al. of 552 patients showed that 32 percent were alive at 24 hours but only 14.9 percent survived until discharge. No patient with sepsis, cancer, or gastrointestinal hemorrhage survived until discharge, and only 3 percent of patients with renal failure survived.[13]

In all these papers, we see a discrepancy between the initial response rate (16 to 45 percent) and survival until discharge (5 to 23 percent overall, with less than 5 percent survival in many groups). Studies that considered the length of survival of patients who were initially resuscitated but died before discharge found that these patients lived an average of 2 to 14 days, usually in an intensive care unit.[11,12,14] The risk of the development of a chronic vegetative state after CPR was 2 percent in the paper by Johnson et al.[13] and 2.7 percent in a paper by Messert and Quaglieri[15] (10 percent of the patients who survived CPR in their study). Thus, although the number of patients who are in a chronic vegetative state after CPR is small, in many disease categories, it approaches the number who survive CPR.

With the above data in mind, let us look again at the case of the young woman with leukemia unresponsive to chemotherapy, bone marrow regenerating with blasts, and lungs affected by a rapidly progressing pneumonia. Despite experimental chemotherapy and treatment with broad-spectrum antibiotics, her condition was rapidly deteriorating. From the medical perspective, was there a "modicum of benefit" to be obtained from CPR? In the light of the data on survival after CPR among patients with cancer, as well as what we know about our ability to reverse the course of this patient's underlying illnesses, we are forced to conclude that her chances of surviving until discharge were virtually nonexistent and could not be improved by CPR. Furthermore, we can see that there are risks involved in performing CPR, including the development of a chronic vegetative state — which many believe is worse than death — or, more likely, survival after the initial resuscitation but with death occurring after an indefinite stay in the intensive care unit. This was what the house staff feared. For them the choice was clear: death on the oncology ward, surrounded by family members and the nurses and doctors who knew the patient well, versus death in the intensive care unit after multiple invasive, painful, and dehumanizing procedures. From the perspective of the patient and her family the choice was less clear. When asked to make their choice, they were not well informed about the likely outcome of CPR. They had never been in an intensive care unit or seen a respirator. For them the choice appeared to be between a chance of life and certain death. When they chose CPR, they were actually choosing something that did not exist — a chance for the patient to live.

Problems like these are not easily solved. Sometimes all that is required is more information about the choices involved. At other times, for a variety of reasons, including guilt and unrealistic hopes for a medical miracle, patients or their families continue to request CPR even when it would clearly be futile. In cases like these, in which CPR offers no conceivable benefit and much possible harm, I believe that patient autonomy cannot be our only guide. The principle of autonomy, which allows patients to refuse any procedure or choose among different beneficial procedures, does not allow them to demand non-beneficial and potentially harmful procedures. On the other hand, if patients continue to request CPR even after being informed of its futility, can we justify the use of CPR on the basis of compassion, the desire not to desert our often desperate patients? Although there may be times when we use CPR for this purpose, we should recognize the patient's impassioned plea for a form of therapy that he or she knows to be futile for what it is — a cry for help, an acute expression of the dying patient's distress at his or her condition. There are usually better ways to deal with this distress than offering CPR as a sort of high-technology placebo; these include listening to the patient's hopes and fears, reassuring him or her that the doctors will continue to be there and provide appropriate therapy,

and if necessary, referring the patient to psychiatric personnel or clergy trained to help patients who are dying.

A closer look at this problem, however, shows us that it is usually not simply a case of a patient demanding something. The young woman with leukemia and her family, for example, were in fact *offered* a choice between CPR and no CPR. Why did the physicians involved even consider CPR an option? What purpose was served by offering the patient a treatment that was known to be of no benefit? If it was done to preserve the patient's autonomy, her autonomy still did not extend to choosing useless procedures. If it was done to relieve her family of guilt, so that they could rest assured that they had really done everything, that purpose could have been better achieved by having the doctors assure the family that everything had been and was being done and that CPR would not add to the therapy. If it was offered to give the family hope, then it was a cruel hope indeed — not only a false hope but a hope that led them to make decisions that could only increase the patient's suffering. Since we were offering her not the chance to survive until discharge but the chance to survive for a couple of days or weeks in the intensive care unit — intubated and sedated and with an arterial line, central line, Foley catheter, and nasogastric tube in place — the choice should have been presented as such, if it had to be presented at all. I believe that the choice should not have been offered. Offering CPR to this patient represented bad faith because doing so implied a potential for benefit when there was none.

What I suggest is a different way of using CPR that takes into account not only the patient's autonomy but also the physician's responsibility to provide care consonant with medical reality. In cases in which CPR has been shown to be of no benefit, as in patients with metastatic cancer, it should not be considered an alternative and should not be presented as such. In these cases physicians could write DNR orders on the chart, with the following type of documentation: "This patient has a condition for which CPR has been shown not to be effective. In case of cardiopulmonary arrest, CPR should not be performed." Because there is a potential for misuse, the type of diagnosis for which such an order could be written should be strictly limited to those for which there is clear documentation of the ineffectiveness of CPR. Consensus needs to be reached, probably on the national level, about what those diagnoses are.

Many cases will not be so clear. Patients with some chronic diseases, such as renal failure, have long-term survival rates after CPR that are low (usually less than 5 percent) but real. In such cases, patient autonomy is the overriding principle and informed consent for CPR should be obtained. Physicians should be strongly encouraged to discuss the preferences of their chronically ill patients with them. The discussions should include the provision of information about the chances of survival after CPR and the risks involved. If a patient's preferences have not been ascertained before cardiac arrest (and it is our responsibility as physicians to see that this seldom happens), CPR should be initiated and continued until the patient's wishes can be ascertained.

Patients who have a cardiac arrest as a result of an acute insult, such as a drug overdose, a complication of a procedure or anesthesia, or an acute myocardial infarction, make up a third category. They are the patients for whom CPR was originally designed and the patients in whom it is most frequently successful. There is usually no question about the appropriateness of CPR in these patients, and CPR should be initiated unless the patient has previously expressed a desire not to have such treatment.

CPR is a desperate technique that works relatively infrequently, and in many types of patients, virtually never. To solve the ethical dilemmas posed by CPR we must first face that medical fact. Furthermore, as we have seen, there is potential harm in CPR in that patients may be kept alive for days to weeks undergoing painful and dehumanizing procedures with no conceivable medical benefits. Because of these facts, we need to reevaluate the ways we use CPR. Too often CPR just happens, without inquiry into the patient's wishes or consideration of its chances of success. Both patient autonomy and physician responsibility are important factors in making decisions regarding CPR. In cases in which CPR has any potential for success, the principle of patient autonomy dictates the patient's right to choose or refuse such treatment. In order for patients to exercise this right, however, two conditions must be met. First, patients need to be given sufficient information concerning the likely outcome of CPR and the risks involved, so that an informed decision can be made. Second, because CPR is attempted unless patients have been asked whether they wish it and have refused it, physicians need to involve their patients earlier and more frequently in the decision to use CPR.

The issue of patient autonomy is irrelevant, however, when CPR has no potential benefit. Here, the physician's duty to provide responsible medical care precludes CPR, either as a routine process in the absence of a decision by a patient or as a response to a patient's misguided request for such treatment in the absence of adequate information. In such cases it is not the physician's responsibility to offer CPR. Both physicians and patients must come to terms with the inability of medicine to postpone death indefinitely.

References

1. Kouwenhoven WB, Jude JR, Knickerbocker GG. Closed-chest cardiac massage. JAMA 1960; 173:1064–7.

2. Talbott JH. Introduction. Jude JR, Elam JO. Fundamentals of cardiopulmonary resuscitation. Philadelphia: F. A. Davis, 1965.

3. Bedell SE, Delbanco TL. Choices about cardiopulmonary resuscitation in the hospital: When do physicians talk with patients? N Engl J Med 1984; 310:1089–93.

4. Charlson ME, Sax FL, MacKenzie R, Fields SD, Braham RL, Douglas RG Jr. Resuscitation: How do we decide? A prospective study of physicians' preferences and the clinical course of hospitalized patients. JAMA 1986; 255:1316–22.

5. Youngner SJ, Lewandowski W, McClish DK, Juknialis BW, Coulton C, Bartlett ET. 'Do not resuscitate' orders: incidence and implications in a medical intensive care unit. JAMA 1985; 253:54–7.

6. Evans AL, Brody BA. The do-not-resuscitate order in teaching hospitals. JAMA 1985; 253:2236–9.

7. Bedell SE, Pelle D, Maher PL, Cleary PD. Do-not-resuscitate orders for critically ill patients in the hospital: How are they used and what is their impact? JAMA 1986; 256:233–7.

8. Brett AS, McCullough LB. When patients request specific interventions: defining the limits of the physician's obligation. N Engl J Med 1986; 315:1347–51.

9. Gulati RS, Bhan GL, Horan MA. Cardiopulmonary resuscitation of old people. Lancet 1983; 2:267–9.

10. Bedell SE, Delbanco TL, Cook EF, Epstein FH. Survival after cardiopulmonary resuscitation in the hospital. N Engl J Med 1983; 309:569–76.

11. Peatfield RC, Sillett RW, Taylor D, McNicol MW. Survival after cardiac arrest in hospital. Lancet 1977; 1:1223–5.

12. Hershy CO, Fisher L. Why outcome of cardiopulmonary resuscitation on general wards is so poor. Lancet 1982; 1:31–4.

13. Johnson AL, Tanser PH, Ulan RA, Wood TE. Results of cardiac resuscitation in 552 patients. Am J Card 1967; 20:831–5.

14. Füsgen I, Summa J-D. How much sense is there in an attempt to resuscitate an aged person? Gerontology 1978; 24:37–45.

15. Messert B, Quaglieri CE. Cardiopulmonary resuscitation: perspectives and problems. Lancet 1976; 2:410–2.

16. Scott RPF. Cardiopulmonary resuscitation in a teaching hospital: a survey of cardiac arrests occurring outside intensive care units and emergency rooms. Anaesthesia 1981; 36:526–30.

17. Hollingsworth JH. The results of cardiopulmonary resuscitation: a 3-year university hospital experience. Ann Intern Med 1969; 71:459–66.

18. Castagna J, Weil MH, Shubin H. Factors determining survival in patients with cardiac arrest. Chest 1974; 65:527–9.

19. Camarata SJ, Weil MH, Hanashiro PK, Shubin H. Cardiac arrest in the critically ill. I. A study of predisposing causes in 132 patients. Circulation 1971; 44:688–95.

20. DeBard ML. Cardiopulmonary resuscitation: analysis of six years' experience and review of the literature. Ann Emerg Med 1981; 10:408–16.

21. Lemire JG, Johnson AL. Is cardiac resuscitation worthwhile? A decade of experience. N Engl J Med 1972; 286:970–2.

Chapter 6

Fetal Survival—What Price

William H. Kirkley, M.D.

Presented at the Forty-Second Annual Meeting of the South Atlantic Association of Obstetricians and Gynecologists, Atlanta, Georgia, Feb. 3–6, 1980. Reprinted, with permission, from *American Journal of Obstetrics and Gynecology* 137(8):873–75, Aug. 15, 1980. Copyright ©1980, C. V. Mosby Co.

William Kirkley, M.D., a physician practicing in Fort Lauderdale, Florida, originally gave this presentation as the presidential address at the 42nd annual meeting of the South Atlantic Association of Obstetricians and Gynecologists in Atlanta, Georgia, in February 1980. Although his data concerning the cost and outcomes of care of low–birth-weight infants are no longer current, the issues he raised and the dilemma he addressed—whose interest is served by the resuscitation of highly compromised infants?—remain painful and controversial more than a decade later.—Editor

Neonatal intensive care units have sprung up all over the country in the last 15 to 20 years. As these centers develop in the United States, there are many physicians who are beginning to question the present-day trend of admitting all live-born infants to an Intensive Care Nursery. What we, as obstetricians and pediatricians, are striving for is a quality product. When one goes into an Intensive Care Nursery, he will almost always find a group of dedicated people who have as their goal survival of the neonate. If they receive a 300 gm infant, they are all very enthusiastic. This is their burning question: "Will this be the smallest baby who ever survived in our unit?" Their every effort is toward that accomplishment. Whether or not the infant has a congenital anomaly is secondary. No thought is given to the fact that it will probably die and the parents will have spent thousands of dollars for naught or, worse still, will have spent thousands of dollars and countless hours in anxiety only to have a less than normal child survive. Somewhere this latter possibility must be taken into consideration.

We are all finally reaching the point of realizing that this country does not have unlimited funds for medical purposes and certainly our patients do not.

Thus priorities must be set, and some thought must be given to economics, even though economics is a very emotional factor when priorities are being set on human life. I am very thankful that during the 1960s I never had to sit on a board that determined who would have renal dialysis and survive, realizing that the ones not selected would die.

At this time I would like to summarize two articles very briefly.

The first article[8] is a report of 75 infants weighing 1,000 gm or less, born between 1973 and 1975. Of these infants, 40% of the survivors appeared normal at 1 to 3 years of age, and 30% had significant physical and/or mental defects. The average cost of the infant who died was $14,236 each. The average cost for the infant who survived was $40,287 each. (The cost actually ranged from $10,700.00 to $106,050.) The cost for a "normal" survivor was found to be $88,058. An additum stated that in 1977 these costs had risen 30%. It is reasonable to assume that they have risen 60% today. Thus the projected cost now would be $64,459 for any survivor and $140,800 for the "normal" child. These were hospital costs only; they did not include the charges made by the doctors involved.

William H. Kirkley, M.D.

The second article[4] deals with the status of infants of 1,000 gm or less and their survival record. The mortality rate was 70%. Of the 43 survivors, 35% had lung problems requiring later hospitalization. If the infant had a diagnosis of chronic lung disease, 86% had significant lung problems the first year and 57% did the second year. Six of 43 underwent major surgery. There were seven cases of retrolental fibroplasia, with two being totally blind. Major neurological defects were present in four children and minor neurological defects were present in 16 others. Thirteen infants or 30% had significant handicaps at age 18 months. Four had severe neurological defects. (In this study, only infants considered capable of survival were included.)

In two other studies, Rush and associates, of John Radford Hospital, Oxford, England, reported a 27% survival rate of infants weighing 1,000 gm or less, and Stewart and associates reported a 32% survival rate of a similar group.[5]

Prior to 1950, most neural tube defects (especially if open and leaking) were managed by "benign neglect" and death occurred rather quickly. In the 1950s a very aggressive early surgical approach was begun, with the result that most of these infants survived.[5-7]

Lorber, of the Department of Child Health of the University of Sheffield (England), has written several articles on the results of this aggressive treatment. The following are some of his quotes: "No person with severe handicaps is likely to be able to earn his living in competitive employment unless his I.Q. is at least 100." (They had very few with IQs above 100.) "With increased technical experience we could save more and more badly handicapped children without increasing the percentage of those less severely affected. Treating all babies without selection has resulted in much suffering for a great number of people in spite of the massive effort of large, dedicated teams. The cost of medical care and of special education of each severely handicapped child exceeded 50,000 pounds by the time they had reached sixteen years of age." He went on to point out the disastrous consequences to the family of such offspring. DeLong,[1] a British neurosurgeon, stated, "Large numbers of spina bifida children kept alive by early closure of the defect and more efficient treatment of the hydrocephalus are now adolescents, most of them painfully aware of their deficiencies." Some of us consider their presence not as a tribute to a medical achievement but as an accusation against misuse of medical power.

Dr. Lorber categorizes survivors by results: In Category 1, no handicap, there were four patients. In Category 2, moderate handicap, there were 20 patients. Of these, five had an IQ of 75 to 79 and the others had a higher IQ. These children had physical handicaps, such as incontinence, paraplegia, hydrocephalus, etc. In Category 3, severe handicaps and normal intelligence, there were 65

patients. Only two were continent, but both of these had severe paraplegia. In Category 4, severe handicaps, with a moderate degree of mental retardation (IQ of 61 to 79), there were 28 patients. In Category 5, profound retardation with gross physical handicaps, there were 16 patients.

Lorber summarized by saying that at most 7% of those treated had less than grossly crippling disabilities and could be considered to have a quality of life consistent with self-respect, earning capacity, happiness, and even marriage.

I believe this aggressive approach to neural tube defects shows what horrors well-intended medical management may produce. If I were a neurosurgeon, looking back on the results such as those just presented, I would have a great deal of guilt and depression in realizing what unfortunate and unhappy products I had produced, not to mention the millions spent on the noble experiment. I fear the thousands of unfortunate neural tube defect survivors will represent only a small percentage of the problems we create with the aggressive treatment of low–birth weight babies.

The present policy of managing all cases of hydrocephaly with the thought of survival is, in my opinion, wrong. Many leading authorities feel that hydrocephalic infants having very large heads with only 4 mm of cortex should be delivered by cesarean section, thus obtaining a very questionable product at a greater risk to the mother. I recently saw one of these children who was markedly retarded. This child was causing severe financial and emotional burdens to his family.

At times, the present concept that everything that is alive (even in utero) has a right to live at all costs, even with greater risks to the mother, bothers most of us who practice obstetrics. We are so intimidated by the hospital administration, legal profession, and, yes, many nurses that we rush all living "things" to the nursery. The ultimate in this stupidity was the case of an anencephalic infant who was sent to the nursery and the support team was proud of the fact that they kept it alive for over 12 hours, although at a significant cost to the parents. Recently one of my partners delivered a grossly abnormal neonate by cesarean section. The pediatrician immediately began to resuscitate it, even though the Apgar score was very low. Fortunately, in a few seconds he looked around very sheepishly and asked if anyone objected to his not resuscitating this baby.

Knowing that prematurity is a leading cause of mental retardation, I feel very uncomfortable with the intentional termination of pregnancy at 30 to 32 weeks for a dropping estriol level or other signs of impending fetal death.

If one takes the average figure in all of the American articles I reviewed, one will find that about 15% of all babies of 2,000 gm or less have physical and/or mental handicaps.

If one treated only 1,500 gm babies in an intensive care unit, I believe we would have a very significant decrease in mental and physical retardation in this country.

The 1,000 gm neonate admitted to an intensive care nursery, loudly crying, with a good Apgar score, etc., has a far better prognosis than a 1,000 gm neonate admitted that must be on a resuscitator to survive. Whether or not the resuscitator should be used in such a case is the question.

It has been pointed out that the "normal" child cannot truly be given this label until it has been in school several years, because subtle learning disabilities and social maladjustments may not be apparent until such time.

Sick neonates who are admitted to a neonatal intensive care unit in a university setting have a better prognosis than those who are not. Those of us who work outside the university have seen neonates who are not doing well and immediately improved after being transferred to a university hospital. Therefore, the facilities available to the neonate unfortunately will influence our management and the ultimate outcome.

I have not heard anyone state that we must take action to limit the tremendous costs in producing these retarded infants or that we must make any recommendations that some selection be made as to who will receive this intensive care. However, the Supreme Court upheld the rights of Dr. Kenneth Edelin to withhold care for a very low–birth weight baby.

So we, as obstetricians, face a real dilemma when we deliver a baby of 1,000 gm or less or when we deliver a child who has significant congenital anomalies. This dilemma is much worse when the child has a low Apgar score at birth. In the past, many times we elected not to resuscitate these babies. At the present time, this is almost impossible. It is my feeling that it is time we address ourselves to this problem and, as a profession, consider taking a stand.

References

1. DeLong, S.: Critical review of the treatment of myelomeningocele, Div. Med. Child Neurol. (Suppl. 32) 16:27, 1974.
2. De La Vega, A.: Is intensive care of newborn really worthwhile? Schweiz. Med. Wochenschr. 109:213, 1979.
3. Franco, S.: Reduction of cerebral palsy by neonatal intensive care, Pediatr. Clin. North Am. 24:3, 1977.
4. Kitchen, W., et al.: A longitudinal study of very low-birthweight infants, Dev. Med. Child Neurol. 20:605, 1978.
5. Lorber, J.: Ethical problems in the management of myelomeningocele and hydrocephalus, J. R. Coll. Physicians Lond. 10:47, 1975.
6. Lorber, J.: Results of treatment of myelomeningocele, Dev. Med. Child Neurol. 13:279, 1971.
7. Lorber, J.: Spina bifida cystica: results of treatment of 270 consecutive cases with criteria for selection for the future, Arch. Dis. Child. 47:854, 1972.
8. Pomerance, J., et al.: Cost of living for infants weighing 1,000 grams or less at birth, Pediatrics 61:908, 1978.
9. Thompson, T., et al.: The results of intensive care therapy for the neonate, J. Perinat. Med. 5:59, 1977.

Chapter 7

Medical Futility: Its Meaning and Ethical Implications

Lawrence J. Schneiderman, M.D., Nancy S. Jecker, Ph.D., and Albert R. Jonsen, Ph.D.

Reprinted, with permission, from *Annals of Internal Medicine* 112(12):949–54, June 15, 1990.

Lawrence J. Schneiderman, M.D., is affiliated with the Department of Community and Family Medicine of the University of California, San Diego, School of Medicine. Nancy S. Jecker, Ph.D., and Albert R. Jonsen, Ph.D., are affiliated with the University of Washington School of Medicine in Seattle.

The notion of medical futility has quantitative and qualitative roots that offer a practical approach to its definition and application. Applying these traditions to contemporary medical practice, we propose that when physicians conclude (either through personal experience, experiences shared with colleagues, or consideration of published empiric data) that in the last 100 cases a medical treatment has been useless, they should regard that treatment as futile. If a treatment merely preserves permanent unconsciousness or cannot end dependence on intensive medical care, the treatment should be considered futile. Unlike decision analysis, which defines the expected gain from a treatment by the joint product of probability of success and utility of outcome, our definition of futility treats probability and utility as independent thresholds. Futility should be distinguished from such concepts as theoretical impossibility, such expressions as "uncommon" or "rare," and emotional terms like "hopelessness." In judging futility, physicians must distinguish between an effect, which is limited to some part of the patient's body, and a benefit, which appreciably improves the person as a whole. Treatment that fails to provide the latter, whether or not it achieves the former, is "futile." Although exceptions and cautions should be borne in mind, we submit that physicians can judge a treatment to be futile and are entitled to withhold a procedure on this basis. In these cases, physicians should act in concert with other health care professionals, but need not obtain consent from patients or family members.

A 62-year-old man with irreversible respiratory disease is in the intensive care unit. He is severely obtunded. During 3 weeks in the unit, repeated efforts to wean him from ventilatory support have been unsuccessful. There is general agreement among his physicians that he could not survive outside of an intensive care setting. They debate whether therapy should include cardiopulmonary resuscitation if the patient has a cardiac arrest or antibiotics if he develops infection. The patient gave no previous indication of his wishes nor executed an advance directive. Some physicians argue that a "do not resuscitate" order may be written without consulting the family, because resuscitation would be futile. Other physicians object, pointing out that resuscitation cannot be withheld on grounds of medical futility, because the patient could survive indefinitely in the intensive care unit. They agree to consult the family on this matter. At first there is considerable disagreement within the family until a son asks whether there is any hope at all that his father might recover. The physicians look at each other. There is always hope. This unites the family. They insist that if the situation is not hopeless, the physicians should continue all measures including resuscitation.

How should these physicians deal with this family's demands? The answer depends on both how the physicians define futility and the weight they give it when patients or surrogates strongly express treatment preferences. Are these issues perhaps too complex or ambiguous to resolve?[1,2] We submit that they are not, and we offer both a theoretical and practical approach to the concept of futility, an approach that we believe serves in this case and more generally in similar cases by restoring a common sense notion of medical duty. We recognize that if futility is held to be nothing more than a vague notion of physician discretion, it is subject to abuse; therefore, we propose specific standards by which this idea can be appropriately invoked. In our view, judgments of futility emerge from either quantitative or qualitative evaluations of clinical situations. Such evaluations determine whether physicians are obligated to offer an intervention. If an intervention is judged to be futile, the duty to present the intervention as an option to the patient or the patient's family is mitigated or eliminated. We recognize—indeed invite—examination and challenge of our proposal.

The Glare of Autonomy

Less than a few decades ago, the practice of medicine was characterized by a paternalism exemplified in the expression, "doctor's orders." Physicians determined by themselves or in consultation with colleagues the usefulness of courses of treatment. The art of medicine was considered to include selectively withholding as well as disclosing information in order to maintain control over therapy. The dramatic shift toward patient self-determination that has taken place in recent decades almost certainly received much of its momentum from society's backlash to this paternalism. In addition, philosophical and political concerns about the rights of individuals and respect for persons elevated the principle of autonomy to a position in ethics that it had not previously held. Today, ethics and the law give primacy to patient autonomy, defined as the right to be a fully informed participant in all aspects of medical decision making and the right to refuse unwanted, even recommended and life-saving, medical care. So powerful has this notion of autonomy become that its glare often blinds physicians (and ethicists) to the validity of earlier maxims that had long defined the range of physicians' moral obligations toward patients. Among these was the maxim, respected in ethics and law, that futile treatments are not obligatory. No ethical principle or law has ever required physicians to offer or accede to demands for treatments that are futile.[3,4] Even the so-called Baby Doe regulations, notorious for their advocacy of aggressive medical intervention, permit physicians to withhold treatment that is "futile in terms of the survival of the infant" or

"virtually futile."[5] Even when this maxim is accepted in theory, however, physicians frequently practice as though every available medical measure, including absurd and overzealous interventions, must be used to prolong life unless patients give definitive directions to the contrary.[6,7] Some physicians allow patients (or surrogates) to decide when a treatment is futile, thereby overriding medical judgment and potentially allowing the patient (or surrogate) to demand treatment that offers no benefit.[8]

Comparison of Effect and Benefit

In the early nineteenth century, all medications were, by definition, effective: They inevitably brought about the effect that their names described. Emetics could be counted on to cause vomiting; purgatives to cause laxation; sudorifics, sweating; and so on.[9] These effects, given the medical theories of the times, were presumed always to be beneficial. Failure to heal was a defect of nature, not of the physician or the treatment. However, one advance of modern medicine, particularly with the introduction of controlled clinical trials, was to clarify by empiric methods the important distinction between effect and benefit. In examining the notion of futility, physicians sometimes fail to keep this distinction in mind.

For example, a recent discussion of futility includes the following: "[Physicians] may acknowledge that therapy is effective, in a limited sense, but believe that the goals that can be achieved are not desirable, as when considering prolonged nutritional support for patients in a persistent vegetative state. Physicians should acknowledge that, in such situations, potentially achievable goals exist. Therapy is not, strictly speaking, futile."[2] On the contrary, we believe that the goal of medical treatment is not merely to cause an effect on some portion of the patient's anatomy, physiology, or chemistry, but to benefit the patient as a whole. No physician would feel obligated to yield to a patient's demand to treat pneumonia with insulin. The physician would rightly argue that (in the absence of insulin-requiring diabetes) such treatment is inappropriate; insulin might have a physiologic effect on the patient's blood sugar, but would offer no benefit to the patient with respect to the pneumonia. Similarly, nutritional support could effectively preserve a host of organ systems in a patient in persistent vegetative state, but fail to restore a conscious and sapient life. Is such nutritional treatment futile or not? We argue that it is futile for the simple reason that the ultimate goal of any treatment should be improvement of the patient's prognosis, comfort, well-being, or general state of health. A treatment that fails to provide such a benefit—even though it produces a measurable effect—should be considered futile.

Lawrence J. Schneiderman, M.D., Nancy S. Jecker, Ph.D., and Albert R. Jonsen, Ph.D.

Approaching a Definition

The word futility comes from the Latin word meaning leaky (*futilis*). According to the *Oxford English Dictionary*, a futile action is "leaky, hence untrustworthy, vain, failing of the desired end through intrinsic defect." In Greek mythology, the daughters of Danaus were condemned in Hades to draw water in leaky sieves. Needless to say, their labors went for nought. The story conveys in all its fullness the meaning of the term: A futile action is one that cannot achieve the goals of the action, no matter how often repeated. The likelihood of failure may be predictable because it is inherent in the nature of the action proposed, and it may become immediately obvious or may become apparent only after many failed attempts.

This concept should be distinguished from etymologic neighbors. Futility should not be used to refer to an act that is, in fact, impossible to do. Attempting to walk to the moon or restore cardiac function in an exsanguinated patient would not be futile acts; they would be physically and logically impossible. Nor should futility be confused with acts that are so complex that, although theoretically possible, they are implausible. The production of a human infant entirely outside the womb, from in-vitro combination of sperm and egg to physiologic viability, may be theoretically possible but, with current technology, is implausible.

Further, futile, because the term is not merely descriptive, but also operational, denoting an action that will fail and that ought not be attempted, implies something more than simply rare, uncommon, or unusual. Some processes that are quite well understood and quite probable may occur only occasionally, perhaps because of their complexity and the need for many circumstances to concur at the same time. For example, successful restoration to health of a drug addict with bacterial endocarditis might require a combination of medical, psychological, social, and educational efforts. These interventions could work but, due to various factors (including limited societal resources), they rarely work. However, they are not futile.

Futility should also be distinguished from hopelessness. Futility refers to the objective quality of an action; hopelessness describes a subjective attitude. Hope and hopelessness bear more relation to desire, faith, denial, and other psychological responses than to the objective possibility or probability that the actions being contemplated will be successful. Indeed, as the chance for success diminishes, hope may increase and replace reasonable expectation. Something plausible is hardly ever hopeless, because hope is what human beings summon up to seek a miracle against overwhelming odds. It is possible then to say in the same breath, "I know this is futile, but I have hope." Such a statement expresses two facts, one about the objective properties of the situation, the other about the speaker's psychological state.

Futility refers to an expectation of success that is either predictably or empirically so unlikely that its exact probability is often incalculable. Without specific data, one might predict futility from closely analogous experience. (For example, one might avoid a trial of a particular chemotherapy for one type of cancer based on failures seen when used for treating similar forms of cancer.) Or one may have accumulated empiric experience insufficient to state precisely the likelihood of success, but sufficient to doubt the likelihood of success. (For example, physicians have had only a few years of experience with a currently popular medication to cure baldness, but sufficient experience to be dubious of its long-term success.)

Reports of one or two "miraculous" successes do not counter the notion of futility, if these successes were achieved against a background of hundreds or thousands of failures. Such rare exceptions are causally inexplicable, because any clinical situation contains a multitude of factors—in addition to treatment—that might affect outcome. As Wanzer and colleagues[10] stated, "The rare report of a patient with a similar condition who survived is not an overriding reason to continue aggressive treatment."

Quantitative and Qualitative Aspects

The futility of a particular treatment may be evident in either quantitative or qualitative terms. That is, futility may refer to an improbability or unlikelihood of an event happening, an expression that is quasi-numeric, or to the quality of the event that treatment would produce. Thus, determining futility resembles using decision analysis—with one important distinction. In decision analysis, the decision to use a procedure is based on the joint product of the probability of success and the quality (utility) of the outcome.[11] Thus, very low probability might be balanced by very high utility. In our proposal of futility, however, we treat the quantitative and qualitative aspects as independent thresholds, as minimal cutoff levels, either of which frees the physician from the obligation to offer a medical treatment.

This independence of futility determinants can be traced back to medical antiquity.[12,13] The perception of futility derived from the Hippocratic corpus might be considered, in modern terms, to be quantitative or probabilistic. A book titled "The Art"[14] enjoins physicians to acknowledge when efforts will probably fail: "Whenever therefore a man suffers from an ill which is too strong for the means at the disposal of medicine, he surely must not even expect that it can be overcome by medicine." The writer further admonishes the physician that to attempt futile treatment is to display an ignorance which is "allied to madness."

Plato's *Republic,*[15] on the other hand, has a qualitative notion of futility, one that emphasizes the inappropriateness of efforts that result in patients surviving, but leading literally useless lives. According to Plato, the kind of medicine "which pampers the disease" was not used by the Asclepian physicians:

Asclepius . . . taught medicine for those who were healthy in their nature but were suffering from a specific disease; he rid them of it . . . then ordered them to live as usual. . . . For those however, whose bodies were always in a state of inner sickness he did not attempt to prescribe a regimen . . . to make their life a prolonged misery. . . . Medicine was not intended for them and they should not be treated even if they were richer than Midas.

Thus, both the quantitative and qualitative aspects of futility are recognized in the most ancient traditions. Hippocrates rejects efforts that are quantitatively or probabilistically unlikely to achieve a cure; Plato objects to a cure consummating (qualitatively) in a life that "isn't worth living." Both quantitative and qualitative aspects relate to a single underlying notion: The result is not commensurate to the effort. The effort is, on the part of the agent, a repeated expenditure of energy that is consistently nonproductive or, if productive, its outcome is far inferior to that intended.

Defining Futility

We propose that, on the basis of these considerations, the noun "futility" and the adjective "futile" be used to describe any effort to achieve a result that is possible but that reasoning or experience suggests is highly improbable and that cannot be systematically produced. The phrase, "highly improbable," implies that a statistical statement about probability might be applicable. In the strict sense, such a statement cannot be made, as proper conditions for determining probability (that is, prospective comparisons of precisely controlled treatment and nontreatment on identically matched subjects) will never be present. We introduce the concept of "systematic" to point out that if a rare "success" is not explicable or cannot be predictably repeated, its causality is dubious, because it is uncertain whether treatment, some extraneous influence, or random variation caused the result.

Quantitative Aspects

In keeping with the quantitative approach to futility, we propose that when physicians conclude (either through personal experience, experiences shared with colleagues,

or consideration of reported empiric data) that in the last 100 cases, a medical treatment has been useless, they should regard that treatment as futile. Technically, we cannot say that observing no successes in 100 trials means that the treatment never works. However, such an observation serves as a point estimate of the probability of treatment success. Although we cannot say with certainty that the point estimate is correct, statistical methods can be used to estimate a range of values that include the true success rate with a specified probability. For example, if there have been no successes in 100 consecutive cases, the clinician can be 95% confident that no more than 3 successes would occur in each 100 comparable trials (3 successes per 100 trials is the upper limit of the 95% CI). This confidence range would narrow as the number of observations increased. If no successes were seen in 200 cases, the upper limit of the 95% CI would be 1.5 successes per 100 cases and, for no successes in 1000 observations, the upper limit would be approximately 0.3 successes per 100 cases. In practical terms, because data from controlled clinical trials can only rarely be called on and applied to a specific case, practitioners usually use their extended experience as the source of their conclusions. Here, speciality practice contributes an essential element; for example, an intensive care pulmonary specialist who sees several hundred patients who have similar disease conditions and receive similar therapy can often group together "futility characteristics" better than a generalist who does not see cases in so focused a manner.

Without systematic knowledge of the various factors that cause a therapy to have less than a 1% chance of success—knowledge that would allow the physician to address these factors—we regard it as unreasonable to require that the physicians offer such therapy. To do so forces the physician to offer any therapy that may have seemed to work or that may conceivably work. In effect, it obligates the physician to offer a placebo. Only when empirically observed (though not understood) outcomes rise to a level higher than that expected by any placebo effect,[16] can a specific therapy be considered to be "possibly helpful" in rare or occasional cases and its appropriateness evaluated according to rules of decision analysis. In the clinical setting, such judgments also would be influenced, of course, by considering such tradeoffs as how cheap and simple the intervention is and how serious or potentially fatal the disease (*see* Exceptions and Cautions).

Although our proposed selection of proportions of success is admittedly arbitrary, it seems to comport reasonably well with ideas actually held by physicians. For example, Murphy and colleagues[17] invoked the notion of futility in their series of patients when survival after cardiopulmonary resuscitation was no better than 2% (upper limit of 95% CI as calculated by authors), and Lantos and colleagues[18] when survival was no better than 7% (upper limit of 95% CI as calculated by authors).

Lawrence J. Schneiderman, M.D., Nancy S. Jecker, Ph.D., and Albert R. Jonsen, Ph.D.

Obviously, as medical data on specific situations are gathered under appropriate experimental conditions, empiric uncertainty can be replaced with empiric confidence.[19] Admittedly, some disorders may be too rare to provide sufficient experience for a confident judgment of futility, even when efforts are made to pool data. We acknowledge this difficulty but adhere to our conservative standard to prevent arbitrary abuse of power. In judging futility, as in other matters, physicians should admit uncertainty rather than impose unsubstantiated claims of certainty. Therefore, our view of futility should be considered as encouraging rather than opposing well conducted clinical trials. Important examples of such work in progress include studies of survival after cardiopulmonary resuscitation[17-24] and use of prognostic measures in patients requiring intensive medical care.[25,26]

Already, data on burn patients[27] and on patients in persistent vegetative state with abnormal neuroophthalmic signs[28] are sufficient to help with decision making. The latter group of patients present a particular challenge to presently confused notions of futility, perhaps accounting in part for why an estimated 5000 to 10 000 patients in persistent vegetative state are now being maintained in medical institutions.[29] The mythologic power of the coma patient who "wakes up" apparently overrides the rarity of documented confirmation of such miraculous recoveries (which have resulted, moreover, in incapacitating mental impairment or total dependence).[28] This point bears on the frequently heard excuse for pushing ahead with futile therapies: "It is only by so doing that progress is made and the once futile becomes efficacious. Remember the futility of treating childhood leukemia or Hodgkin lymphoma." These statements hide a fallacy. It is not through repeated futility that progress is made, but through careful analysis of the elements of the "futile case," followed by well designed studies, that advances knowledge. We also point out that our proposal is intended for recognized illness in the acute clinical setting. It does not apply to preventive treatments, such as immunizations, estrogen prophylaxis for hip fractures, or penicillin prophylaxis for rheumatic heart disease and infectious endocarditis, all of which appear to have lower rates of efficacy because they are purposely administered to large groups of persons, many of whom will never be at risk for or identified with the particular diseases that their treatments are intended to prevent.

Qualitative Aspects

In keeping with the qualitative notion of futility we propose that any treatment that merely preserves permanent unconsciousness or that fails to end total dependence on intensive medical care should be regarded as nonbeneficial and, therefore, futile. We do not regard futility as "an elusive concept."[2] It is elusive only when effects on the patient are confused with benefits to the patient or when the term is stretched to include either considerations of 5-year survival in patients with cancer (not at all pertinent to the notion of futility) or the "symbolic" value to society of treating handicapped newborns or patients in persistent vegetative state (which rides roughshod over patient-centered decision making).[2]

Here is the crux of the matter. If futility is qualitative, why should the patient not always decide whether the quality achieved is satisfactory or not? Why should qualitatively "futile" results not be offered to the patient as an option? We believe a distinction is in order. Some qualitatively poor results should indeed be the patient's option, and the patient should know that they may be attainable. We believe, however, that other sorts of qualitatively poor results fall outside the range of the patient's autonomy and need not be offered as options. The clearest of these qualitatively poor results is continued biologic life without conscious autonomy. The patient has no right to be sustained in a state in which he or she has no purpose other than mere vegetative survival; the physician has no obligation to offer this option or services to achieve it. Other qualitatively poor results are conditions requiring constant monitoring, ventilatory support, and intensive care nursing (such as in the example at the beginning of our paper) or conditions associated with overwhelming suffering for a predictably brief time. Admittedly, these kinds of cases fall along a continuum, and there are well known examples of the most remarkable achievements of life goals despite the most burdensome handicaps. However, if survival requires the patient's entire preoccupation with intensive medical treatment, to the extent that he or she cannot achieve any other life goals (thus obviating the goal of medical care), the treatment is effective but not beneficial; it need not be offered to the patient, and the patient's family has no right to demand it.

Specifically excluded from our concept of futility is medical care for patients for whom such care offers the opportunity to achieve life goals, however limited. Thus, patients whose illnesses are severe enough to require frequent hospitalization, patients confined to nursing homes, or patients with severe physical or mental handicaps are not, in themselves, objects of futile treatments. Such patients (or their surrogates) have the right to receive or reject any medical treatment according to their own perceptions of benefits compared with burdens.

Some observers might object, as a matter of principle, to excluding patient input from assessments of qualitative futility. Others might be concerned that such exclusion invites abuse, neglect, and a retreat to the paternalistic "silent world" of the past in which doctors avoided communication with their patients.[30] In response to the latter objection, we acknowledge that potential for abuse is present and share this concern. We would deplore the use of our proposal to excuse physicians from engaging patients in ongoing informed dialogue. Nonetheless, the alternative is also subject to abuse (for example, when legal threats made by patients and surrogates cow hospitals into providing excessive care). We reiterate that the distinction between medical benefit and effect justifies excluding patients from determination of qualitative futility. Physicians are required only to provide medical benefits to patients. Physicians are permitted, but not obligated, to offer other, non-medical benefits. For example, a physician is not obligated to keep a patient alive in an irreversible vegetative state, because doing so does not medically benefit the patient. However, as noted below, a physician may do so on compassionate grounds, when temporary continuance of biologic life achieves goals of the patient or family.

Exceptions and Cautions

We have attempted to provide a working definition of futility. We also have drawn attention to the ethical notion that futility is a professional judgment that takes precedence over patient autonomy and permits physicians to withhold or withdraw care deemed to be inappropriate without subjecting such a decision to patient approval. Thus, we regard our proposal as representing the ordinary duties of physicians, duties that are applicable where there is medical agreement that the described standards of futility are met. We recognize, however, that the physician's duty to serve the best interests of the patient may require that exceptions to our approaches be made under special circumstances.

An exception could well be made out of compassion for the patient with terminal metastatic cancer who requests resuscitation in the event of cardiac arrest to survive long enough to see a son or daughter who has not yet arrived from afar to pay last respects. Such an exception could also be justified to facilitate coping and grieving by family members, a goal the patient might support.[32-36] Although resuscitation may be clearly futile (that is, would keep the patient alive in the intensive care unit for only 1 or 2 more days), complying with the patient's wishes would be appropriate, provided such exceptions do not impose undue burdens on other patients, health care providers, and the institution, by directly threatening the health care of others. We hasten to add, however, that our notion of futility does not arise from considerations of scarce resources. Arguments for limiting treatments on grounds of resource allocation should proceed by an entirely different route and with great caution in our present open system of medical care, as there is no universally accepted value system for allocation[31] and no guarantee that any limits a physician

imposes on his or her patients will be equitably shared by other physicians and patients in the same circumstances.[37,38]

Admittedly, in cases in which treatment has begun already, there may be an emotional bias to continue, rather than withdraw, futile measures.[10] If greater attention is paid at the outset to indicating futile treatments, these situations would occur less frequently; however, the futility of a given treatment may not become clear until it has been implemented. We submit that physicians are entitled to cease futile measures in such cases, but should do so in a manner sensitive to the emotional investments and concerns of caretakers.

What if a hospitalized patient with advanced cancer demands a certain medication (for example, a particular vitamin), a treatment that the physician believes to be futile? Several aspects of this demand support its overriding the physician's invocation of futility. Certain death is expected and, although an objective goal such as saving the patient's life or even releasing the patient from the hospital might be unachievable, the subjective goal of patient well-being might be enhanced (a placebo-induced benefit). In this particular situation, the effort and resources invested to achieve this goal impose a negligible burden on the health care system and do not threaten the health care of others. Thus, although physicians are not obligated to offer a placebo, they occasionally do. For example, Imbus and Zawacki[27] allowed burn patients to opt for treatment even when survival was unprecedented. In this clinical situation, compassionate yielding imposes no undue burden, because survival with or without treatment is measured in days. In contrast, yielding to a surrogate's demand for unlimited life-support for a patient in persistent vegetative state may lead to decades of institutional care.

Acknowledgments: The authors thank two anonymous reviewers and Robert M. Kaplan, Ph.D., for their helpful comments.

References

1. Younger, SJ. Who defines futility? *JAMA.* 1988;260:2094–5.
2. Lantos JD, Singer PA, Walker RM, et al. The illusion of futility in clinical practice. *Am J Med.* 1989;87:81–4.
3. President's Commission for the Study of Ethical Problems in Medicine and Biomedical and Behavioral Research. *Deciding to Forego Life-Sustaining Treatment: A Report on the Ethical, Medical, and Legal Issues in Treatment Decisions.* Washington DC: U.S. Government Printing Office; 1983:60–89.
4. Jonsen AR. What does life support support? *Pharos.* 1987; 50(1):4–7.
5. *Child Abuse and Neglect Prevention and Treatment.* Washington, DC: U.S. Department of Health and Human

Services, Office of Human Development Services; 1985: Federal Register 50:14887–8.

6. Blackhall LJ. Must we always use CPR? *N Engl J Med.* 1987; 317:1281–5.

7. Tomlinson T, Brody H. Ethics and communication in do-not-resuscitate orders. *N Engl J Med.* 1988;318:43–6.

8. Lo B. Life-sustaining treatment in patients with AIDS: challenge to traditional decision-making. In: Juengst ET, Koenig BA, eds. *The Meaning of AIDS.* v 1. New York: Praeger; 1989:86–93.

9. Rosenberg CE. The therapeutic revolution: medicine, meaning, and social change in nineteenth-century America. *Perspect Biol Med.* 1977;20:485–506.

10. Wanzer SH, Adelstein SJ, Cranford RE, et al. The physician's responsibility toward hopelessly ill patients. *N Engl J Med.* 1984;310:955–9.

11. Weinstein MC, Fineberg HV. *Clinical Decision Analysis.* Philadelphia: W.B. Saunders; 1980.

12. Amundsen DW. The physician's obligation to prolong life: a medical duty without classical roots. *Hastings Cent Rep.* 1978;8:23–30.

13. Jonsen AR. *The Old Ethics and the New Medicine.* Cambridge: Harvard University Press; 1990.

14. Hippocratic corpus, the art. In: Reiser SJ, Dyck AJ, Curran WJ, eds. *Ethics in Medicine: Historical Perspectives and Contemporary Concerns.* Cambridge, Massachusetts: MIT Press; 1977:6–7.

15. Plato. In: Grube GM, transl. *Republic.* Indianapolis: Hackett Publishing; 1981:76–7.

16. Beecher HK. The powerful placebo. *JAMA.* 1955;159:1602–6.

17. Murphy DJ, Murray AM, Robinson BE, Campion EW. Outcomes of cardiopulmonary resuscitation in the elderly. *Ann Intern Med.* 1989;111:199–205.

18. Lantos JD, Miles SH, Silverstein MD, Stocking CB. Survival after cardiopulmonary resuscitation in babies of very low birth weight. *N Engl J Med.* 1988;318:91–5.

19. Freiman JA, Chalmers TC, Smith H Jr, Kuebler RR. The importance of beta, the type II error and sample size in the design and interpretation of the randomized control trial. Survey of 71 "negative" trials. *N Engl J Med.* 1978;299:690–4.

20. Bedell SE, Delbanco TL, Cook EF, Epstein FH. Survival after cardiopulmonary resuscitation in the hospital. *N Engl J Med.* 1983;309:569–76.

21. Gordon M, Hurowitz E. Cardiopulmonary resuscitation of the elderly. *J Am Geriatr Soc.* 1984;32:930–4.

22. *Life-Sustaining Technologies and the Elderly.* Washington, DC: U.S. Congress, Office of Technology Assessment; 1987: publication OTA-BA-306, 167–201.

23. Johnson AL, Tanser PH, Ulan RA, Wood TE. Results of cardiac resuscitation in 552 patients. *Am J Cardiol.* 1967;20:831–5.

24. Taffet GE, Teasdale TA, Luchi RJ. In-hospital cardiopulmonary resuscitation. *JAMA.* 1988;260:2069–72.

25. Knaus WA, Draper EA, Wagner DP, Zimmerman JE. APACHE II: a severity of disease classification system. *Crit Care Med.* 1985;13:818–29.

26. Knaus WA, Draper EA, Wagner DP, Zimmerman JE. An evaluation of outcome from intensive care in major medical centers. *Ann Intern Med.* 1986;104:410–8.

27. Imbus SH, Zawacki BE. Autonomy for burned patients when survival is unprecedented. *N Engl J Med.* 1977;297:308–11.

28. Plum F, Posner JB. *The Diagnosis of Stupor and Coma.* 3d ed. Philadelphia: F. A. Davis; 1980.

29. Cranford RE. The persistent vegetative state: the medical reality (getting the facts straight). *Hastings Cent Rep.* 1988;18:27–32.

30. Katz J. *The Silent World of Doctor and Patient.* New York: Free Press; 1984.

31. Emery DD, Schneiderman LJ. Cost-effectiveness analysis in health care. *Hastings Cent Rep.* 1989;19:8–13.

32. Yarborough M. Continued treatment of the fatally ill for the benefit of others. *J Am Geriatr Soc.* 1988;36:63–7.

33. Perkins HS. Ethics at the end of life: practical principles for making resuscitation decisions. *J Gen Intern Med.* 1986;1:170–6.

34. Miles SH. Futile feeding at the end of life: family virtues and treatment decisions. *Theor Med.* 1987;8:293–302.

35. Jecker NS. Anencephalic infants and special relationships. *Theor Med.* 1990.

36. Jecker NS. The moral status of patients who are not strict persons. *J Clin Med.* 1990.

37. Schneiderman LJ, Spragg RG. Ethical decisions in discontinuing mechanical ventilation. *N Engl J Med.* 1988;318: 984–8.

38. Daniels N. Why saying no to patients in the United States is so hard: cost containment justice, and provider autonomy. *N Engl J Med.* 1986;314:I380–3.

Chapter 8

Cost Containment and the Physician

Marcia Angell, M.D.

Marcia Angell, M.D., is executive editor for The New England Journal of Medicine, *Waltham, Massachussetts.*

The United States is now spending about $450 billion a year on health care, or approximately $2,000 for every man, woman, and child. This is almost four times more than the British pay per capita for health care and 1½ times what the Swedish pay. Furthermore, expenditures for health care are rising rapidly, much faster than the gross national product. Not surprisingly, this situation is alarming to many economists and other experts, and professional journals are filled with suggestions for curbing the rise in health care costs.

The Call for Rationing

One solution that has been put forward is to ration health care. Rationing in this context usually means deliberately limiting access to certain types of expensive medical care—for example, organ transplantation or intensive care in special units. Proponents of rationing point out that much of this care is already limited by circumstances, but in a haphazard way that tends to favor the wealthy. Shouldn't we cut down on the availability of expensive care in order to lower costs, and then allocate the remaining care in a just and systematic manner?

Just who would do the rationing is not clear from the literature. Often the proposed rationers are referred to vaguely as policymakers or "decision makers." Presumably they include third-party payers, government leaders, and health economists. The role of physicians is more problematic. Some see physicians as advisors to policymakers, offering their expertise to help inform the rationing process. Others believe that physicians should be directly involved in rationing, in the sense that costs should influence their decisions in caring for patients. It was pointed out in one article[1] promoting this view that very few patients pay their own medical bills; most of the expense is borne by society as a whole, in the form of taxes and insurance premiums. Therefore, it was argued, physicians have obligations not only to their patients but also to society, and these obligations may conflict when very expensive care is at issue. Whether this is a proper conclusion is an important issue, one that I will return to later.

The Premise of Rationing

Most of the discussion about rationing contains the premise that more medical care is better than less. The problem, then, is simply that we cannot afford to provide all the care that would be beneficial. This assumption is particularly apparent in the writings of economists and other nonphysicians, although some physicians also accept it. According to their view, medical care is like most commodities—the more, the better. To be sure, most people who hold this view acknowledge that there is a "flat of the curve," that is, an intensity of medical care beyond which additional care yields only very small increments of benefit. However, they believe that on the whole medical care is useful, so that to cut costs significantly, we must limit benefits. The premise that medical care is almost entirely beneficial to patients is important to the argument for rationing, here defined as limiting the availability of beneficial health care, and it explains the painful nature of the prescription for rationing.[2]

Is More Medical Care Better?

But is this view correct? Is it true that more care is better care, and that it will therefore be necessary to ration medical care to control costs? I think not. Far from being beneficial, much of the medical care in this country is unnecessary—by which I mean that it is of no demonstrated value to those who receive it—and some of it is harmful. In the face of the spectacular successes of the American medical system, this is a difficult concept to accept, particularly for nonphysicians who have become accustomed to media accounts of medical miracles. I intend here to argue that until serious attempts are made to identify and control unnecessary medical care, the call for rationing is not only premature but inappropriate.

Types of Unnecessary Medical Care

Unnecessary medical care may be considered in three categories. The first consists of laboratory tests and x-ray films—termed "little-ticket items"—that are performed without medically valid indications. Little-ticket items account for about 25% of the costs of both hospital and ambulatory care, and they are the most rapidly swelling component of health care costs.[3,4] Almost certainly many of these tests and x-ray films are unnecessary.[5] One study showed that laboratory tests in a teaching hospital could be cut by 47% without any apparent loss in the quality of patient care.[6] Although more testing may occur at teaching hospitals than at other hospitals, if we extrapolate the findings only to teaching hospitals, the annual savings in 1985 dollars would be about $10 billion. Another recent study demonstrated that routine admission chest x-ray films, even in a population at high risk for heart and lung disease, are of almost no benefit. The authors estimated that the nationwide savings from eliminating routine admission chest x-ray films would be $1.5 billion each year.[7]

The second category of unnecessary medical care consists of expensive operations and procedures—termed "big-ticket items"—that are used in circumstances in which they are of no known value. The large variations among geographic regions in the rates of certain operations, such as prostatectomy, suggest that many may not be necessary, although data on outcome are wanting.[8] Similar variations in the rate of hospitalization itself suggest that

this very large expense, too, is often incurred unnecessarily. In general, big-ticket items come into widespread use without a clear understanding of their indications or benefits. Consider two examples: coronary artery bypass grafting and carotid endarterectomy. Last year about 200,000 patients underwent coronary artery bypass grafting, at a cost of $4 billion (*Boston Globe,* Jan 14, 1985, p 5). I have asked several leading cardiologists to estimate how many of these operations are performed in the absence of valid indications. The consensus was that about 25% of the operations are not indicated. This estimate is supported by results of the Coronary Artery Surgery Study.[9] Carotid endarterectomy is done for 50,000 asymptomatic patients each year, at a cost of about a quarter of a billion dollars.[10,11] Yet, this procedure is of no known benefit in asymptomatic patients, and it carries an operative risk of death or stroke of about 10%.

The third category of useless medical care consists of the aggressive treatment of terminally ill patients for whom treatment other than palliative care is no longer appropriate. These patients suffer greatly at the hands of high-technology medicine. This tragic practice is well illustrated by the case of William Bartling, a Californian with severe emphysema and lung cancer who was, as George Annas[12] has said, sentenced to spend the rest of his life in an intensive care unit after a biopsy specimen confirmed the diagnosis of inoperable lung cancer. During that procedure, Mr Bartling's lung collapsed and he was artificially ventilated. When he asked that it be stopped, the hospital refused. Mr Bartling hired an attorney and went to court to have the mechanical respiration ended. Incredibly, the hospital fought his request and prevailed, despite the fact that Mr Bartling's competence was never questioned. He spent five months being mechanically ventilated before he finally died—still being ventilated. The cost of those five months of medical care was $500,000.[13]

There are undoubtedly many such patients in hospitals across the country (although, obviously, they don't all go to court), patients whose every organ is treated maximally, despite the fact that medicine no longer has anything to offer except palliation—ironically, the one thing that is often withheld at this point.[14] Last year, in a large teaching hospital in New York, 10% of the hospital budget was spent on the final admissions of the 4% of patients who died in the hospital (*New York Times,* Jan 14, 1985, pp B1, B4). If these figures represent the general practice throughout the country, the hospital care of the dying accounts for $20 billion of our health care expenditures each year. Of course, it is not always clear in advance that a patient is dying, and aggressive treatment may be especially appropriate when it is not clear. However, about 40% of the patients dying in the New York hospital had diagnoses such as cancer that would suggest that, by their final admission, their terminal status was clear. If this approximates the percentage throughout the country, then about $8 billion each year is spent on the final admissions of patients known to be dying. Treating these patients much less aggressively and directing the treatment toward their comfort would in most cases be kinder, and it would secondarily result in very large savings.

Obviously, my estimates for the frequency and costs of the above examples of unnecessary medical care are very rough. Some of the cost estimates ignore such issues as distinguishing between marginal and average costs or the offsetting costs of possible alternative care. In general, adequate data are not available to justify more refined calculations, and attempts to do so suggest a spurious degree of accuracy. My purpose is simply to *suggest* the magnitude of the expenditures involved in just a few examples of unnecessary medical care, representing only a part of the wasteful practice in our system.

The Growth of Unnecessary Medical Care

It has been argued that even if health care expenditures were reduced considerably by eliminating unnecessary medical care, this would be only a one-time saving, since costs would continue to increase at their current rate and very soon reach and pass their original levels. However, this argument fails to recognize that costs are rising not just because useful new technologies are being added, but also because of an increasing application of both old and new technologies, useful and useless. Expenditures for unnecessary medical care are an inherent part of the American medical system, and they are growing just as our technology is growing. There are three major reasons for this.

First, our peculiar fee schedules reward physicians preferentially for performing tests and procedures. This is not to say that physicians do unnecessary tests and procedures simply to make money, although some may, but rather that any doubt tends to be resolved in favor of the test or procedure. Furthermore, too many physicians are in specialties characterized by high-technology care. It may be that medical students are drawn to these specialties because of the favorable fee schedules. Whatever the reason, specialists tend to generate their own business.

Second, the specter of the malpractice suit further tips the balance toward tests and procedures. The heavy use of tests adds an aura of meticulousness to medical care that may help to fend off accusations of negligence. In addition, recent confused messages from the courts have made physicians particularly reluctant to withhold aggressive treatment from terminally ill patients, regardless of how inappropriate it is.[15]

The third reason for the growth of unnecessary medical care, I think, is that we Americans learn early to believe that any problem has a solution, often a technological one. We are loath to stop testing and treating, even when we have no reason to expect any benefit or when the patient is clearly beyond medical help. And as our technology grows, so grows our ability to apply it indiscriminately.[16] Thus, if unnecessary medical care were largely eliminated, not only would the cost of medical care be reduced, but the rate of increase of that cost would be reduced.

Expensive but Beneficial Medical Care

Compare the unnecessary medical care discussed above with another type of medical care—high-technology medical treatment that is very expensive but almost certainly beneficial to those who receive it. This is the type of medical care that is the focus of much of the discussion about rationing. The best example is transplantation of vital organs, with most of the attention these days being given to heart and liver transplantations. These forms of treatment are so extreme that they almost certainly are not done unless the patients would die without them. Without treatment, then, the mortality would be close to 100%. The two-year survival after heart transplantation is now about 78%, and the one-year survival after liver transplantation is about 60%.[17] Thus, these procedures are clearly life saving. They make the same difference to patients as, say, the treatment of childhood leukemia, an undisputed medical triumph.

The problem is their costs. The fully allocated average cost of heart transplantation is roughly $150,000. It has been estimated that if heart transplantations were performed on all who needed them, limited only by the availability of donors, about 50,000 would be required each year, at a cost of about $7.5 billion,[17] although much lower estimates have also been given.[18] The fully allocated average cost of liver transplantation is about $200,000, and it has been estimated that 4,500 might be needed each year, at a cost of less than $1 billion.[17] Compare these costs for highly effective treatments with our earlier estimates—probably totaling over $15 billion—for selected examples of care of no demonstrated benefit. Furthermore, as we develop more experience with these very new technologies, it can be expected that survival will increase and, perhaps, costs will decrease.

Another example of expensive but beneficial medical care is long-term dialysis, provided for all who need it by the Medicare-funded end-stage renal disease program. We now spend about $2 billion each year to maintain over 70,000 people undergoing long-term dialysis. Because this is a far greater number of patients than was anticipated when the program was instituted, the end-stage renal disease program has become a symbol of expensive medical care run amok.[19] I agree with those who believe that we probably dialyze too many patients, not because of the costs, but because dialysis may in some cases prolong dying rather than add to the quality of life. Nevertheless, when dialysis is used appropriately, it is a life-saving procedure.

Distinguishing Unnecessary From Beneficial Medical Care

The crucial point here is the importance of differentiating medical care that is both useful and expensive from medical care that is merely expensive. I believe that in many instances the distinction is clear. For example, no one should have any trouble distinguishing between the usefulness of the medical care given to William Bartling and that given to Jamie Fiske, the little girl who received a liver transplant after her father made a well-publicized appeal to a meeting of the American Academy of Pediatrics.[20]

Between these two extreme types of care—exemplified by the cases of William Bartling and Jamie Fiske—is a large gray area, in which a great deal of expensive medical care is often provided on the basis of very little information about benefits. Such care includes coronary artery bypass surgery, carotid endarterectomy, neonatal and adult intensive care, invasive monitoring, and costly new imaging techniques, along with a large number of older practices and procedures, such as hysterectomy, tonsillectomy, and chemotherapy for some of the most common cancers. The data concerning the indications and medical risks and benefits of many of these procedures and practices are simply inadequate. In the absence of data, the tendency is to act rather than to refrain from acting, as pointed out earlier.

In 1979, the Health Care Financing Administration set up the National Center for Technology Assessment to try to develop accurate information on the risks and benefits of new technologies. It had an annual budget of about $4 million—hardly a princely amount when compared with the costs of the technologies it was to assess—but even that was considered too much. It was abolished in the early part of the first Reagan administration. Other attempts at technology assessment, for example, by the National Institutes of Health Consensus-Development Program and by the Congressional Office for Technology Assessment, have had to rely on existing data. They are not funded to do their own studies, but merely to review the literature and to reach some consensus on the basis of that. It seems to me that our approach to technology assessment has been worse than inadequate, and it has certainly been a false economy.

Cost Containment Through Preventive Health Care?

It is often argued that any analysis of high-technology medical care misses the mark, that the very best way to improve our health and lower costs is to concentrate on preventive measures. Advocates of this approach point out that if we ate better and exercised more, didn't smoke and didn't drink too much, and drove more carefully, our medical costs would be much lower, and problems of technology assessment would seem relatively unimportant.

It is probably true that preventive measures would do more to improve the health of the population than does curative medical care, although whether it would lower medical costs in the long run is not clear in view of the fact that we all die of something at some age.[21] However, the changes in habits that would be required for prevention cannot be commanded by the medical system. The means to influence our habits are primarily educational, social, and political. Physicians can, for example, recommend that their patients not smoke cigarettes, but it is unlikely that these efforts will be very successful in a society in which the tobacco industry is so heavily subsidized and advertised. Furthermore, patients do not usually come to physicians for advice about how to live; they come because they are sick. It may seem disproportionate for the medical system to offer so much, say, to young adults with Hodgkin's disease, while doing relatively little about accidents, homicide, and suicide—the three leading causes of death in young adults. But victims of accidents, homicide, and suicide do not usually seek medical care in advance, nor are we equipped to do much about it if they did. These are complicated problems that have to do with the kind of society in which we live. Physicians can contribute, as citizens with specialized knowledge, to debates about social and legal reforms, but they can do very little for individual members of society. In contrast, they can do a great deal for patients with Hodgkin's disease.

I do not wish to imply that preventive care has no place in medical practice or in the allocation of medical resources. On the contrary, physicians should do everything they can to influence their patients to adopt healthier habits, and fee schedules should be revised to reflect the importance of preventive care. Preventive care and curative care are not mutually exclusive. However, physicians will by and large be more successful at the latter, and our new awareness of the importance of healthy habits should not be used as an excuse to limit the availability of beneficial medical care for people who need it—that is, patients for whom prevention is too late.

The Role of Physicians in Containing Medical Costs

If preventive care is not the answer to the problem of rising health care costs, what is? What can individual physicians do to contain costs, and what can we do as a profession? There are steps we should take and steps we should not take.

As individual physicians, we must do the very best we can for each patient. The patient rightly expects his physician to act single-mindedly in his best interests. If very expensive care is indicated, then the physician should do his utmost to obtain it for the patient. As Levinsky[22] pointed out, the physician cannot serve two masters—his patient and society's coffers. If society is spending more than it can afford on medical care (and this has yet to be demonstrated), then that is all the more reason for the physician to abide by his commitment to be an uncompromising advocate for his patient's needs.

Nevertheless, the physician should not engage in unnecessary tests and procedures. Sometimes patients themselves suggest them in the belief that high-technology medicine is good medicine. When this happens, the physician must take the time to talk with the patient about the general overemphasis on testing, as well as to explain why the particular test or procedure would not be worth the risks (including the risk of a false-positive result). In terminal illness, the goal should be to ensure the patient's maximal comfort, not to eke out his days, unless this is what the patient wishes. The physician should be honest with the patient when he has nothing medically to offer, and not continue to test and treat to avoid the issue or suggest the opposite. Finally, although the concern about the risk of malpractice charges is a real one and the individual physician can do little to alter the litigiousness of our society, this concern must not come to outweigh the concern for the patient's best interests.

What can we do as a profession? It is crucial that we support the revision of fee schedules so that they no longer reward the use of tests and procedures. This is perhaps the single most important reform to be made in the present system. Although it would involve some dislocations within the profession, the long-term benefits would be more than worth the adjustments. Fee schedules and salaries must be as neutral toward technology as possible, so that physicians are unbiased in deciding what should be done for their patients. Obviously, it is very difficult to set up a truly technology-neutral fee schedule within our present system, but we can do a great deal better than we have. Many of the present attempts to solve the problem, including prospective reimbursement, have merely substituted an incentive to undertreat for one to overtreat.

Second, the profession should press for adequate funding of careful technology assessment, so that we have some way of knowing when and how to use tests and procedures of uncertain benefits. Relman[23] has suggested that private and federal third-party insurers earmark less than 1% of their health care expenditures for this purpose. Careful technology assessment will take time, as well as money and effort. In the meantime, aggressive peer review by random spot-checking might help to bring practice styles into conformity with the best available infor-

mation. An important focus of attention should be the discretionary use of hospital care for conditions that could be treated in an outpatient setting.

The problem of malpractice suits must be addressed by both the medical and legal professions, as well as by the state legislatures. Clearly, we need to curb the incentive of lawyers without depriving patients of their rights. This is a complicated problem, beyond the scope of this article, but a useful first step for the medical profession would be to regulate itself more stringently, so that the public would not regard the courts as the only safeguard against incompetent physicians.

Cost Containment Without Rationing

Now I would like to suggest what we should not do. I believe that we should not accept a role in devising schemes for limiting the availability of beneficial medical care. I say this for two reasons. First, there is so much unnecessary medical care that curtailing it should be the thrust of our cost-containment efforts. For the profession to take part in limiting benefits before dealing with waste is unseemly, at best. Cost containment should be seen as a matter of directing funds and services away from unnecessary care and toward beneficial care, even though the unit costs of the latter may be high. From this perspective, the problem with liver transplantation is not that Jamie Fiske had one, but that others who need it do not, and there is only a rudimentary system for helping them.

The second reason physicians should not be involved in rationing is that any role in limiting useful medical care is inconsistent with our role as advocates for the health of our patients, as pointed out by Boyle.[24] It is often argued that some sort of rationing is inevitable and that if the medical profession does not accept a role in planning how best to do it, rationing will be thrust upon us by people outside the profession who are even less informed than we are. But physicians, of all people, should be skeptical of the notion that we have no choice but to ration health care. Consider the source of the calls for rationing. By and large, they have come neither from physicians nor from patients, but from third parties—business leaders, economists, and some government leaders. These fiscal experts have been responding to the rapidly growing cost of health care as one of a number of budgetary items. Their concern is to cut wherever they can cut with the least resistance. If health care is regarded in that light, as one of many competing claims, then it seems to me that our task as a profession is to argue our claim, not to acquiesce, and certainly not to lead the retreat.

In a country that is this year spending about $300 billion on defense and $25 billion on tobacco, and in which $500,000 is spent for a 30-second television advertisement during the Super Bowl, we should be prepared to argue for spending whatever is necessary for effective medical care. Our responsibility as individuals is to each patient; our responsibility as a profession is to the value of health.

References

1. Leaf A: The doctor's dilemma—and society's too. *N Engl J Med* 1984;310:718–720.

2. Aaron HJ, Schwartz WB: *The Painful Prescription: Rationing Hospital Care.* Washington, DC, The Brookings Institute, 1984.

3. Scitovsky AA: Changes in the use of ancillary services for 'common' illness, in Altman SH, Blendon R (eds): *Medical Technology: The Culprit Behind Health Care Costs?* publication (PHS) 79-3216. US Dept of Health, Education, and Welfare, 1979.

4. Moloney TW, Rogers DE: Medical technology: A different view of the contentious debate over costs. *N Engl J Med* 1979;301:1413–1419.

5. Lundberg GD: Perseveration of laboratory test ordering: A syndrome affecting clinicians. *JAMA* 1983;249:639.

6. Martin AR, Wolf MA, Thibodeau LA, et al: A trial of two strategies to modify the test ordering behavior of medical residents. *N Engl J Med* 1980;903:1330–1336.

7. Hubbell FA, Greenfield S, Tyler JL, et al: The impact of routine admission chest x-ray films on patient care. *N Engl J Med* 1985;312:209–213.

8. Wennberg JE, McPherson K, Caper P: Will payment based on diagnosis-related groups control hospital costs? *N Engl J Med* 1984;311:295–300.

9. Coronary Artery Surgery Study (CASS): A randomized trial of coronary artery bypass surgery. *Circulation* 1983;68:939–950.

10. Dyken ML, Pokras R: The performance of endarterectomy for disease of the extracranial arteries of the head. *Stroke* 1984;15:948–950.

11. Brott T, Thaliner K: The practice of carotid endarterectomy in a large metropolitan area. *Stroke* 1984;15:950–955.

12. Annas GJ: Prisoner in the ICU: The tragedy of William Bartling. *Hastings Center Rep* 1984;14:28–29.

13. Rust M: Key ruling awaited on terminating treatment. *Am Med News* 1984;27:1, 29–30.

14. Angell M: The quality of mercy. *N Engl J Med* 1982;306:989.

15. Suber DG, Tabor MJ: Withholding of life-sustaining treatment from the terminally ill, incompetent patient: Who decides? *JAMA* 1982;248:2250–2251, 2431–2432.

16. Barondess JA: The health policy agenda for the American people. *JAMA* 1983;249:2073–2074.

17. Annas GJ: *Report of the Massachusetts Task Force on Organ Transplantation.* Boston, Boston University School of Public Health, 1984.

18. Austen WG, Cosimi AB: Heart transplantation after 16 years. *N Engl J Med* 1984;311:1436–1438.

19. Evans RW: Health care technology and the inevitability of resource allocation and rationing decisions. *JAMA* 1983;249:2208–2219.

20. Gunby P: Media-abetted liver transplants raise questions of 'equity and decency.' *JAMA* 1983;249:1973–1974, 1980–1982.

21. Eisenberg L: Barriers to care. *Can J Psychiatry* 1984;29:452–460.

22. Levinsky NG: The doctor's master. *N Engl J Med* 1984;311:1573–1575.

23. Relman AS: Assessment of medical practices. *N Engl J Med* 1980;303:153–154.

24. Boyle JF: Should we learn to say no? *JAMA* 1984;252:782–784.

Chapter 9

Outcomes Research, Cost Containment, and the Fear of Health Care Rationing

John E. Wennberg, M.D., M.P.H.

Reprinted, with permission, from *The New England Journal of Medicine* 323(17):1202–4, Oct. 25, 1990. Adapted from a presentation given at a Featured Research Symposium of the American Federation of Clinical Research, the American Society of Clinical Investigation, the American Association of Physicians, and the Society of General Internal Medicine, Washington, D.C., on May 4, 1990.

John E. Wennberg, M.D., M.P.H., is on the staff of the Department of Community and Family Medicine at Dartmouth Hitchcock Medical Center, Lebanon, New Hampshire.

Expectations are high for the Agency for Health Care Policy and Research, established by the 101st Congress to promote research on medical outcomes and develop guidelines for practice. Physicians and patients expect that such research will make it possible to sort out what works in medicine and learn how to make clinical decisions that reflect more truly the needs and wants of individual patients. Many business leaders, third-party payers, and policy makers believe that this effort will lead to the development of practice guidelines, which in turn will reduce the pressure for growth and produce a leaner, trimmer health care economy.

The decision to fund assessment teams that will have continuing responsibility for the study of specific common conditions is an important step in positioning the agency for early success. The priorities include a focus on six conditions—angina pectoris, benign prostatic hyper-

trophy, gallstones, arthritis of the hip, conditions of the uterus, and low back pain—the treatment options for which account for more than half of inpatient surgery. For many patients with these conditions, there are other common but less invasive treatments that are also consistent with contemporary standards of care.

The experience of the assessment team studying benign prostatic hypertrophy over the past four years shows that this approach can be used to test the spectrum of alternative treatments, establish the probabilities for the outcomes that matter to patients, and gain wide support, cooperation, and participation from practitioners. The response of the urologists participating in the Maine Medical Assessment Foundation made it possible to conduct the initial research.[1] The leadership of the American Urological Association has responded very positively to the challenges of our findings, leading to a plan for a 20-center randomized clinical trial to evaluate mortality after prostatectomy, as well as the effects of new treatment options such as balloon dilation and drugs on symptoms, functional status, and the incidence of complications.[2]

Perhaps the most important conclusion so far is that for individual patients with benign prostatic hypertrophy, rational choices among treatments depend on attitudes about risks and benefits—on how patients view their predicaments.[1,3,4] Men differ in their degree of concern about the symptoms of benign prostatic hypertrophy. Even some severely symptomatic patients are not bothered very much by their condition and prefer watchful waiting to surgery. Indeed, no objective data derived from physical examination, clinical history, or careful quantification of symptoms can accurately predict the preferences

John E. Wennberg, M.D., M.P.H.

of individual patients for surgery or watchful waiting. A rational choice depends on the patient's active involvement in the decision, because the patient's attitudes and values are the key to making the right decision. Since the only way to find out what patients actually want is to ask them, practice guidelines that take the form of prescriptive rules will not work.

The research agenda of the Agency for Health Care Policy and Research is also focused on evaluating the costly differences in patterns of use among hospitals. For historical reasons unrelated to the needs of populations or even to different theories about the role of hospital beds in effective treatment, the number of hospital beds per capita varies considerably among communities. Bostonians, for example, use 4½ beds per 1000 members of the population, as compared with fewer than 3 beds per 1000 for New Haven. Per capita expenditures for hospitalizations in Boston are consistently about double those in New Haven. Most of the difference in resources used is invested in the care of patients listed as having medical conditions for which there is high variation in use rates and for which the rules or policies physicians use to determine the need for hospitalization—their clinical thresholds—depend on the supply of beds.[5] The rules governing the use of hospitals for such conditions are thus determined more by behavioral accommodations to the available supply than by recognized medical theory. Indeed, clinicians in New Haven do not believe they are withholding valuable care and have defended their low use of hospitals as cost effective.[6]

If we learn what works in medicine—not in all situations or conditions, but in those that now contribute most to the striking variations in use and cost among hospital markets—will the amount of services demanded by informed patients and physicians be less than, about the same as, or more than what is used now? When the answers are in for the big-ticket items that are the priorities for the new agency, will we be faced with the need to ration effective services, or will we find that current investments are more than are needed to provide the services that patients want and can benefit from?

Some in the health policy community believe we have reached the point at which beneficial health care must be rationed, because medical progress and patients' demands are rapidly exceeding the capacity to pay for effective care. Indeed, in Oregon the legislature has already moved to withhold treatment from Medicaid patients with diseases for which there are effective but expensive treatments. Coby Howard, a young Medicaid patient with leukemia, was denied access to bone marrow transplantation with the explanation that the state needed to spend its limited resources on more cost-effective treatments—namely, a program for prenatal care. His death is the first I know of that can be attributed to explicit rationing by the state on the basis of cost-effectiveness analysis.

Outcomes research holds out hope for those who want to believe that full entitlement to effective health care is attainable within the limits of our national willingness to fund medical care. The fear that rationing will be needed is based on the assumption that current levels of use of expensive treatments such as bypass surgery or intensive care reflect consumer demand and the pace of medical progress. But we really don't know much about what patients demand of the health care market, nor are we clear about how the rates of use reflect medical progress.[7] Although we are now more sophisticated about the role of untested theory and supplier-induced demand in determining the rates of use of services, we have not had the opportunity to learn what the level of demand would be if patients were fully informed of their options and if the probabilities of the various outcomes were presented to them comprehensively. Outcomes research provides this opportunity for the first time, and we have much to learn about our assumptions regarding theories of treatment and the behavior of patients when they are fully informed about their options.

This line of research will reveal, I predict, that for most conditions rational choices among treatments require that individual patients understand the predicaments they face. The predicaments arise because there is seldom a single correct answer to a medical problem. Most conditions or illnesses entail a number of morbidities, symptoms, and disabilities. Outcomes research will clarify the probabilities of the various outcomes for the various treatments, showing many to be effective in some respects that are important to patients. Learning what the demand for any given treatment truly is depends on asking patients what they want in a fashion that disentangles the preferences of the patient from those of the physician. As we improve in our ability to do this, patients will be shown to differ in their degree of concern about their predicament, and the outcomes they want will differ accordingly; they will also differ in the risk they are willing to take to get what they want.

I want to suggest two reasons why the proportion of the gross national product now invested in health may exceed the proportion required to fund fully the caring and effective services that patients want. First, my belief that the current rates of use of invasive, high-technology medicine could well be higher than patients want is based on the hypothesis that, particularly when risks must be taken to reduce symptoms or improve the quality of life, patients tend to be more averse to risks than physicians. Given an option, patients will on average select less invasive strategies than physicians. If so, then disentangling the preferences will lead to lower demand. The early results of our experiments in informing patients about their options in the treatment of benign prostatic hypertrophy support this hypothesis. The growing interest in advance directives and the concern about terminal care suggest that when faced with the inevitability of death, in many situations patients may prefer less rather than more. Better information about outcomes and an improved discourse between patients and physicians over options may therefore lower the demand for more costly treatment. And if not, at least we shall know that patients really do want more and that medical progress and patients' demands are at the heart of the cost-containment problem.

The second reason is the possibility that we have over-invested in the use of hospitals for the treatment of patients with medical conditions for which there is high variation in use.[8] With a concerted effort on the part of the agency and the research community, it will be possible to test thoroughly the hypothesis that an increase in the supply of hospital beds above the numbers seen in low-use areas such as New Haven produces no discernible reduction in mortality or morbidity and no important gains in the symptom state or functional status of the resident population.

The opportunities for redirection of priorities and reallocation of resources are truly astounding. I am fascinated by the prospects. In 1982, the 685,000 residents of Boston incurred about $300 million more in hospital expenditures (in 1982 dollars) and used 795 more hospital beds than would have been the case if the use rates of New Haven had applied.[6] If the hypothesis holds, the hospital resources now allocated to Boston are sufficient for a population twice that city's size. There are many other communities in the United States with use profiles like that of Boston, just as there are many with profiles like that of New Haven. If the hypothesis holds, resources will have been identified to meet many unmet priorities in health care, including access to effective but high-cost treatment such as the bone marrow transplantation needed by Coby Howard. Funds will also have been identified to help fund long-term care.

How can the opportunities for reallocation be realized? Assume that within three or four years outcomes research identified many inefficiencies in the current deployment of resources: is it reasonable to expect that the effort to persuade physicians to practice cost-effective medicine will lead to the correction of these inefficiencies? Put another way, will the pressures placed on the doctor-patient relationship by managed care and practice guidelines exert sufficient influence on the supply to achieve the needed reallocations in fee-for-service markets?

Everything I have learned about the peculiar relations among medical theory, the supply of resources, and the practice styles of physicians in fee-for-service markets warns me that this cannot be so. Although I am confident that the priorities of the new agency ensure that assessments can be completed for big-ticket treatment options for common conditions, efforts to micromanage the doctor-patient relationship and teach physicians to practice cost-

effective care do not really address the issue of capacity. In a market with an increasing supply of resources and particularly of physicians themselves, one should not underestimate the ability of physicians to come up with new ideas. The inventive nature of the medical mind, the endless possibilities for plausible theories, and the urge all physicians feel to work for and be helpful to their patients combine to make it impossible for outcomes research to keep up with the flow of new medical ideas.

Reaching the levels of use that outcomes research suggests are right from the patient's point of view will require policies that deal directly with the capacity of the system. Saving money by reducing the number of medical hospitalizations with widely varying use rates will require a reduction in the number of beds and in the number of employees in the hospital industry—not their redeployment to provide yet another untested treatment, such as programs for the inpatient treatment of alcoholism and drug abuse. Saving money by reducing the number of treatments to that demanded by patients will require a reconsideration of the number and types of physicians we need. This will require policies directed toward medical schools and residency programs. The current circumstances of increasing supply, subsidization of high-cost markets by those living in low-cost markets (through insurance transfer payments),[9] and easy availability of new ideas ensure opportunities for unwanted variations and continuing increases in the costs and amount of care provided. The key to the preservation of fee-for-service markets, as the Canadians seem to recognize, is not the micromanagement of the doctor-patient relationship but the management of capacity and budgets. The American problem is to find the will to set the supply thermostat somewhere within reason. This is not a problem that outcomes research will solve.

References

1. Wennberg JE, Mulley AG Jr, Hanley D, et al. An assessment of prostatectomy for benign urinary tract obstruction: geographic variations and the evaluation of medical care outcomes. JAMA 1988; 259:3027–30.
2. Winslow R. Avoiding the knife: prostate patients get choice of treatments that obviate surgery. Wall Street Journal. February 7, 1990: 1.
3. Barry MJ, Mulley AG Jr, Fowler FJ, Wennberg JE. Watchful waiting vs immediate transurethral resection for symptomatic prostatism: the importance of patients' preferences. JAMA 1988; 259:3010–7.
4. Fowler FJ Jr, Wennberg JE, Timothy RP, Barry MJ, Mulley AG Jr, Hanley D. Symptom status and quality of life following prostatectomy. JAMA 1988; 259:3018–22.
5. Wennberg JE. Small area analysis and the medical care outcome problem. In: AHCPR conference proceedings: research methodology: strengthening causal interpretations

of nonexperimental data, May 1990. Department of Health and Human Services, Agency for Health Care Policy and Research, 1990:177–206.

6. Wennberg JE, Freeman JL, Culp WJ. Are hospital services rationed in New Haven or over-utilised in Boston? Lancet 1987; 1:1185–9.

7. Wennberg JE. Which rate is right? N Engl J Med 1986; 314: 310–1.

8. Wennberg JE, Freeman JL, Shelton RM, Bubolz TA. Hospital use and mortality among Medicare beneficiaries in Boston and New Haven. N Engl J Med 1989; 321:1168–73.

9. Wennberg JE. Should the cost of insurance reflect the cost of use in local hospital markets? N Engl J Med 1982; 307: 1374–81.

Chapter 10

Why Saying No to Patients in the United States Is So Hard

Norman Daniels, Ph.D.

Reprinted, with permission, from *The New England Journal of Medicine* 314(21):1380–83, May 22, 1986. Supported by grants from the Retirement Research Foundation and the National Endowment of the Humanities. This paper is based on the Truman Collins Memorial Lecture delivered to the Portland, Oregon, Academy of Medicine in December 1984.

Norman Daniels, Ph.D., is a professor of philosophy at Tufts University, Medford, Massachusetts.

Cost Containment, Justice, and Provider Autonomy

If cost-containment measures, such as the use of Medicare's diagnosis-related groups (DRGs), involved trimming only unnecessary health care services from public budgets, they would pose no moral problems. Instead, such measures lead physicians and hospitals to deny some possibly beneficial care, such as longer hospitalization or more diagnostic tests, to their own patients—that is, at the "micro" level.[1] Similarly, if the "macro" decision not to disseminate a new medical procedure, such as liver transplantation, resulted only in the avoidance of waste, then it would pose no moral problem. When is it morally justifiable to say no to beneficial care or useful procedures? And why is it especially difficult to justify saying no in the United States?

Justice and Rationing

Because of scarcity and the inevitable limitation of resources even in a wealthy society, justice—however we elucidate it—will require some no-saying at both the macro and micro levels of allocation. No plausible principles of justice will entitle an individual patient to every potentially beneficial treatment. Providing such treatment might consume resources to which another patient has a greater claim. Similarly, no class of patients is entitled to whatever new procedure offers them some benefit. New procedures have opportunity costs, consuming resources that could be used to produce other benefits, and other classes of patients may have a superior claim that would require resources to be invested in alternative ways.

How rationing works depends on which principles of justice apply to health care. For example, some people believe that health care is a commodity or service no more important than any other and that it should be distributed according to the ability to pay for it. For them, saying no to patients who cannot afford certain services (quite apart from whether income distribution is itself just or fair) is morally permissible. Indeed, providing such services to all might seem unfair to the patients who are required to pay.

In contrast, other theories of justice view health care as a social good of special moral importance. In one recent discussion,[2] health care was seen to derive its moral importance from its effect on the normal range of opportunities available in society. This range is reduced when disease or disability impairs normal functioning. Since we have social obligations to protect equal opportunity, we also have obligations to provide access, without financial or discriminatory barriers, to services that adequately protect and restore normal functioning. We must also weigh new technological advances against alternatives, to judge the overall effect of their introduction on equal opportunity. This gives a slightly new sense to the term "opportunity cost." As a result, people are entitled only to services that are part of a system that on the whole protects equal opportunity. Thus, even an egalitarian theory that holds health care as of special moral importance justifies sometimes saying no at both the macro and micro levels.

Saying No in the British National Health Service

Aaron and Schwartz have documented how beneficial services and procedures have had to be rationed within the British National Health Service, since its austerity budget allows only half the level of expenditures of the United States.[3] The British, for example, use less x-ray film, provide little treatment for metastatic solid tumors, and generally do not offer renal dialysis to the elderly. Saying no takes place at both macro and micro levels.

Rationing in Great Britain takes place under two constraints that do not operate at all in the United States. First, although the British say no to some beneficial care, they nevertheless provide universal access to high-quality health care. In contrast, over 10 percent of the population in the United States lacks insurance, and racial differences in access and health status persist.[4,5] Second, saying no takes place within a regionally centralized budget. Decisions about introducing new procedures involve weighing the net benefits of alternatives within a closed system. When a procedure is rationed, it is clear which resources are available for alternative uses. When a procedure is widely used, it is clear which resources are unavailable for other uses. No such closed system constrains American decisions about the dissemination of technological advances except, on a small scale and in a derivative way, within some health maintenance organizations (HMOs).

These two constraints are crucial to justifying British rationing. The British practitioner who follows standard practice within the system does not order the more elaborate x-ray diagnosis that might be typical in the United States, possibly even despite the knowledge that additional information would be useful. Denying care can be justified as follows: Though the patient might benefit from the extra service, ordering it would be unfair to other patients in the system. The system provides equitable access to a full array of services that are fairly allocated according to professional judgments about which needs are most important. The salve of this rationale may not be what the practitioner uses to ease his or her qualms about denying beneficial treatment, but it is available.

A similar rationale is available at the macro level. If British planners believe alternative uses of resources will produce a better set of health outcomes than introducing coronary bypass surgery on a large scale, they will say no to a beneficial procedure. But they have available the following rationale: Though they would help one group of patients by introducing this procedure, its opportunity cost would be too high. They would have to deny other patients services that are more necessary. Saying yes instead of no would be unjust.

These justifications for saying no at both levels have a bearing on physician autonomy and on moral obligations to patients. Within the standards of practice determined by budget ceilings in the system, British practitioners remain autonomous in their clinical decision making. They are obliged to provide the best possible care for their patients within those limits. Their clinical judgments are not made "impure" by institutional profit incentives to deny care.

The claim made here is not that the British National Health Service is just, but that considerations of justice are explicit in its design and in decisions about the allocation of resources. Because justice has this role, British rationing can be defended on grounds of fairness. Of course, some no-saying, such as the denial of renal dialysis to elderly patients, may raise difficult questions of justice.[2] The issue here, however, is not the merits of each British decision, but the framework within which they are made.

Saying No in the United States

Cost-containment measures in the United States reward institutions, and in some cases practitioners, for delivering treatment at a lower cost. Hospitals that deliver treatment for less than the DRG rate pocket the difference. Hospital administrators therefore scrutinize the decisions of physicians to use resources, pressuring some to deny beneficial care. Many cannot always act in their patients' best interests, and they fear worse effects if DRGs are extended to physicians' charges.[6] In some HMOs and preferred-provider organizations, there are financial incentives for the group to shave the costs of treatment—if necessary, by denying some beneficial care. In large HMOs, in which risks are widely shared, there may be no more denial of beneficial care than under fee-for-service reimbursement.[7] But in some capitation schemes, individual practitioners are financially penalized for ordering "extra" diagnostic tests, even if they think their patient needs them. More ominously, some hospital chains are offering physicians a share of the profits made in their hospitals from the early discharge of Medicare patients.

When economic incentives to physicians lead them to deny beneficial care, there is a direct threat to what may be called the ethic of agency. In general, granting physicians considerable autonomy in clinical decision making is necessary if they are to be effective as agents pursuing their patients' interests. The ethic of agency constrains this autonomy in ways that protect the patient, requiring that clinical decisions be competent, respectful of the patient's autonomy, respectful of the other rights of the patient (e.g., confidentiality), free from consideration of the physician's interests, and uninfluenced by judgments about the patient's worth. Incentives that reward physicians for denying beneficial care clearly risk violating the fourth-mentioned constraint, which, like the fifth, is intended to keep clinical decisions pure—that is, aimed at the patient's best interest.

Rationing need not violate the constraint that decisions must be free from consideration of the physician's interest. British practitioners are not rewarded financially for saying no to their patients. Because our cost-containment schemes give incentives to violate this constraint, however, they threaten the ethic of agency. Patients would be foolish to think the physician who benefits from saying no is any longer their agent. (Of course, patients in the United States traditionally have had to guard against unnecessary treatments, since reimbursement schemes provided incentives to overtreat.)

American physicians face a problem even when the only incentive for denying beneficial care is the hospital's, not theirs personally. For example, how can they justify sending a Medicare patient home earlier than advisable? Can they, like their British peers, claim that justice requires them to say no and that therefore they do no wrong to their patients?

American physicians cannot make this appeal to the justice of saying no. They have no assurance that the resources they save will be put to better use elsewhere in the health care system. Reducing a Medicare expenditure may mean only that there is less pressure on public budgets in general, and thus more opportunity to invest the savings in weapons. Even if the savings will be freed for use by other Medicare patients, American physicians have no assurance that the resources will be used to meet the greater needs of other patients. The American health care system, unlike the British one, establishes no explicit priorities for the use of resources. In fact, the savings from saying no may be used to invest in a procedure that may never provide care of comparable importance to that the physician is denying the patient. In a for-profit hospital, the profit made by denying beneficial treatment may be returned to investors. In many cases, the physician can be quite sure that saying no to beneficial care will lead to greater harm than providing the care.

Saying no at the macro level in the United States involves similar difficulties. A hospital deciding whether or not to introduce a transplantation program competes with other medical centers. To remain competitive, its directors will want to introduce the new service. Moreover, they can point to the dramatic benefit the service offers. How can opponents of transplantation respond? They may (correctly) argue that it will divert resources from other projects—projects that are perhaps less glamorous, visible, and profitable but that nevertheless offer comparable medical benefits to an even larger class of patients. They insist that the opportunity costs of the new procedure are too great.

This argument about opportunity costs, so powerful in the British National Health Service, loses its force in the United States. The alternatives to the transplantation program may not constitute real options, at least in the climate of incentives that exists in America. Imagine someone advising the Humana Hospital Corporation, "Do not invest in artificial hearts, because you could do far more good if you established a prenatal maternal care program in the catchment area of your chain." Even if correct, this appeal to opportunity costs is unlikely to be persuasive, because Humana responds to the incentives society offers. Artificial hearts, not prenatal maternal-care programs, will keep its hospitals on the leading technological edge, and if they become popular, will bring far more lucrative reimbursements than the prevention of low–birth-weight morbidity and mortality. The for-profit Humana, like many nonprofit organizations, merely responded to existing incentives when it introduced a transplantation program during the early 1980s, at the same time prenatal care programs lost their federal funding. Similarly, cost-containment measures in some states led to the cutting of social and psychological services but left high-technology services untouched.[8] Unlike their British colleagues, American planners cannot say, "Justice requires that we forgo this procedure because the resources it requires will be better spent elsewhere in the system. It is fair to say no to this procedure because we can thereby provide more important treatments to other patients."

The failure of this justification at both the micro and macro levels in the United States has the same root cause. In our system, saying no to beneficial treatments or procedures carries no assurance that we are saying yes to even more beneficial ones. Our system is not closed; the opportunity costs of a treatment or procedure are not kept internal to it. Just as important, the system as a whole is not governed by a principle of distributive justice, appeal to which is made in decisions about disseminating technological advances. It is not closed under constraints of justice.

Some Consequences

Saying no to beneficial treatments or procedures in the United States is morally hard, because providers cannot appeal to the justice of their denial. In ideally just arrangements, and even in the British system, rationing beneficial care is nevertheless fair to all patients in general. Cost-containment measures in our system carry with them no such justification.

The absence of this rationale has important effects. It supports the feeling of many physicians that current measures interfere with their duty to act in their patients' best interests. Of course, physicians should not think that duty requires them to reject any resource limitations on patient care. But it is legitimate for physicians to hope they may act as their patients' advocate within the limits allowed by the just distribution of resources. Our cost-containment measures thus frustrate a legitimate expectation about what duty requires. Eroding this sense of duty will have a long-term destabilizing effect.

The absence of a rationale based on justice also affects patients. Resource constraints mean that each patient can legitimately expect only the treatments due him or her under a just or fair distribution of health care services. But if beneficial treatment is denied even when justice does not require or condone it, then the patient has reason to feel aggrieved. Patients will not trust providers who put their own economic gain above patient needs. They will be especially distrustful of schemes that allow doctors to profit by denying care. Conflicts between the interests of patients and those of physicians or hospitals are not a necessary feature of a just system of rationing care. The fact that such conflicts are central in our system will make patients suspect that there is no one to be trusted as their agent. In the absence of a concern for just distribution, our cost-containment measures may make patients seek the quite different justice afforded by tort litigation, further destabilizing the system.

Finally, these effects point to a deeper issue. Economic incentives such as those embedded in current cost-containment measures are not a substitute for social decisions about health care priorities and the just design of health care institutions. These incentives to providers, even if they do eliminate some unnecessary medical ser-vices, will not ensure that we will meet the needs of our aging population over the next several decades in a morally acceptable fashion or that we will make effective—and just—use of new procedures. These hard choices must be faced publicly and explicitly.

References

1. Diagnosis-related groups (DRGs) and the Medicare program: implications for medical technology. Washington D.C.: U.S. Congress, 1983. (Office of Technology Assessment OTA-TM-H-17.)
2. Daniels N. Just health care. New York: Cambridge University Press, 1985.
3. Aaron HJ, Schwartz WB. The painful prescription: rationing hospital care. Washington D.C.: The Brookings Institution, 1984.
4. President's Commission for the Study of Ethical Problems in Medicine and Biomedical and Behavioral Research. Securing access to health care: ethical implications of differences in the accessibility of health services. Vol. I. Washington D.C.: Government Printing Office, 1983.
5. Iglehart JK. Medical care of the poor—a growing problem. N Engl J Med 1985; 313:59–63.
6. Jencks SF, Dobson A. Strategies for reforming Medicare's physician payments: physician diagnosis-related groups and other approaches. N Engl J Med 1985; 312:1492–9.
7. Yelin EH, Hencke CJ, Kramer JS, Nevitt MC, Shearn M, Epstein WV. A comparison of the treatment of rheumatoid arthritis in health maintenance organizations and fee-for-service practices. N Engl J Med 1985; 312:962–7.
8. Cromwell J, Kanak J. The effects of prospective reimbursement on hospital adoption and service sharing. Health Care Financ Rev 1982; 4:67.

Part III

Dilemmas in the Patient–Provider Relationship

The issue of autonomy looms large in the language and practice of ethics. Providers, both institutional and individual, believe that only through jealously guarding their autonomy can they serve patients without being compromised by conflicting motives. Increasingly, patients are seeking greater autonomy in making decisions about when, how, and where to accept or refuse care. Interest groups—for example, those infected with human immunodeficiency virus (HIV), women with breast cancer, ethnic or cultural subgroups—complain that the health care system denies them autonomy in order to serve its own interests. Alexis de Tocqueville wrote, 150 years ago, that the conflict between liberty and equality was the basic tension of the American heart; health care is proving him right yet again.

In this section, some of these conflicts are explored. George Annas, J.D., looks at the state of patient–provider relations in care of the terminally ill and the continuing fight over the use of technology and life-prolonging techniques. David Jackson, M.D., Ph.D., and Stuart Youngner, M.D., offer some caveats regarding termination of treatment and patient decision making, warning that there are situations when heeding patient requests to end treatment can constitute abandonment of the patient. Ronald Bayer, Ph.D., offers a penetrating analysis of the conflict that erupted between the gay community and American medicine as the AIDS epidemic spread; he reminds us that health care can represent a promise, a threat, or both to the sick. And Kate Brown, Ph.D., probes the increasingly important issue of cross-cultural ethics and the need for providers to come to grips with demographic changes and their implications for the provision of care.

Chapter 11

High-Tech Death: Using Law and Ethics to Humanize Dying in American Hospitals

George J. Annas, J.D., M.P.H.

George J. Annas, J.D., is Utley Professor of Health Law, Boston University Schools of Medicine and Public Health, Boston.

American medicine is high-tech medicine, and the American way of death is high-tech death.[1] It is a cliché that health care providers often concentrate more on medical technology and procedures than on the patient. Sometimes we seem to act as if medical technologies such as ICUs and ventilators have rights to be used, and patients have an obligation to use them. In the face of a terminal or serious medical condition, and in a high-tech hospital environment, patients often feel powerless and alienated. Americans worry about this and fear an impersonal death in a hospital because of loss of control, isolation, and pain. The central irony and tragedy of American health care is that with millions of uninsured citizens denied care they desperately need, we continue to force others to endure expensive and invasive treatment they do not want. How did we get where we are, and how can we reempower patients and recapture the human dimensions of dying?

Medical Technology

Medical technology has become our new religion and is so accepted as religion that we routinely speak of innovation in medicine as "medical miracles." The ultimate miracle was the resurrection—and our ultimate goal seems to be to abolish death. As novelist Don DeLillo has one of his characters in *White Noise* say to a friend who is worried about death: You can deny it, you can put your faith in religion, or

... you can put your faith in technology. It got you here, it can get you out. This is the whole point of technology. It creates an appetite for immortality on the one hand. It threatens universal extinction on the other....

It's what we invented to conceal the terrible secret of our decaying bodies. But it's also life, isn't it? It prolongs life, it provides new organs for those that wear out. New devices, new techniques every day. Lasers, masers, ultrasound. Give yourself up to it.... They'll insert you in a gleaming tube, irradiate your body with the basic stuff of the universe.... Light, energy, dreams. God's own goodness.[2]

Physicians are not immune from such magical thinking. As psychiatrist Jay Katz has noted, when medical science seems impotent to fight the claims of nature, "all kinds of senseless interventions are tried in an unconscious effort to cure the incurable magically through a 'wonder drug,' a novel surgical procedure, or a penetrating psychological interpretation."[3] This quest for miracles, like a trip to Lourdes, has brought us media events such as the Jarvik-7 artificial heart and Baby Fae—experiments that were objectively doomed to failure from the start.

Perhaps this is why the movement to insist that patients have the right to refuse medical treatment is often simply called the "right to die." This slogan wrongly implies that death is optional and that individuals actually achieve some political or practical victory by having their inevitable end legally recognized. Nonetheless, the slogan does confront us with the reality of death itself, a reality we spend most of our lives fleeing. Medicine cannot ultimately save lives, it can only (sometimes) postpone death. Most people recognize what many medical care providers refuse to face: There are fates worse than death, and death is not always the enemy.

The Case of Karen Ann Quinlan

The story of Karen Ann Quinlan is a modern parable. Severely brain-damaged in an accident, Ms. Quinlan was "successfully" resuscitated in a hospital emergency department and put on a mechanical ventilator that breathed for her. When it became clear that she would never regain consciousness, her parents asked her physician to remove the ventilator and let her die. Worried about possible civil and criminal liability, her physician asked her parents to obtain legal immunity for him in court. A lower court refused, but in 1976 the New Jersey Supreme Court ruled that if she were competent, Ms. Quinlan would have a constitutional right to refuse continued medical treatment and that her parents could exercise this right on her behalf.[4] Ms. Quinlan's ventilator was thereafter removed — although she survived another decade in a coma, able to breath on her own.

Almost all Americans have said, "I never want to be like Karen Ann Quinlan." We intuitively, if not rationally, recognize that such expensive and intensive medical intervention is both pointless for us and cruel for our families. Since 1976, more than 50 courts in almost 20 states have reviewed cases dealing with the right to refuse treatment. All but two have agreed with the basic analysis and conclusion of the New Jersey Supreme Court. The two that disagreed merit comment because these exceptions illuminate the reasons for existing legal rules.

The Case of Mary O'Connor

The first is a New York case in which the state's highest court rejected the previously expressed wishes of a 77-year-old widow to refuse a nasogastric tube proposed to deliver nourishment to her body. Mary O'Connor was severely demented and profoundly incapacitated as a result of a series of strokes that left her bedridden, paralyzed, unable to care for herself, and with no hope of any significant improvement. Her husband had died of brain cancer, and the last two of her nine brothers had also died of cancer. A former hospital administrator, she had visited them regularly when they were hospitalized and had cared for them at home. During this time, she had several con-

versations with hospital co-workers and her daughters, saying among other things, that it was "monstrous to keep someone alive . . . by using machines and things like that when they were not going to get better" and that she "would never want any sort of intervention, any sort of life-support system."[5] Her two daughters, both nurses, had no doubt that their mother would not want the nasogastric tube. Nonetheless, the hospital went to court to force treatment.

The lower court denied the hospital's petition, but the New York Court of Appeals, in a cruel opinion, granted the hospital's request on the basis that Ms. O'Connor had not been specific enough in expressing her desires. For example, the court noted that her husband and brothers had died of cancer, whereas she "is simply an elderly person who as a result of several strokes suffers certain disabilities. . . ." The court also observed that almost everyone has made similar statements: "Her comments . . . are in fact, no different than those that many of us might make after witnessing an agonizing death."

The fact that almost everyone has made similar statements is no reason to ignore them all; indeed, it is *the* reason to take them all seriously. It is precisely because medical technology is being used indiscriminately that most elderly citizens have had to witness the painfully and pointlessly prolonged dying process of friends and relatives and have consequently expressed their wishes not to be similarly abused. My guess is that most of us would rather have our courts err on the side of protecting our liberty rather than on the side of prolonging our lives in similar situations. In this regard, death, Patrick Henry's "second choice," remains preferable to being treated as an inanimate object without personality, family, or history.

The Case of Nancy Cruzan

The second aberrant case, that of Nancy Cruzan, is more important because it was decided by the U.S. Supreme Court. This case is essentially identical to the case of Karen Ann Quinlan, with one exception: Nancy Cruzan, a young woman in a permanent coma as a result of an automobile accident, required only tube feeding (rather than a mechanical ventilator and tube feeding) to continue to survive. Her parents believed she would not want to have the tube feeding continued in such circumstances, and she herself had said that she would not want to continue to live if she could not be "at least halfway normal." Unlike *Quinlan,* however, the trial court granted the family's request to have their daughter's tube feeding discontinued, and the Supreme Court of Missouri reversed on the ground that Nancy herself had not left "clear and convincing evidence" of her wishes regarding tube feeding.[6]

This opinion was affirmed by the U.S. Supreme Court in 1990.[7] In the Court's words, the question in *Cruzan* was "whether the U.S. Constitution forbids a state from requiring clear and convincing evidence of a person's expressed decision while competent to have hydration and nutrition withdrawn in such a way as to cause death." The Court concluded that the Constitution did not prohibit this procedural requirement. Four basic reasons were given. The first reason was that this heightened evidentiary standard promotes the state's legitimate interest "in the protection and preservation of human life." The second was that "the choice between life and death is a deeply personal decision. . . ." The third was that abuses can occur in the case of incompetent patients who do not have "loved ones available to serve as surrogate decision-makers." And the fourth reason was that the state may properly "simply assert an unqualified interest in the preservation of human life. . . ."

There is no mathematical formula for the "clear and convincing" standard of proof, which is somewhere between the usual civil standard of "preponderance of the evidence" and the criminal standard of "beyond a reasonable doubt." The use of this strict standard of proof was justified primarily by the same argument the Missouri Supreme Court used, that it is better to make an error on the side of continuing treatment:

An erroneous decision not to terminate results in a maintenance of the status quo; the possibility of subsequent developments such as advancements in medical science, the discovery of new evidence regarding the patient's intent, changes in the law, or simply the unexpected death of the patient despite the administration of life-sustaining treatment, at least create the potential that a wrong decision will eventually be corrected or its impact mitigated. An erroneous decision to withdraw life-sustaining treatment, however, is not susceptible of correction.

The Court held that Missouri could require clear and convincing evidence of Cruzan's wishes before permitting surrogates to authorize the termination of treatment. Even though Nancy Cruzan's mother and father are "loving and caring parents," Missouri may "choose to defer" only to Nancy Cruzan's wishes and ignore both the parents' own wishes and their views about what their daughter would want.

Justice William Brennan wrote for three of the four dissenting members of the Court. Justice Brennan asserted that the Missouri restriction is irrational, because it probably would lead to more deaths than would current medical practice. This is because medical measures to sustain life, once begun, cannot now be terminated without clear and convincing evidence of the patient's wishes as long as continued treatment prolongs life. Trials of therapy are thus effectively discouraged by the Missouri rule, a result

that is irrational. Justice Brennan also argued that the only legitimate interest the state can assert in Nancy Cruzan's case is an interest in accurately determining her wishes. In his view, the Missouri rules were designed not to determine her wishes, but to frustrate them.

Finally, Justice Brennan argued that the Missouri rules are simply out of touch with reality: people do not write elaborate documents about all the possible ways they might die and the various interventions doctors might have available to prolong their lives. Friends and family members are most likely to know what the patient would want. By ignoring such evidence of a person's wishes, the Missouri procedure "transforms [incompetent] human beings into passive subjects of medical technology."

But there was some good news in the opinion as well. Although it was technically not part of the holding, the majority of the Court found that competent adults have a fundamental constitutional right (under the liberty interest in the Fourteenth Amendment) to refuse medical treatment, and six of the nine justices explicitly found that there was no distinction between artificially delivered fluids and nutrition and other forms of medical treatment.[8]

Nancy Cruzan died on December 26, 1990, approximately two weeks after Judge Charles E. Teel ruled again (as he had in 1988) that her parents could order the feeding tubes removed from their daughter's body. There were three major differences in the 1990 hearing. First, three of Nancy's friends testified that Nancy had told them she would never want to live "like a vegetable" on medical machines. Second, her attending physician, James C. Davis, testified that continued treatment was no longer in Nancy's best interests. And third, the state of Missouri withdrew from the case, leaving no one with legal standing to oppose the family's petition or appeal the judge's finding that "clear and convincing evidence" demonstrated that Nancy would not have wanted tube feeding continued.

Post-Cruzan Developments

Every state has a durable-power-of-attorney law that permits individuals to designate another to make decisions for them after they become incapacitated.[9] Although these statutes were enacted primarily to permit the agent to make financial decisions, no court has ever invalidated a durable power of attorney specifically designed for health care decisions. Moreover, in her concurring opinion in *Cruzan*, Justice Sandra Day O'Connor advised individuals to utilize this device. She also observed that *Cruzan* "does not preclude a future determination that the Constitution requires the States to implement the decisions of a duly appointed surrogate."[10] The *Cruzan* case energized the "health care proxy," just as the *Quinlan* case had previously energized the living will. Physicians are legally and ethically bound to respect the directions of a patient set forth in a living will. But living wills are limited, because no one can accurately foretell the future, and interpretation may be difficult. Attempts to make the living will less ambiguous by developing comprehensive checklists with alternative scenarios may be too confusing and abstract to be useful to either patients or health care providers, although opinions on this differ.[11]

The current trend in the United States is for states to enact proxy laws that deal specifically with health care, although this is *not* legally required in any state (because of existing durable-power-of-attorney laws). Such health care proxy laws generally specify the information that must be included in the proxy form and the standards by which treatment decisions must be made and grant "good faith" immunity for all involved in carrying out the treatment decision. (Two of the best-written proxy laws became effective in New York in January 1991 and in Massachusetts in December 1990.) The New York law is based on a recommendation of the New York State Task Force on Life and the Law, and that group's publication of its rationale is still the best introduction to the health care proxy concept.[12] The Massachusetts health care proxy law is largely modeled on the New York law.

The heart of both laws (and of all proxy laws) is the same: enabling a competent adult (the "principal") to choose another person (the agent) to make treatment decisions for him if he becomes incompetent to make them himself. The agent has the same decision-making authority the patient would have if competent. Instead of being faced with a document to decipher, the physician is able to discuss treatment options with a person who has the legal authority to grant or withhold consent on behalf of the patient. The manner in which the agent must exercise this authority is also crucial. The agent must make decisions consistent with the wishes of the patient, if known, or otherwise consistent with the patient's best interests.

Proxy laws also permit the principal to specify in the document any limits in the agent's authority (for example, no authority to refuse CPR or tube feeding). However, the more limitations the principal puts on the agent, the more the health care proxy resembles a living will. In addition, because every limitation is subject to interpretation, the likelihood of a dispute arising about the meaning of the document is increased with each limitation. One compromise is to give blanket decision-making authority to the agent and to give the agent a private letter detailing one's values and wishes with as much precision as possible. The agent could use this letter when relevant to the actual decision and keep it private when it was not relevant.

The goal of the health care proxy is to simplify decision making by increasing the likelihood that the patient's wishes will be followed, not to complicate existing problems. If hospitals and hospital lawyers cooperate, this goal will be attained because the vast majority of physicians will welcome the opportunity to discuss treatment options with a person chosen by the patient who has the legal authority to give or withhold consent. Hospitals can help their patients by making a simple form available; by educating their medical, nursing, and social service staff about the health care proxy; and by supporting decisions based on it.

It should be stressed that the health care proxy does not substantively change existing law; it merely makes it procedurally easier for a person to designate an agent to make whatever health care decision the person could legally make if competent and gives health care providers legal immunity for honoring such decisions. The patient can, for example, give the agent the authority to refuse any and all medical care; but the agent has no more legal authority than the principal to demand assisted suicide or to demand a lethal injection. The proxy mechanism also solves the problem of a dispute among family members concerning treatment, as the agent has the legal and ethical right and responsibility to make the decision. When the long-lost relative arrives and demands that "everything be done or I'll sue," the physician can refer that person to the agent, rather than try to get all the relatives to agree on what the patient would want.[13]

Limits of the Proxy

The health care proxy only applies to competent adults who actually execute the document. Given that fewer than 10 percent of Americans have either living wills or organ donor cards, few may use this mechanism. It has no application to children, the mentally retarded, and others unable to appreciate the nature and consequences of their decisions. Treatment decisions for these populations will continue to be governed by the vague "best interest" standard, which is the functional equivalent of "reasonable medical care," "appropriate medical care," and "indicated medical care." Many people will not have a friend or relative they trust enough to act as their agent, and for them the living will remains their best strategy. The health care proxy will also be of limited use in the emergency department, although there may be rare cases in which the health care agent arrives with the principal and there is time for consultation and informed consent before a specific intervention is tried. Nor will the proxy mechanism solve problems of "futility." Physicians will retain the right not to offer treatment they believe is contraindicated, useless, or futile.

Because many individuals will not designate an agent, states will pass statutes designed to legally authorize specific family members to make decisions for their loved ones. Such decisions will not always be precisely those that the patient would have made. Nonetheless, the overwhelming majority of Americans will agree that it is more likely that family members' decisions will be consistent with their wishes and best interests than that state officials' decisions which will be made in the interests of the state, will be congruent with their personal interests. Not only should such statutes be passed (to prevent a "*Cruzan* disaster" from being legislatively imposed), but the standard for challenging family decisions under such statutes should be the reverse of the *Cruzan* "clear and convincing evidence" standard,[14] that is, the state must demonstrate by clear and convincing evidence that the decision of the authorized family member is *not* consistent with the wishes of the individual (or, if these are unknown, is not in the individual's best interests) in order to interfere with it.

Related Issues

Americans fear not only loss of control but also isolation and pain in dying. The widespread public reaction to Jack Kevorkian's "suicide machine" and to the publication of Derek Humphrey's do-it-yourself suicide manual, *Final Exit,*[15] makes it clear that most Americans favor physician-assisted suicide. A national public opinion poll done in late 1991, for example, indicated that 64 percent of Americans favor physician-assisted suicide and euthanasia for terminally ill patients who request it.[16] Nonetheless, when Washington state residents voted on Initiative 119 in November 1991, it went down to defeat by a margin of 56 to 44 percent.[17] Even in defeat, however, Initiative 119, which would have given physicians legal immunity for killing competent, terminally ill patients upon request, indicates profound disgust by almost half of the population with the way people currently die in America's hospitals.

It is now settled constitutional law (and in most states statutory and common law as well) that competent patients have a right to refuse *any* treatment, life-sustaining or not, and a right to name another person to exercise this legal authority on their behalf. There is no right to assisted suicide. But if hospitals and other health care providers do not respond as constructively as the hospice movement has to the anguish of the pain and isolation of technologically driven death, Americans increasingly will take matters into their own hands, not only by committing suicide at home, but also by insisting that physicians kill them.

Conclusions and Recommendations

- All hospitals and other health care providers must not only provide patients with the informtion on

their rights required by the Patient Self-Determination Act, but they also must recognize and honor the legal and ethical right of competent patients (those who understand the facts needed for informed consent) to refuse *any* treatment. It should be made clear to patients *throughout their stay* at the hospital that their wishes will be respected as a matter of course.
- Ethics committees and patient advocates should actively educate the medical and nursing staff on the rights of patients, with special attention to the right to refuse treatment.
- Hospitals should take advantage of the publicity elicited by the Nancy Cruzan case, *Final Exit,* and the Patient Self-Determination Act to encourage patients and others to discuss death and medical treatment issues with their families and physicians so that physicians know what relatives and patients want regarding medical treatment. The more specific such discussions can be, the better. People should not have to guess about what patients and relatives would decide in various circumstances; they should know.
- Hospitals and other providers should actively encourage everyone—patients, employees, and others—to appoint someone they trust, through a document called a durable power of attorney, or health care proxy, to make health care decisions on their behalf if they are unable to make them for themselves.
- Hospitals and nursing homes should go beyond the letter of the Patient Self-Determination Act and make living will (written statement of directions regarding treatment in the event of incompetency) and health care proxy forms routinely available to all patients prior to or upon admission, so that thinking about dying and making decisions about treatment during incompetency become matters that *must* be confronted and are seen as the personal responsibility of each of us.
- Health care providers must routinely provide patients with sufficient pain medication to keep them pain-free. Patients have no obligation to suffer, and doctors do have an obligation to alleviate suffering, even if doing so shortens life.
- Health care providers should be *required* to honor a patient's directions regarding treatment refusals (or to quickly find another physician who will) under penalty of license revocation for unethical and unprofessional conduct and malpractice charges.
- Refusal of treatment by family members on behalf of incompetent patients should be honored unless the health care providers believe such requests are contrary to the patient's wishes and are willing to obtain a court order to continue treatment.

George J. Annas, J.D., M.P.H.

Medical technology is a good servant but a cruel and heartless master. We have acted as if medical technologies had a right to be used. It's past time to recognize that people have rights, including a right to decide whether to use the modern miracles of high-tech medicine. Death may never be seen as desirable, but it is inevitable, and caring for the dying in ways that respect their dignity, personhood, and autonomy can humanize death and restore the dying process to the world of the living.

Notes

1. Portions of this chapter are based on Annas, G. J. Life, liberty and death, *Health Management Quarterly,* first quarter 1990, pp. 5–8.
2. DeLillo, D. *White Noise.* New York City: Penguin, 1986, p. 285.
3. Katz, J. *The Silent World of Doctor and Patient.* New Haven, CT: Yale University Press, 1984, p. 151.
4. *In re Quinlan,* 70 N.J. 10, 355 A.2d 647 (1976).
5. *In the Matter of Mary O'Connor,* 72 N.Y.2d 517 (1988).
6. *Cruzan v. Harmon,* 760 S.W.2d 408 (Mo. 1988)(en banc).
7. *Cruzan v. Director, Missouri Dept of Health.* 110 S. Ct. 2841 (1990).
8. See, generally, Annas G. J. The long dying of Nancy Cruzan. *Law, Medicine & Health Care* 19(1–2):52–59, 1991.
9. Sabatino, C. P. *Health Care Powers of Attorney.* Chicago: American Bar Association, 1990.
10. *Cruzan v. Director, Missouri Dept. of Health* (1990).
11. Emanuel, L. L., Barry, M. J., Stoeckle, J. D., Ettelson, L. M., and Emanuel, E. J. Advance directives for medical care: A case for greater use. *New England Journal of Medicine* 324:889–95, Mar. 1991.
12. New York State Task Force on Life and the Law. *Life-Sustaining Treatment: Making Decisions and Appointing a Health Care Agent.* New York City: N.Y. State Task Force on Life and the Law, 1990.
13. Annas, G. J. The health care proxy and the living will. *New England Journal of Medicine* 324:1210–13, Apr. 25, 1991.
14. *Cruzan v. Harmon* (1988).
15. Humphrey, D. *Final Exit.* Eugene, OR: The Hemlock Society, 1991.
16. Knox, R. A. "Poll: Americans favor mercy killing." *Boston Globe,* Nov. 3, 1991, p. 1.
17. Merz, B. Despite defeat of state's suicide initiative, issue still unsettled. *American Medical News,* Nov. 18, 1991, p. 1.

Chapter 12

Patient Autonomy and "Death with Dignity": Some Clinical Caveats

David L. Jackson, M.D., Ph.D., and Stuart Youngner, M.D.

Reprinted, with permission, from *The New England Journal of Medicine* 301(8):404–8, Aug. 23, 1979.

From the Division of Clinical Pharmacology and Critical Care Medicine, the Medical Intensive Care Unit, Department of Medicine, and the Consultation Liaison Service, Department of Psychiatry, Case Western Reserve University, University Hospitals of Cleveland. Supported in part by a grant (MH 15022-02) from the National Institute of Mental Health.

The rapid advance in medical technology over the past two decades has raised serious questions about patient autonomy and the right to die with dignity. This article will attempt to examine psychologic issues affecting decision making in these areas. Attempts to answer these questions have come from many quarters: legal, ethical and religious, as well as medical. The lay public and press have also participated actively in this dialogue.

Both legislatures and the courts have attempted to clarify these issues. Many states have enacted laws providing for "living wills"— legal documents that give patients the right to refuse heroic measures for their care when in a "terminal" condition.[1] Such laws also protect physicians from legal action by family members when they comply with such "wills." Both the courts and some state legislatures have recently attempted to provide legal definitions of death.[2] The courts have also ruled on who should make the final decisions when patients are not competent. Most recently, in the Saikewicz case,[3,4] the

Supreme Court of Massachusetts asserted that all decisions about the institution or termination of life-prolonging measures must be made by the courts if the patient is not legally competent.

Physicians have approached the difficult problem of decision making for critically ill patients in various ways. Attempts have been made to establish reliable clinical criteria for predicting outcome in critically ill patients. This effort has been most successful in defining brain death, where clear-cut clinical criteria can predict with certainty a fatal outcome.[2] Efforts at predicting outcome in "vegetative" brain states and other serious "terminal" conditions have been less successful.

Another approach has been to develop systems for classifying patient-care categories.[5-7] This triage approach is designed to permit direction of maximal effort toward the care of "viable" patients, stressing daily re-evaluation of medical status and treatment options and open communication among medical personnel, patient and family.

Many hospitals have established ethics or "optimal-care" committees that serve in an advisory capacity to physicians, patients and families when difficult decisions arise about stopping or withholding life-support systems.[8]

Imbus and Zawacki[8] described an approach for patients with "burns so severe that survival is unprecedented." When given a choice between "ordinary" care or "full treatment measures," 21 of 24 patients chose the former. The authors make a strong argument for an aggressive approach to preserve patient autonomy. They ask, "Who is more likely to be totally and lovingly concerned with the patient's best interest than the patient himself?"

David L. Jackson, M.D., Ph.D., and Stuart Youngner, M.D.

Little has been written, however, about the specific clinical and psychologic problems that may complicate the concept of patient autonomy and the right to die with dignity. Cassem[9] has noted that in clinical situations where pain and depression are prominent features, "the physician ethically could proceed against the will of the patient." Rabkin and his colleagues[10] warn that "caution should be exercised that a patient does not unwittingly 'consent' to an ONTR [order not to resuscitate], as a result of temporary distortion (for example, from pain, medication or metabolic abnormality) in his ability to choose among available alternatives." They go on to say that "it may be inappropriate to introduce the subject of withholding cardiopulmonary resuscitation efforts to certain competent patients when, in the physician's judgment, the patient will probably be unable to cope with them psychologically." Unfortunately, the authors do not develop this concept in a detailed manner and therefore leave it open to criticism.[8]

The issues of patient autonomy and the right to die with dignity are without question important ones that require further discussion and clarification by our society as a whole. However, there is a danger that in certain cases, preoccupation with these dramatic and popular issues may lead physicians and patients to make clinically inappropriate decisions—precisely because sound clinical evaluation and judgment are suspended. This article will attempt to illustrate this concept by use of clinical examples from a medical intensive-care unit. Each case will demonstrate a specific clinical situation where concerns about patient autonomy and the right to die with dignity posed a potential threat to sound decision making and the total clinical (medical, social and ethical) basis for the "optimal" decision.

Case Reports

Case 1—Patient Ambivalence

An 80-year-old man was admitted to the Medical Intensive-Care Unit (MICU) with a three-week history of progressive shortness of breath. He had a long history of chronic obstructive lung disease. He had been admitted to a hospital with similar problems four years earlier and had required intubation, mechanical respiratory support and eventual tracheostomy. The patient remained on the respirator for two months before weaning was successfully completed. During the four years after discharge, his activity had been progressively restricted because of dyspnea on exertion. He required assistance in most aspects of self-care.

On admission, he was afebrile, and there was no evidence of an acute precipitating event. Maximum attempts at pulmonary toilet, low-flow supplemental oxygen and treatment of mild right-sided congestive heart failure and

bronchospasm were without effect. After four days of continued deterioration, a decision had to be made about whether to intubate and mechanically ventilate the patient. His private physician and the director of the MICU discussed the options with this fully conversant and alert patient. He initially decided against intubation. However, 24 hours later, when he became almost moribund, he changed his mind and requested that respiratory support be initiated. He was unable to be weaned from the respirator and required tracheostomy—a situation reminiscent of his previous admission. Two months later, he had made no progress, and it became obvious that he would never be weaned from respiratory support.

Attempts were made to find extended-care facilities that could cope with a patient on a respirator. Extensive discussions with the patient and his family about the appropriate course to follow revealed striking changes of mind on an almost daily basis. The patient often expressed to the MICU staff his wish to be removed from the respirator and said, "If I make it, I make it." However, when his family was present, he would insist that he wanted maximal therapy, even if it meant remaining on the respirator indefinitely. The family showed similar ambivalence. The patient was regularly the center of conversation at the MICU weekly interdisciplinary conference (liaison among medical, nursing, social-work and psychiatric staff). There was great disagreement among MICU staff members concerning which side of the patient's ambivalence should be honored. Ultimately (after 4½ months on the respirator), the patient contracted a nosocomial pulmonary infection, became hypotensive and experienced ventricular fibrillation. No efforts were made at cardiopulmonary resuscitation. In this difficult case, the concept of patient "autonomy" became impossible to define.

Case 2—Depression

A 54-year-old married man with a five-year history of lymphosarcoma was admitted to the hospital intensive-care unit for progressive shortness of breath and a one-week history of nausea and vomiting. Over the past five years, he had received three courses of combination-drug chemotherapy, which resulted in remission. His most recent course occurred four months before admission. On admission, x-ray examination of the chest showed a diffuse infiltrate, more on the left than on the right. Eight hours after admission, he was transferred to the MICU because of hypotension and increasing dyspnea. Initially, it was not clear whether these findings indicated interstitial spread of lymphosarcoma or asymmetric pulmonary edema. Physical findings were compatible with a diagnosis of congestive heart failure, and he was treated for pulmonary edema, with good response. His neurologic examination was normal, except for a flat, depressed affect. Deep-tendon reflexes were 2+ and symmetric.

Laboratory examination revealed only a mildly elevated blood urea nitrogen, with a normal creatinine and a slightly elevated calcium of 11.8 mg per deciliter (2.95 mmol per liter). There were no objective signs of hypercalcemia. His respiratory status improved rapidly.

The patient refused his oncologist's recommendation for additional chemotherapy. Although his cognitive abilities were intact, he steadfastly refused the pleas of his wife and the MICU staff to undergo therapy. Over the first six days in the MICU with treatment by rehydration, his calcium became normal, his nausea and vomiting slowly improved, and his affect brightened. At that time, he agreed to chemotherapy, stating that, "Summer's coming and I want to be able to sit in the backyard a little longer." During this course of chemotherapy, the patient discussed his previous refusal of therapy. In his opinion, the nausea and vomiting had made "life not worth living." No amount of reassurance that these symptoms were temporary could convince him that it was worthwhile to continue his fight. Only when this reassurance was confirmed by clinical improvement did the patient overcome his reactive depression and concur with the reinstitution of vigorous therapy.

Case 3 — Patient Who Uses a Plea for Death with Dignity to Identify a Hidden Problem

A 52-year-old married man was admitted to the MICU after an attempt at suicide. He had retired two years earlier because of progressive physical disability related to multiple sclerosis during the 15 years before admission. He had successfully adapted to his physical limitations, remaining actively involved in family matters with his wife and two teenage sons. However, during the three months before admission, he had become morose and withdrawn but had no vegetative symptoms of depression. On the evening of admission, while alone, he ingested an unknown quantity of diazepam. When his family returned six hours later, they found the patient semiconscious. He had left a suicide note.

On admission to the MICU, physical examination showed several neurologic deficits, including spastic paraparesis, right-arm monoparesis, cortical sensory deficits, bilateral ophthalmoplegia and bilateral cerebellar dysfunction. This picture was unchanged from recent neurologic examinations. The patient was alert and fully conversant. He expressed to the MICU house officers his strong belief in a patient's right to die with dignity. He stressed the "meaningless" aspects of his life related to his loss of function, insisting that he did not want vigorous medical intervention should serious complications develop. This position appeared logically coherent to the MICU staff. However, a consultation with members of the psychiatric liaison service was requested.

During the initial consultation, the patient showed that the onset of his withdrawal and depression coincided with a diagnosis of inoperable cancer in his mother-in-law. His wife had spent more and more time satisfying the needs of her terminally ill mother. In fact, on the night of his suicide attempt, the patient's wife and sons had left him alone for the first time to visit his mother-in-law, who lived in another city. The patient had "too much pride" to complain to his wife about his feelings of abandonment. He was able to recognize that his suicide attempt and insistence on death with dignity were attempts to draw the family's attention to his needs. Discussions with all four family members led to improved communication and acknowledgment of the patient's special emotional needs. After these conversations, the patient explicitly retracted both his suicidal threats and his demand that no supportive medical efforts be undertaken. He was discharged, to have both neurologic and psychiatric follow-up examinations.

Case 4 — Patient Demands Out of Fear That Treatment Be Withheld or Stopped

An unmarried 18-year-old woman, 24 weeks pregnant and with a history of chronic asthma, was admitted to the hospital with a two-day history of increasing shortness of breath. She was found to have a left lobar pneumonia and a gram-negative urinary-tract infection. She was transferred to the MICU for worsening shortness of breath and hypoxia resistant to therapy with supplemental oxygen. Despite vigorous pulmonary toilet and antiasthmatic and antibiotic therapy, her condition continued to deteriorate. She was thought to require intubation for positive end-expiratory pressure respiratory therapy. Initially, she refused this modality of treatment. She was alert, oriented and clearly legally competent. After several discussions with physicians, nurses, family and friends, she openly verbalized her fears of the imposing and intimidating MICU equipment and environment. She was able to accept reassurance and consented to appropriate medical therapy. She showed slow but progressive improvement and was discharged eight days later.

Case 5 — Family's Perception Differs from Patient's Previously Expressed Wishes

A 76-year-old retired man was transferred to the MICU four days after laparotomy for diverticulitis. Before hospitalization, he had enjoyed good health and a full and active life-style. He sang regularly in a barbershop quartet until one week before admission. The patient's hospital course was complicated by a urinary-tract infection, with sepsis and aspiration pneumonia requiring orotracheal intubation to control pulmonary secretions.

Before intubation, he had emphasized to the medical staff his enjoyment of life and expressed a strong desire to return, if possible, to his previous state of health. After intubation, he continued to cooperate vigorously with his daily care, including painful procedures (e.g., obtaining

David L. Jackson, M.D., Ph.D., and Stuart Youngner, M.D.

samples of arterial-blood gas). However, he contracted sepsis and became delirious, and at this time his wife and daughter expressed strong feelings to the MICU staff that no "heroic" measures be undertaken. Thus, serious disagreement arose concerning the appropriate level of supportive care for this patient. The professional staff of the MICU felt that the medical problems were potentially reversible and that the patient had both explicitly and implicitly expressed a wish to continue the struggle for life. Because this view conflicted with the family's wishes, the MICU visiting physician called a meeting of the Terminal Care Committee (a hospital committee with broad representation that meets at the request of any physician, nurse or family member who would like advice concerning the difficult decision to initiate, continue, stop or withhold intensive care for critically ill patients). Meeting with the committee were the private physician, the MICU attending physician, as well as representatives from the MICU nursing and house-officer teams. The family was given the opportunity to attend but declined. The committee supported the judgment of the MICU staff that because of the patient's previously expressed wishes and the medical situation, vigorous supportive intervention should be continued. A meeting was then held between medical staff and the patient's family, during which it was agreed by all that appropriate medical intervention should be continued but that the decision would be reviewed on a daily basis. Five days later, the patient contracted a superinfection that did not respond to maximal antibiotic therapy. He became transiently hypotensive and showed progressive renal failure. In the face of a progressing multilobe pneumonia and sepsis caused by a resistant organism, the decision to support the patient with maximum intervention was reviewed. The family concurred with the professional staff's recommendation that cardiopulmonary resuscitation should not be attempted if the patient suffered a cardiopulmonary arrest. On the 18th day in the MICU, the patient died.

Decision making in this case became more difficult because the patient's deteriorating condition made him unable to participate. The advice of the Terminal Care Committee was critically important in this situation, where the family's perception of death with dignity conflicted not only with the patient's own wishes but also with the professional judgment of the MICU staff.

Case 6 — Misconception by Some of MICU Staff of Patient's Concept of Death with Dignity

A 56-year-old woman was receiving chemotherapy on an outpatient basis for documented bronchogenic carcinoma metastatic to the mediastinal lymph nodes and central nervous system when she had a sudden seizure, followed by cardiorespiratory arrest. Resuscitation was accomplished in the outpatient department, and she was transferred to the MICU. She had been undergoing combination-drug chemotherapy as an outpatient for six months but continued to work regularly.

In the MICU, her immediate management was complicated by "flail chest" and a tension pneumothorax requiring tube drainage of the chest. She was deeply comatose and hypotensive. Several MICU staff members raised questions about the appropriateness of continued intensive care. After initial medical stabilization, including vasopressor therapy and mechanical respiration, her clinical status was reviewed in detail with the family. Because of the patient's ability to continue working until the day of admission, her excellent response to chemotherapy and her family's perception of her often-stated wish to survive to see the birth of her first grandchild (her daughter was seven months pregnant), maximal efforts were continued. She remained deeply comatose for three days. Her course was complicated by recurrent tension pneumothoraces, gram-negative sepsis caused by a urinary-tract infection and staphylococcal pneumonia. She gradually became more responsive and by the seventh hospital day was able to nod "yes" or "no" to simple questions. Her hospital course was similar to that of many critically ill patients. As soon as one problem began to improve, a major setback occurred in another organ system. With each setback, there was growing dissension among the MICU staff about the appropriate level of supportive care. The vast majority of the MICU staff felt strongly that continued maximum intervention was neither warranted nor humane. A smaller group of staff, supported by the patient's daughter and (once she was able to communicate) the patient herself, felt that as long as there was any chance for the patient to return to the quality of life she had enjoyed before cardiorespiratory arrest, maximum therapy was indicated.

The patient was the subject of many hours of debate and was a regular topic of conversation at the weekly interdisciplinary conference. She survived all her medical complications and was discharged home after seven weeks in the MICU, awake, alert and able to walk and engage in daily activities around her home without limitation. She saw the birth of her granddaughter, and spent Thanksgiving, Christmas and New Year's Day at home with her family. She died suddenly at home 11 weeks after discharge.

Discussion

Our purpose is not to refute the importance of patient autonomy or discredit the more complex concept of death with dignity. Rather, we have attempted to provide a specific clinical perspective that may help clarify the difficult and often conflicting factors underlying the decisions made daily at the bedsides of critically ill patients.

Veatch[11] has effectively argued that many of the decisions regarding the withholding or stopping of life-support systems are ethical, not medical and therefore not the exclusive responsibility of the physician. Capron and Kass[12] state, "Physicians *qua* physicians are not expert on these philosophic questions, nor are they experts on the question of which physiological functions decisively identify the 'living human organism.'" However, careful examination of the legal guidelines suggested by these authors or the living-will statutes enacted by several states reveals vague terms, such as "irreversible,"[11,12] "hopeless"[13] and "terminal condition."[14] As Cassem has pointed out,[9] "In most cases in intensive care units, the confidence with which these label(s) [sic] can be applied depends entirely on the clinical judgment of the primary doctor, along with the best consultations he is able to acquire." Public policy can establish useful guidelines when medical evidence is clear, when exact physiologic measurement is possible and when disease outcome is accurately predictable (e.g., criteria for brain death[2] or Imbus and Zawacki's burn patients[9]). But rigid guidelines are not useful in most clinical situations, where separation of medical from social or ethical responsibility is difficult or artificial.

We heartily support the plea by Imbus and Zawacki[8] for "more and earlier communication with the patient." However, their question, "Who is more likely to be totally and lovingly concerned with the patient's best interest than the patient himself?" may be somewhat naive and, in certain clinical situations, potentially dangerous. Physicians must not use "professional responsibility" as a cloak for paternalism, but they must be alert not to let the possibility of abuse keep them from the appropriate exercise of professional judgment. Physicians who are uncomfortable or inexperienced in dealing with the complex psychosocial issues facing critically ill patients may ignore an important aspect of their professional responsibility by taking a patient's or family's statement at face value without further exploration or clarification.

The cases presented in this article illustrate specific situations in which superficial preoccupation with the issues of patient autonomy and death with dignity could have led to inappropriate clinical and ethical decisions. They suggest a checklist that may aid the clinician in evaluating such difficult situations.

Case 1 — Patient Ambivalence

One must be cautious not to act precipitously on the side of the patient's ambivalence with which one agrees, while piously claiming to be following the principle of patient autonomy. Ambivalence may not be detected if communication is not a continuing feature of the situation or if the physician makes clear to the patient the answer he expects to hear. Ideally, one hopes for resolution of the ambivalence through clarification of the issues or changes in the course of the illness. However, in some instances, ambivalence may not resolve despite a protracted course and maximal communicative efforts.

Case 2 — Depression

A patient's refusal or request for cessation of treatment may be influenced by depression. If the depression is adequately treated or, as is more frequently encountered, is reactive to physical discomfort that can be relieved, the patient may well change his or her mind. The astute clinician must be alert for a history of endogenous depression, vegetative signs of depression and any acute conditions to which the patient may be reacting. Vigorous attempts to treat the causes of the depression should be made before automatically acquiescing to the patient's wishes.

Case 3 — Patient Who Uses a Plea for Death with Dignity to Identify a Hidden Problem

As demands for autonomy and death with dignity become acceptable and even popular, patients may use them to mask other less "acceptable" problems or complaints. As Case 3 illustrates, a thorough psychosocial history and clinical interview with the patient and family may identify the real problem. If the MICU team can deal effectively with the underlying "real" problems, the plea for death with dignity may radically change.

Case 4 — Patient Demands Out of Fear That Treatment Be Withheld or Stopped

Situations do exist in which fear is rational, unshakable and ultimately a reasonable basis for refusing treatment. On the other hand, fear is often transient and based on misperception or misinformation. When a patient refuses treatment, the physician should try to identify any fears that may underlie the refusal of therapy. The physician can attempt to overcome the fear by means of honest, open explanation and reassurance and by efforts from family, friends and members of the health-care team.

Case 5 — Family's Perception Differs from Patient's Previously Expressed Wishes

Case 5 illustrates this difficult problem. In the absence of a legal document specifically expressing the patient's wishes, who has the right to decide? Clearly, the family represents the interest of the patient, but must a physician comply if both his medical judgment and his assessment of the patient's wishes conflict with the family's view? Of course, the issue could be decided in court. Fortunately, in this case, consultation with the ethics committee of the hospital led to a compromise satisfactory to both family and the MICU staff.

Case 6 — Misconception by Some of MICU Staff of Patient's Concept of Death with Dignity

In Case 6, some of the MICU staff assumed that a comatose patient with metastatic cancer would not want intensive "heroic" treatment. They were mistaken. This patient's will to live was revealed in her desire to see her grand-

David L. Jackson, M.D., Ph.D., and Stuart Youngner, M.D.

child born. In such cases, efforts must be made to ascertain the patient's wishes, rather than to make assumptions by the test "what would I want." Questioning family or waiting until the patient can communicate are methods of discovering the wishes of the patient. Supportive therapy must be continued until this information can be gathered.

This checklist describes six patients we have seen in a busy MICU. It is by no means complete but we hope it will help to clarify situations in which superficial and automatic acquiescence to the concepts of patient autonomy and death with dignity threaten sound clinical judgment. As physicians, we strongly support the principles of patient autonomy and death with dignity and welcome any dialogue that promotes them. Spencer[15] highlighted the importance of judiciously balancing the role of patient and family input into these often difficult decisions with the exercise of sound professional judgment. We must continue to emphasize our professional responsibility for thorough clinical investigation and the exercise of sound judgment. Living up to this responsibility can only enhance the true autonomy and dignity of our patients.

References

1. Zucker KW: Legislatures provide for death with dignity. J Leg Med 5(8):21–24, 1977
2. Black PM: Brain death. N Engl J Med 299:338–344, 393–401, 1978
3. Curran WJ: The Saikewicz decision. N Engl J Med 298:499–500, 1978
4. Relman AS: The Saikewicz decision: judges as physicians. N Engl J Med 298:505–509, 1978
5. Grenvik A, Powner DJ, Snyder JV, et al: Cessation of therapy in terminal illness and brain death. Crit Care Med 6:284–290, 1978
6. Tagge GF, Adler D, Bryan-Brown CW, et al: Relationship of therapy to prognosis in critically ill patients. Crit Care Med 2:61–63, 1974
7. Critical Care Committee of the Massachusetts General Hospital: Optimum care for hopelessly ill patients. N Engl J Med 295:362–364, 1976
8. Imbus SH, Zawacki BE: Autonomy for burned patients when survival is unprecedented. N Engl J Med 297:308–311, 1977
9. Cassem N: When to disconnect the respirator. Psychiatr Ann 9:84–93, 1979
10. Rabkin MT, Gillerman G, Rice NR: Orders not to resuscitate. N Engl J Med 295:364–366, 1976
11. Veatch RM: Death, Dying, and the Biological Revolution. New Haven, Yale University Press, 1976
12. Capron AM, Kass LR: A statutory definition of the standards for determining human death: an appraisal and a proposal. University of Pennsylvania Law Review 121:87–118, 1972
13. Taylor LF: A statutory definition of death in Kansas. JAMA 215:296, 1971
14. West's Annotated California Codes: Health and Safety Code. Section SS7185, Vol 39A. Accumulated pocket part for use in 1979, page 46
15. Spencer SS: "Code" or "no code": a nonlegal opinion. N Engl J Med 300:138–140, 1979

Chapter 13

AIDS and the Gay Community: Between the Specter and the Promise of Medicine

Ronald Bayer, Ph.D.

Reprinted, with permission, from *Social Research* 52(3):581–606, Autumn 1985. Copyright ©1985 *Social Research*.

Ronald Bayer, Ph.D., is professor of sociomedical sciences at Columbia University, New York City. Professor Bayer is a long-time chronicler of the course and implications of the AIDS epidemic. This was an early essay (1985), and his data on the spread of the disease have been supplanted by newer and even more tragic statistics. However, the underlying lessons of why society, the gay community, and medicine clashed over the epidemic, and the essential tension between nonmainstream populations and mainstream medicine may never be more clearly outlined.— Editor

The advances of the biological sciences and of medical technology in the past three decades have held out the promise of greater understanding of disease, the alleviation of human suffering, and the extension of life itself. Against the dictates of nature, a promethean vision has sought to liberate us from the ravages of illness. But the very promise of medicine, born of its increasing power, has provided the grounds for dread as well. Would medicine seek to establish its hegemony by bringing within its orbit every dimension of human existence? Would the positivist dream be fulfilled by the flattening out of all moral discourse under the aegis of medicine? Would medical authority and state power be merged, posing a threat to privacy and liberty?

The specter of medicine—the other side of its promise—became the subject of social criticism in the mid-1960s. By the early 1970s, the attack upon medical authority had become part of the broader assault on professional authority in the United States. Thomas Szasz had prefigured this challenge by his narrower but trenchant questioning of the cultural and institutional power of psychiatry.[1] Ivan Illich's more far-reaching critique sought to force a retreat upon the entire medical establishment.[2]

Less strident, but deriving from the same sense of disquiet, were the challenges posed by biomedical ethics as it took form as an intellectual undertaking in the mid-1960s. Because of America's individualistic cultural tradition, the abuse of medical authority, even when exercised for benign social ends, became a primary concern.[3] Against researchers and clinicians, it was argued, subjects and patients needed protection. Autonomy and privacy thus became the central moral categories of bioethics. The risks associated with the dominance of medicine as a social and cultural institution required that the integrity of moral and political discourse be asserted.

At the same moment that these liberal themes were being developed in the critique of the power of medicine, a second and very different set of concerns was being put forward. A commitment to protection against the abuses of medicine could not obscure the demands of social justice; the structural barriers to health care had to be eliminated. Human need, not ability to pay, it was argued, should drive the health care system.

As medicine has been called upon to respond to the public health crisis posed by AIDS, the tension between the specter of medicine and its promise has informed the complex social debate. In these debates, the central concerns of biomedical ethics have surfaced as the gay community has been forced to confront medicine, government, and itself. Because the gay community has so much to gain from the understanding and ultimate control of AIDS, it has been drawn by the promise of medicine. Because it has been so fearful of how medical authority might be abused, it has sought to invoke protections enunciated in the liberal tradition of biomedical ethics.

Typically, the issues of biomedical ethics have been argued among philosophers, physicians, social scientists, and attorneys. Though the voices of individual patients and research subjects have been heard, their concerns generally have been represented by professionals acting as surrogates. Because of the level of political and social organization within the gay community, however, the interests, hopes, and fears of patients and subjects have been given direct collective expression in the case of AIDS. The thematic concerns of biomedical ethics are thus given a unique and important rendering, and are placed in a sociopolitical context from which they have in the past been too frequently separated.

The Epidemiology of AIDS

Four years ago the Centers for Disease Control (CDC) began to report the appearance, in previously healthy gay men, of diseases that had occurred only in individuals whose immune systems had been severely compromised. In June 1981, *Morbidity and Mortality Weekly Reports,* CDC's publication, described an outcropping of five cases of pneumocystis carinii pneumonia in Los Angeles. Terming this occurrence "unusual," the *Reports* suggested the possibility of "an association between some aspect of homosexual lifestyle or disease acquired from sexual contact and pneumocystis pneumonia in this population."[4]

The next month, CDC reported that in the prior two and a half years Kaposi's sarcoma, a malignancy unusual in the United States, had been diagnosed in twenty-six gay men. Eight of those patients had died within two years of diagnosis. In each of these cases, two factors were striking: the youth of the victims—in the past, Kaposi's had been reported only in elderly Americans—and its "fulminant" course.[5]

During the next year the CDC continued to record the toll of what was now called acquired immune deficiency syndrome (AIDS). By May 28, 1982, 355 cases of Kaposi's sarcoma, pneumocystis pneumonia, and other opportunistic infections among those who had not been previously diagnosed with immune suppressed conditions had been reported. Of these, 79 percent were either gay or bisexual. Among the heterosexual patients, the dominant feature was illicit intravenous drug use. Though

there was no definitive explanation of how AIDS spread, there was increasingly suggestive evidence that some factor transmitted through sexual contact or the sharing of needles by drug users was involved. Why recent immigrants from Haiti seemed to be overrepresented among the heterosexual AIDS cases was a mystery.

In the first year of AIDS reporting, the pattern of morbidity and mortality seemed largely limited to three distinct groups—gay and bisexual men, drug users, and Haitians. The population at large seemed unaffected. In July 1982, however, CDC reported AIDS in three heterosexuals with hemophilia.[6] Two had died, one was critically ill. These cases suggested the possibility that the disease could be transmitted by blood or blood products. These fears were confirmed when the case of a twenty-month-old infant with an unexplained cellular immune deficiency along with opportunistic infection was reported. The child had received multiple transfusions after birth. One of these had come from a donor who, though apparently in good health at the time of his donation, had subsequently developed the first symptoms of AIDS.[7]

Each year, since the first reports of AIDS were made by the CDC, the number of cases has mounted. By April 1985, 9,400 cases had come to the attention of public health authorities. There had been more than 4,500 deaths. The overall mortality of just less than 50 percent conceals the course of the disease and its toll. Of those reported in 1981 and earlier, 85 percent were dead by April 1985. This was true of 70 percent of those reported in 1982, 63 percent of those reported in 1983, and 47 percent of those reported in the first six months of 1984.[8]

It is a grim fact about the statistics on AIDS that these numbers will be painfully outdated by the time this article is read. Though just fewer than 9,000 cases had been reported as of December 1984, there is little doubt that there will be an additional 9,000 cases in 1985. With the long-hoped-for "flattening of the epidemiological curve" still elusive, some have suggested that there may be as many as 40,000 new cases within the next two years.[9] Though some small progress has been made in treatment, there is little reason to believe that the mortality figures will show much improvement.

Despite the increase in numbers, the distribution of AIDS among various subgroups in the population has remained relatively constant (Table 1). Haitians, it will be noted, have been eliminated as a designated risk group, ostensibly for statistical reasons.[10] What remains uncertain at this point is how deeply AIDS will penetrate the at-risk populations, and whether the relatively circumscribed features of the current epidemiological pattern will be maintained.

A recently developed antibody test for HTLV-III/LAV, the virus now believed to be causative of AIDS, makes it possible to estimate the level of viral exposure and

Table 1. Distribution of AIDS Cases in April 1985

Homosexual or bisexual men	73.6 percent
Intravenous drug users	16.9
Transfusion-associated	1.3
Heterosexual contact	0.9
Hemophiliacs	0.7
No officially designated risk group	6.6

provides some indication of the dimensions of the problem. In one study it was found that virtually all hemophiliacs examined were antibody-positive. In San Francisco 65 percent of homosexual patients attending a clinic for sexually transmissible diseases were antibody-positive in 1984. In the same year 87 percent of the intravenous drug users admitted to a detoxification program in New York were antibody-positive.[11] James Curran of the CDC has estimated that overall between 500,000 and 1 million Americans may already have been exposed to the virus.[12] It is unknown at present how many of those who are antibody-positive will actually develop full-blown AIDS. Epidemiologists suggest, however, that the figure may be as high as 5–20 percent. Summarizing the complex and uncertain data, one recent report concluded: "Given what is already known about the high and rising sero prevalence of HTLV-III in known risk groups and the potential for spread to other populations, the implications of the presence of this virus in a community are staggering."[13]

The Public Reaction

The reaction to AIDS, as well as the debate over how to resolve the pressing ethical issues that have emerged as a result of that reaction, have been indelibly affected by the unique social distribution of the disease. With more than 90 percent of reported cases coming from those of marginal social status (gay and bisexual men, intravenous drug users, Haitians), it is hardly surprising that the fears associated with a deadly disease of unknown etiology have merged with those associated with contamination from below and without.

The response of the public to AIDS was slow to take form.[14] With few exceptions, there was little media interest in the unique and troubling pattern of disease that at first seemed to affect only male homosexuals. What reporting of the nascent AIDS epidemic there was tended to focus on technical medical issues, with little concern evidenced for the impact upon the gay community. As long as AIDS was restricted to intravenous drug users, to Haitians, to homosexual and bisexual males, it seemed unworthy of broad attention. One former *New York Times* reporter, commenting on the behavior of her own news-

paper in the early years of the epidemic, stated, "I think that the story was ignored in all of its aspects for a long time because of who was being affected."[15]

Silence in the press was for the gay community an indication of prevailing homophobia. It represented an unwillingness to respond to the suffering of gays, a refusal to marshal the medical and technical resources for the tasks of discovering the causes of AIDS, of developing preventive strategies, and of providing clinical interventions that could interrupt the course of the disease. But at the same time there were those in the gay community who feared the consequence of too much public discussion of a disease that was so closely identified with male homosexuals. Might not such discussion provoke fears about a "gay plague"? Might it not provoke a backlash that would threaten the very important though modest advances made in the prior decade of efforts to advance the legal and social status of homosexuals?[16]

Fears of what form a broadened public awareness might take were in fact confirmed. As one analysis of the press coverage of AIDS has noted: For one and a half years it seemed that no one was suffering at all. Suddenly, in late 1982, the press began to warn that everyone could fall victim.[17] Discussions that glided from what was suspected about sexual contact in the spread of AIDS to references about "intimate" and then "close" contact provoked fears about the risks of contagion and of the possible spread of the disease by casual public encounters with members of high-risk groups. Reports began to appear that detailed the refusal of prison guards, undertakers, garbage collectors, and even health care workers to perform their duties with those suspected of having AIDS as well as with AIDS patients themselves.[18]

These reactions were punctuated by the extreme responses from those who sought to use the occasion of public consternation over AIDS to underscore their own antipathy to homosexuality and to what they viewed as the disastrous social consequence of greater social tolerance in sexual matters. The *Moral Majority Report*[19] featured a front-cover photograph of a family wearing surgical masks to introduce a story entitled "AIDS: Homosexual Disease Threatens American Families." Jerry Falwell demanded strong action against the homosexual carriers of AIDS: "If the Reagan administration does not put its full weight against what is now a gay plague in this country, I feel a year from now [the President] personally will be blamed [when this] awful disease breaks out among the innocent American public."[20] Invoking the image of divine retribution for sexual licentiousness, the Moral Majority leader asserted that AIDS represented a "spanking": "Herpes, AIDS, venereal disease . . . are a definite form of judgment of God upon society."[21] Patrick Buchanan, the conservative political columnist and now White House director of communications, invoked a naturalistic vision of the punishment of gays when he wrote in the *New York Post,* "The poor homosexuals—they have declared war upon Nature, and now Nature is exacting an awful retribution."[22]

In the most extreme cases, there were calls for the incarceration of homosexuals "until and unless they can be cleansed of their medical problems."[23] Even the traditionally sacrosanct public commitment to the medical treatment of the sick was not spared the assault of those who viewed AIDS as emblematic of the moral degradation of society: "What I see is a commitment to spend our tax dollars on research to allow these diseased homosexuals to go back to their perverted practices."[24] These declamations, typically though not exclusively expressed in the idiom of religious fundamentalism, were amplified by and at times fueled the broader public consternation about the threat of AIDS.

What accounts for the shift from the relative silence of the first year or so of AIDS reporting to the dramatic attention of the subsequent period? Both the rise in the number of cases and the rising mortality certainly played a role. In all of 1981, there had been 255 reported cases. There were more than that number in the first six months of 1982. In the last six months of the year there were 625 new cases—more than had been reported in the prior year and a half. But more was clearly involved. The emergence of AIDS cases among hemophiliacs dependent upon Factor VIII—the clotting agent derived from large numbers of blood donations—and the occurrence of cases among blood-transfusion recipients, and especially among infants and children, provoked a sense of dread about the spread of a deadly disease to "vulnerable" and "innocent" bystanders. In the very act of responding to the possible spread of AIDS the community expressed not only its fears about contagion but also its moral judgment. Gay males and drug users were victims, but were implicated by their own behavior, in the onset of the disease. Those in need of transfusions and Factor VIII were "innocents" who could do little to protect themselves.

Time magazine typified the sense of alarm provoked by fears of transfusion-associated cases of AIDS when it asserted that "a majority of experts believe that what was once known as the 'gay plague' will enter the general population" and that the most likely route of entry would be through blood.[25] On one widely watched television program the newscaster, Geraldo Rivera, urged that those who might be in need of transfusions "store up" their own blood.[26] Others urged a break with the important social practice of drawing appropriately matched blood products from the general public, and argued for directed donations from family and friends believed to be safe.

The debate that swirled around the necessity of developing appropriate blood practices in the face of AIDS was emblematic of those that were to emerge in the next two years over every dimension of public health policy and the response to AIDS. On the one hand, there

was a realization that the welfare of the community required the development of measures designed to inhibit spread of AIDS. On the other hand, gays and their political allies feared that incautiously crafted policies might stigmatize the homosexual community, thus adding scientific and medical fuel to the social antipathy directed at those who had so recently succeeded in making strides toward social toleration, if not integration.

In early 1983, the National Hemophilia Foundation moved to gain agreement from commercial plasma companies to ban donations from all male homosexuals. Gay leaders, aware of the symbolic significance of being excluded from the blood donor pool and fearful of the stigma that might well be associated with the charge of "bad blood," urged that efforts be made to exclude only those homosexuals who it was believed were at specially high risk—those who had engaged in sexual relations with many partners. An overriding concern was the protection of the gay community from rashly designed medical policies that would serve as a subterfuge for antihomosexual prejudice. Central to that effort was the determination that no official policy of exclusion be enunciated. Rather, gays should exercise prudence and discretion, imposing upon themselves appropriate restrictions.[27] But with increasing recognition that gays could inadvertently contaminate the blood supply, it was only a matter of time before the Public Health Service (PHS) would issue its first exclusionary recommendations. In March 1983, the PHS called upon members of all high-risk groups, including "sexually active homosexual or bisexual men with multiple partners,"[28] to refrain from blood donations. Those responsible for collecting blood were to inform all potential donors of those federal standards. These were the most liberal of what were to be an increasingly restrictive series of recommendations. Eventually, virtually all homosexual males were to be excluded from the donor pool. In its recommendations of December 1984, the PHS urged the exclusion of "all males who have had sex with more than one male since 1979, and males whose male sex partner has had sex with more than one male since 1979."[29]

Sexuality and the Fears of Medicalization

The debate over the nation's blood supply was set against the background of a far broader set of concerns within the gay community, responsive to the troubling recognition that homosexuality was once again becoming the focus of medical attention, debate, scrutiny, and policy. A central feature of the contemporary struggle for gay liberation had been a long and acrimonious debate centering on the demedicalization of homosexuality.[30] Against psychiatry, which had classed homosexuality as a disease, the homophile movement of the 1960s had sought to demonstrate that a pseudoscientific ideology had masked the moral strictures that had long dominated Western attitudes toward sexual activity among those of the same sex. Prodded by a well-organized challenge that was at once political, theoretical, and moral, the American Psychiatric Association was forced to confront its own diagnostic presuppositions. After a bitter intraprofessional encounter that entailed reconsideration of the scope of the concept "disease," America's psychiatrists yielded to gay pressures in 1973 by removing homosexuality from their official classification of mental disorders. Now, a decade later, faced by the threat of disease and death, the power of medicine was being brought into intimate contact with the gay community. The power of medicine was at once the sole hope for halting the spread of the disease that threatened to devastate the homosexual community and the specter threatening to subvert the achievements of the prior twenty years. Not only was there a risk that medical justifications would be used to reverse the public victories won as the result of great organizational efforts, but that every dimension of private sexual expression would become the target of medical scrutiny, diagnosis, and challenge.

As gays had forced psychiatry to confront itself, now medicine was compelling the gay community to examine its own behavior. Within the gay community, the epidemiological linkage that had been suggested by researchers between "fast lane" behavior and the enhanced risk for contracting AIDS forced a reflection upon the most intimate dimensions of sexual behavior. Some suggested that AIDS might be the consequence of repeated assaults on the immune system that resulted from certain sexual acts, including anal intercourse. Others argued that indiscriminate sexual contact with large numbers of anonymous partners simply enhanced the prospect of being exposed to the disease-bearing agent.

Joseph Sonnabend, a physician who cares for AIDS patients and former medical director of the AIDS Medical Foundation, has emerged as the leading advocate of the immunological-overload theory. "There is such a thing as sexual excess, though to say that sounds like some throwback to Victorian morality," he has asserted. "Put simply, I believe one of the biggest risks is to be exposed anally to semen from many different partners, especially in a large urban area where the risks of coming into contact with cytomegalovirus, which I think is a causative agent somehow, is very high." Sonnabend was especially critical of physicians who, because of political and social concerns, recoiled from the implications of these data: "Gay men have been poorly served by their doctors in the last decade. There was no clear and positive message about the dangers of promiscuity. We must admit that our desire to be nonjudgmental has interfered with our primary commitment to our patients."[31]

For many gay physicians, Sonnabend's unvarnished challenge passed beyond the bounds of appropriate clin-

ical and professional discourse. Writing in the *Journal of the American Medical Association,* Neil Schram and Dennis McShane, of the American Association of Physicians for Human Rights, asserted:

> It is important to note that terms such as *profound promiscuity,* when used by medical personnel to describe multiple sex partners, have a strong judgmental quality, and, as such, are not suitable to the scientific and medical literature. Those physicians caring for homosexual males with or without AIDS have been encouraged to be supportive of their patients. It is terms like "promiscuity" that make many homosexuals reluctant to discuss their sexual orientation with their medical care providers, even though doing so clearly improves the quality of medical care.[32]

But however the scientific issues were framed, a clear message was derived from the earliest scientific evidence. "Safe" sexual practices, sexual moderation, and caution were necessary. Lawrence Mass, a physician active in gay circles, writing in the *New York Native,* emphasized this point. While rejecting the moralistic undertones of the religious challenge to homosexual practice, he cautioned prudence upon his readers: "A major priority at this time is to discourage sexual lifestyles that involve many different, especially anonymous, partners."[33] Some gay men perceived this message as a challenge to their behavior, adopting an extremely harsh perspective on their own past activities. Others, using a hydraulic image, sought to argue that an excessive preoccupation with sexuality had poorly served their community. Michael Callen, who has AIDS, and who is an ally of Dr. Sonnabend, thus asserted: "All the great sex we've been having for the past ten years has syphoned off our collective anger that might otherwise have been translated into social and political action."[34]

The calls for restraint, for the observance of "immunological Lent," and even for monogamy, were not, however, always greeted so enthusiastically. Some viewed them as representing a thinly disguised scientific call for a return to sexual conventionality. Once again, physicians were seeking to establish their dominance over homosexuality, a dominance that so recently had been discarded. Writing in the *Body Politic,* a Canadian gay journal, Michael Lynch stated: "Gays are once again allowing the medical profession to define, restrict, pathologize us." To follow the advice of physicians would involve renunciation of "the power to determine our own identity," and would represent "a communal betrayal of gargantuan proportions" of gay liberation founded upon a "sexual brotherhood of promiscuity."[35] Doubting the scientific validity of the data on the basis of which the cautionary advice was being proferred, another wrote, "I feel that what we are being advised to do involves all of the things

I became gay to get away from. . . . So we have a disease for which supposedly the cure is to go back to all the styles that were preached at us in the first place. It will take a lot more evidence before I'm about to do that."[36] In a particularly vitriolic attack upon Jonathan Lieberson's essay on AIDS that appeared in the *New York Review of Books*, John Rechy wrote, "How eagerly do even *perhaps* 'good heterosexuals' impose grim sentences of abstinence on others."[37]

Bathhouses and Quarantine: The Fears of State Power

While the encounter with medicine over sexual behavior centered on how its cultural authority could affect the personal and private choices of gay men, the controversy surrounding the operation of gay bathhouses focused on medicine's interaction with government. Here the possibility that medical and epidemiological evidence might be used by the public health authorities as a justification for imposing the power of the state in the effort to interrupt the spread of AIDS was central. The gay bathhouse has emerged as a powerful symbol of the struggle for greater social toleration for homosexuality. The existence of such establishments reflects not only the willingness of certain cities to tolerate the flourishing of gay social institutions but the willingness to accept the existence of commercial establishments in which homosexual activity occurs. It is therefore not surprising that suggestions that these centers be closed would provoke an enormous political controversy.

For those who have advocated the closing of the baths the logic has been rather straightforward. Since the bathhouse exists to facilitate sexual encounters among strangers, any public health strategy committed to prophylaxis requires that it be eliminated. For civil libertarians, efforts to move in such a direction represented potential infringement on privacy and on the right of individuals to congregate. Some gay leaders, though by no means all, feared that the baths would be the first target of those committed to an assault on the communal institutions of the gay world. Shrouded in the mantle of medicine, protected from scrutiny by the ideology of public health, such an attack, some have believed, would ultimately extend to gay bars, businesses, and the employment possibilities of homosexual men.[38] Given this perspective, it is not surprising that at least on one occasion outrage took the form of a hyperbolic comparison between efforts to close the baths and the Nazi assault on Jewish cultural institutions.[39]

Not all public health officials have supported bathhouse closure. Their arguments have been moral and political as much as they have been medical. Dr. David Sencer, the commissioner of health in New York City, thus

opposed Dr. Mervyn Silverman of San Francisco, who had sought to close his city's baths,[40] stating:

I can see no reason why we would close the bathhouses. I don't think that changing the habitat is necessarily going to change the behavior. There are other places people can go and have indiscriminate sexual relations if they want to. To try to legislate change in lifestyle has never been effective. Public education through the routes of organized groups who are at risk is the most important thing.[41]

Others within and outside the gay community have seen the refusal or the inability of public health officials to close the baths as a capitulation in the face of irresponsible political pressure. The community's interests were thus sacrificed in an effort to appease those who did not understand the critical importance of removing the aura of public toleration from establishments that so unmistakably symbolized anonymous sexual activity. In an interview published in *San Francisco Magazine*, an AIDS patient thus said: "I was at a friend's house, a doctor, and he was just furious that they were thinking about closing the baths—that it was taking away gay rights. Well, you know, when there are hundreds of lives involved, gay rights go right out the window, as far as I am concerned."[42]

While the debate over the baths captured public attention, a far more critical matter regarding the relationship between medical and state authority was being considered—quarantine. Once a central feature of the public health response to contagious disease, the isolation of individuals during the infectious period of illness had fallen into desuetude. Now with AIDS perceived as a threat to the public health, the legitimacy of quarantine received renewed attention. But unlike earlier discussions of this extreme measure that centered on matters of necessity and efficacy, the debate now took on an essentially political character. Given the vulnerable social status of the population at risk and the contemporary anxiety in liberal public health circles about the potential abuses of state authority, the debate could not have been different.

When, if ever, would it be appropriate to consider the isolation of those with AIDS to prevent the spread of the disease? Would a refusal to desist from sexual activity on the part of an individual who had AIDS warrant state intervention? Should prostitutes with AIDS be held in custody to prevent them from contaminating those with whom they might engage in sexual contact? Should women with AIDS be permitted to have children?

Like the bathhouse controversy, the quarantine debate took on its most salient form in California. In December 1983, James Chin, chief of the infectious disease section of the California Department of Health, proposed a course of action designed to provide control over the "recalcitrant" AIDS patient.[43] "Modified isolation" would be invoked if such an individual, after due warning, refused to abstain from sexual activities, which "could transmit a possible AIDS agent to sexual contacts who were unaware that he had AIDS." If such efforts failed to produce compliance with the behavior deemed medically necessary by the authorities, they would be permitted to proceed with the quarantine of the patient's residence by "posting a placard at his residence which indicates that a person with a communicable disease which can be spread by intimate contact resides in the household." Though California did not proceed with this proposal, Dr. Chin's office was informed that statutory authority already existed to charge with a misdemeanor any individual with an infectious disease who willfully exposed another person. Since special authorization was thus unnecessary to control "recalcitrant" AIDS patients, only a symbolic provocative public health gesture would have been involved in forcing the issue of quarantine.

Connecticut did adopt a quarantine statute that could include those with AIDS. That move resulted in expressions of outrage from those who viewed it as an unwarranted medicopolitical threat against both civil liberties and the rights of gay men.

The executive director of the Connecticut Civil Liberties Union asserted that the new statute would permit the state to "sweep a person off the streets on mere suspicion."[44] Dr. Alvin Novick, who has been active in gay medical circles, stated:

Quarantine is such a devastating blow to someone's life. If it were invoked for someone with AIDS, it would forever after deprive them of jobs . . . social life. It would be used as a statement of official oppression that is not unknown in our society, but that today is hardly tolerable. People in public health are not precluded from being ignorant or evil, and there are people in public health who are evil and ignorant.[45]

Epidemiology and the Threat to Privacy

That the debate over bathhouse closure and quarantine would have directly engaged gay political leaders is not surprising. More unusual has been their close and watchful involvement in the conduct of public and private research into the etiology, course, and epidemiology of AIDS. Fear of being labeled, of being incarcerated, and of being deprived of access to employment and insurance has marked the ongoing conflict between the representatives of the gay community concerned with privacy and researchers who have asserted that the public health requires the conduct of epidemiological studies based upon the most intimate details about AIDS patients' lives

and identities. The conflict arose early as the Centers for Disease Control sought the names of AIDS patients reported to public health authorities throughout the country. Recognizing the critical importance of longitudinal studies to a broad research program, gay leaders were nevertheless fearful that providing federal health officials with such data would create the circumstances for the deprivation of the civil rights of gay men, intravenous drug users, and undocumented aliens. For them, the technical requirements of research had to be viewed within a broad political and ethical context.

How much did federal researchers need to know? Could codes be substituted for names? Were codes inviolable? Could the CDC's professional scientists be trusted to protect the confidentiality of their data? What were the links between public health researchers and public health enforcers? These were the questions that proved so troublesome.

Doubts about the capacity or willingness of federal researchers to protect the privacy interests of AIDS patients came from many sources. The commissioner of health in the District of Columbia thus stated:

I wouldn't trust the CDC one moment not to give up information to the FBI, the CIA, or the Social Security Administration. The CDC is a federal agency. You and I both know that federal agencies do exchange information, and they will always do that on what they understand to be an appropriate need-to-know basis. And they will not consider that a breach of confidentiality.[46]

Virginia Apuzzo, executive director of the National Gay Task Force, underscored the social context of the confidentiality debate:

In this country we [gays] are illegal in half of the states. We can't serve in the armed forces, we can't raise our own kids in many states, and we sure as hell can't teach other people's kids. When you tell us you're interested in our social security numbers, when we know we are not permitted to have security clearance, we would . . . be naive, at best, not to ask "What will you do with the information? Can we trust you enough?"[47]

The dilemma posed for gay leaders was pinpointed by Jeff Levi of the National Gay Task Force: "We could not be more interested in the gathering of accurate information about AIDS, but we also firmly believe that reporting mechanisms must guarantee confidentiality."[48]

While some believed that no tension existed between the imposition of ironclad protections and the conduct of epidemiological research, others felt it imperative to note that, while it was possible to strike a compromise position, all such efforts involved trade-offs in the speed and ease with which data could be gathered and subjected to analysis. The *New York Native,* a gay newspaper, soberly observed:

> Confidentiality and epidemiology may not be as mutually compatible as some gay leaders would have us think. Confidentiality and epidemiology are matters of tense negotiation, not marriage. We are in a gray area in which abuses on both sides could occur. On the one hand, someone could illegally obtain a list of people with AIDS and try to create havoc. On the other hand, some well-intentioned gay leaders who think that AIDS is primarily a civil liberties issue may be endangering research.[49]

In a remarkable and quite unusual process, representatives of gay organizations entered into a complex set of negotiations over the nature of the confidentiality protections that were to be afforded to AIDS research subjects. Out of this process of negotiation and confrontation, compromises were fashioned for the protection of confidentiality. While some have asserted that the interests of public health have been sacrificed, others have acknowledged that the volatile setting of AIDS research required such adjustments. A refusal to yield would have produced inadequate or inaccurate reporting. James Allen of the CDC thus noted, "It clearly is a compromise position, which will make it more difficult to do our work. But if we are not getting reports, we can't do it either."[50]

The issue of confidentiality and of potential risks to the subjects of AIDS research surfaced in a particularly focused form in 1984, as efforts to create a test for the presence of the antibody to HTLV-III were moving to success. Developed primarily to screen blood donations in order to limit the still-troubling problem of the transfusion-associated cases of AIDS, the antibody test was also viewed as providing an important source of data for researchers seeking to determine the extent to which those exposed to the HTLV-III virus actually developed full-blown cases of AIDS. Because it was feared that the results of the tests would not be protected from scrutiny of private insurers, law enforcement officials, and employers, and because it was assumed that the test would serve as a surrogate marker for homosexuality, an extraordinary effort was mounted by gay leaders to discourage individuals from being tested by private practitioners.[51] More significantly, they called upon members of the gay community to refuse participation in crucial research studies unless the guarantees of confidentiality were made more explicit.[52] Thus Nancy Langer of the Lambda Legal Defense Fund stated, "We don't want to be a roadblock to government research into AIDS; indeed, the opposite is true. But we don't want research to boomerang and

become *the* major threat to the rights of gays and lesbians in this decade."[53] Once again, compromise and negotiation of an unprecedented kind resulted in additional protections for those who would be the subjects of research.

Research, Medical Care, and the Fears of Neglect

Despite the enormous consternation generated by the threat of the abuse of medical authority, those who have been most active in the medical politics surrounding AIDS have consistently and forcefully challenged the federal government, state officials, and the scientific community to increase drastically the resources available for research into the disease. A sense of despair has imbued the repeated calls for an enhanced research commitment and the critique of what has been done thus far. For gay leaders the "torpid" federal[54] response to AIDS was but another indication of a homophobia that discounted the lives and suffering of homosexuals.

Government officials, including the secretary of health and human services, have repeatedly asserted that research into AIDS has been given the highest priority. Gay leaders and their political allies within the scientific bureaucracies have viewed these assertions as cynical efforts to mask an unwillingness to treat AIDS as a true crisis. Dr. Donald Francis, CDC's AIDS coordinator for laboratory resources, thus wrote in April 1983: "The time wasted pursuing money from Washington . . . has sandwiched those responsible for research and control between mass pressure to do what is right and an unmovable wall of inadequate resources . . . our government's response to this disaster has been far too little."[55] This personal observation was buttressed in the same year by a report of the Committee on Government Operations of the House of Representatives. In "The Federal Response to AIDS,"[56] the Committee charged that inadequate funding had hampered Public Health Service efforts to "fight the AIDS epidemic." Two years later the Office of Technology Assessment found a similar pattern of inadequate funding, noting in addition that administration requests had been consistently below the levels deemed necessary by the Congress.[57]

The irony of being dependent upon more research into AIDS, while dreading the potential social consequences of efficiently organized and well-funded undertakings, was never really lost from view. Dennis Altman, a perceptive and trenchant analyst of gay politics, thus noted: "The very research demanded by the gay movement mean[t] greater surveillance and possible controls over us."[58]

Not only was this irony manifested in the discussions of research, however. The enormous costs generated by the medical care of AIDS patients (about $150,000 per patient from the moment of diagnosis) has provoked fears that those who were the victims of this illness would become the victims of neglect as well. For years gays had struggled to protect themselves against the ministrations of physicians who had defined their sexuality as pathological; now they feared that their pathologies would be ignored because they were homosexual.

Because health insurance in the United States is typically linked to employment, those who are chronically or even temporarily unemployed often find themselves without protection. Those who are so unprotected are sometimes treated as charity cases, more often by public hospitals. Studies of the health care system make it clear, however, that a lack of insurance coverage results in great hardships for those in need of care. Since patients with AIDS, especially in its advanced stages, cannot work, they often confront economic difficulties when seeking access to the health care system, especially when outpatient care is involved.

Concerned about the personal financial burden of needed medical attention and about the willingness of government to provide the resources for such care, gay leaders have been forced to confront the inequities of the American health system. Some have attempted to construe the problem narrowly by suggesting that federally underwritten categorical programs be expanded to protect AIDS patients. Others have argued that the problems faced by those with AIDS simply underscore the necessity of a more far-reaching reform of the American health care system: "The real point is that access to health care in the United States is not equally distributed. The poor, the nonwhite, the old, also die of neglect."[59]

AIDS thus forced a confrontation with the most basic question of justice and the health care system.

Hope and Fear

In October 1984, New York's gay newspaper, *The Native*, published two editorials, the juxtaposition of which exquisitely exhibits the tensions posed for those desperate to bring an end to AIDS as they confront both the promise and specter of medicine.[60] The first editorial, entitled "What Curran Should Do," was a denunciation of the inadequate funding of research into AIDS: "The time has come for [James] Curran [head of CDC's AIDS task force] to commit the bravest, most powerful act of his career: to call a press conference on the steps of Congress and announce that he is considering resignation because he will no longer be the front man for an ineffective, often homophobic public health response to a national emergency." The second editorial, "Don't Take This Test," was a warning to gays about the risks that would attend the availability of the antibody test for HTLV-III: "Will test

results be used to identify the sexual orientation of millions of Americans? Will a list of names be made? How can such information be kept truly confidential? Who will be able to keep the list out of the hands of insurance companies, employers, landlords, and the government itself?"

Spurred by the hopes evoked by medicine's power and by the fears about how that power might be used, the gay community has sparked an important debate that will test the capacity of American society to respond effectively and humanely to an unfolding tragedy. To this point the confluence of political and social forces that has emerged in the public encounter with AIDS has permitted a sympathetic hearing of the moral concerns that have been central to bioethics. Whether the social crisis that will be created if the spread of AIDS continues unabated will provide so hospitable a setting for those liberal values within which privacy and voluntarism are so important is far from certain.

References

1. Thomas Szasz, *The Myth of Mental Illness,* rev. ed. (New York: Harper & Row, 1974).
2. Ivan Illich, *Medical Nemesis* (New York: Pantheon Books, 1975).
3. See, for example, Henry Beecher, "Consent in Clinical Experimentation—Myth and Reality," *Journal of the American Medical Association,* Jan. 3, 1966, pp. 124–125.
4. U.S. Department of Health and Human Services, *Morbidity and Mortality Weekly Reports (MMWR),* June 5, 1981.
5. *MMWR,* July 3, 1981.
6. *MMWR,* July 16, 1982.
7. *MMWR,* Dec. 10, 1982.
8. Telephone interview, Centers for Disease Control.
9. "Perspectives on the Future of AIDS," *Journal of the American Medical Association,* Jan. 11, 1985, p. 247.
10. For discussions of the debate over whether Haitians should constitute a special risk group, a debate in which Haitians had argued that such a designation represented a scientifically unwarranted stigmatization, see the *New York Times,* July 29, 1983, and the *Los Angeles Times,* Sept. 5, 1983.
11. Sheldon Landesman, Harold Ginzburg, Stanley Weiss, "The AIDS Epidemic," *New England Journal of Medicine,* Feb. 21, 1985, p. 521.
12. J. Silberner, "AIDS: Disease, Research Efforts Advance," *Science News,* Apr. 27, 1985, p. 260.
13. Landesman, Ginzburg, Weiss, "The AIDS Epidemic," p. 522.
14. Harry Schwartz, Appendix to *Science in the Streets,* Report to the Twentieth Century Fund Task Force on the Communication of the Scientific Risk, 1984.
15. Julius Genachowski, "Press Covering AIDS," *Broadway,* Sept. 15, 1983, p. 11.
16. See, in general, Dennis Altman, "The Politicization of an Epidemic," *Socialist Review,* November/December 1984.
17. Genachowski, "Press Covering AIDS."

18. See, for example, "Morticians Balk at AIDS Victims," *Washington Post,* June 18, 1983.
19. *Moral Majority Report,* July 1983.
20. *Washington Post,* July 6, 1983.
21. *Ibid.*
22. *New York Post,* May 24, 1983.
23. *New York Times,* Aug. 7, 1983.
24. Cited in Genachowski, "Press Covering AIDS," p. 14.
25. *Time,* Mar. 28, 1983.
26. *Newsweek,* July 4, 1983, p. 21.
27. Discussed in Ronald Bayer, "Gays and the Stigma of Bad Blood," *Hastings Center Report,* April 1983, pp. 5–7.
28. U.S. Department of Health and Human Services, Memorandum from the Director, Office of Biologics, National Center for Drugs and Biologics, "Recommendations to Decrease the Risk of Transmitting Acquired Immune Deficiency Syndrome from Plasma Donors," Mar. 24, 1983.
29. U.S. Department of Health and Human Services, Memorandum from Acting Director, Office of Biologics Research and Review, "Research Recommendations to Decrease the Risk of Transmitting an Immunodeficiency Syndrome (AIDS) from Blood and Plasma Donors," Dec. 14, 1984.
30. Ronald Bayer, *Homosexuality and American Psychiatry: The Politics of Diagnosis* (New York: Basic Books, 1981).
31. *American Medical News,* Jan. 20, 1984, p. 3.
32. *Journal of the American Medical Association,* Jan. 20, 1984, p. 341.
33. Lawrence Mass, "The Case Against Medical Panic," *New York Native,* Jan. 17–30, 1983, p. 23.
34. Jonathan Lieberson, "Anatomy of an Epidemic," *New York Review of Books,* Aug. 18, 1983, p. 20.
35. *Ibid,* p. 19.
36. *Ibid,* p. 22.
37. John Rechy, Letter to the *New York Review of Books,* Oct. 13, 1983, p. 43.
38. Kenneth W. Payne and Stephen J. Risch, "The Politics of AIDS," *Science for the People,* September/October 1984, p. 23.
39. Charles Krauthammer, "The Politics of a Plague," *The New Republic,* Aug. 1, 1983, p. 19.
40. David Black, "The Plague Years," *Rolling Stone,* Apr. 25, 1985, p. 44.
41. Lieberson, "Anatomy of an Epidemic," p. 21.
42. Frank Cron, "Conversation with a Victim," *San Francisco Magazine,* April 1985, p. 66.
43. "AIDS—A New Reason to Regulate Homosexuality," *Journal of Contemporary Law,* 1984, pp. 340–341.
44. Black, "The Plague Years," p. 60.
45. *Ibid.*
46. *Washington Post,* July 18, 1983, p. 4.
47. *Washington Post,* July 18, 1983.
48. "'Confidentiality' Issue May Cloud Epidemologic Studies of AIDS," *Journal of the American Medical Association,* Oct. 21, 1983, p. 1945.
49. *New York Native,* Nov. 7–20, 1983.
50. *Washington Post,* July 18, 1983.
51. *New York Times,* Oct. 12, 1984.
52. "Why You Should Not Be Tested for HTLV-III," *New York Native,* Oct. 8–21, 1984.
53. "Consent Form for AIDS Research Urged on Brandt," *The Advocate,* Oct. 16, 1984.
54. Lieberson, "Anatomy of an Epidemic," p. 18.
55. Judith Randal, "Too Little for AIDS," *Technology Review,* August/September 1984, p. 10.
56. U.S. House of Representatives, Committee on Government Operations, "The Federal Response to AIDS," Nov. 30, 1983.
57. U.S. Congress, Office of Technology Assessment, *Review of the Public Health Services' Response to AIDS: A Technical Memorandum* (Washington, D.C., February 1985).
58. Altman, "Politicization of an Epidemic," p. 107.
59. *Ibid.,* p. 108.
60. *New York Native,* Oct. 8, 1984.

Chapter 14

Death and Access:
Ethics in Cross-Cultural Health Care

Kate Brown, Ph.D.

Kate Brown, Ph.D., is the assistant director for the Center for Health Policy and Ethics at Creighton University in Omaha, Nebraska.

Hard choices are the dark side of new medical technologies. These technologies present new options for responding to the age-old stuff of medicine: birth, illness, suffering, and death. Now, for instance, amniocentesis can reveal features about a fetus early in a pregnancy. A pregnant woman can decide whether to carry to term or abort a fetus, depending on the results of this test. Arguments can be made for either option, but is one choice best? Who will decide? What if the significant test result is the sex of the fetus? What if the test shows a profound genetic problem? Should such findings provide the basis for decisions?

The exponential rate and success of technological innovation in health care over the past 30 years have exploded the range of potential care options and increased the complexity of questions facing us all. Furthermore, there has been an expansion in the number of opinions that seem reasonable to consider in the debates surrounding the use of these new technologies. The voices of practitioners, ethicists, lawyers, patients, and administrators are all heard in the din. Even full-time advocates with no relation to patients make it their business to express opinions regarding patient care. But any journal, newspaper, or talk show reveals that there is little consensus about what is the "right thing" to do in response to given and future options in medical care.

Whom should we listen to? What are their reasons? Is there a "really" right answer? Are we to accept a cacophony of disparate voices or should we look for consensus? I propose that these voices are not just individual opinions but expressions of different cultural values, meanings, expectations, and standards of judgment through which we see and make sense of medical events. This position raises additional questions: Should each cultural group do its own thing, or is it okay to impose a dominant position on everyone? What are good cultural reasons? Who decides?

The United States is a nation of many cultures, and consequently there are many different opinions about what is ethical in health care. Thus it is necessary for health care professionals to develop a sympathetic appreciation of the cultural "rationality" supporting these differences and in so doing become more sensitive to the influence culture plays in the construction of their own moral choices. Such sensitivity and critical self-reflection can go a long way toward teasing out solutions to the interpersonal and institutional challenges facing professionals who work in cross-cultural clinical settings.

Culture and Ethics

Using an anthropological definition of culture, it is possible to view just about every medical interchange as cross-cultural to some extent. This is because culture, in this technical sense, refers to more than its usual association with ethnic identity. Culture forms around other affinities as well, such as national heritage, occupation, political persuasion, religion, or neighborhood. The attributes of social class, sex, and even age give rise to different cultural frameworks (as any middle-aged person who lives with a teenager knows). Certainly anyone in health care can recognize identifiable physician and nursing cultures.[1]

Culture refers to the shared ideas, meanings, and assumptions that shape what human groups believe reality to be. Our relationships to ourselves, each other, the environment, and the supernatural world make sense because of the influence of culture in our lives. Culture informs our notions of what is right or wrong medical practice; it gives meaning to illness and suffering; culture even defines what is life and death. Culture delimits the nature of our selves, our capacities, our biologies, our desires, and our relationships to others—and all of this has bearing on what we consider to be appropriate and ethical in the context of health care. Less abstractly, it is culture that leads us, for instance, to choose a physician instead of a shaman for the relief of pain. Similarly, it is culture that allows some of us to expect that a terminal prognosis will be withheld from a patient, that a fetus will be granted the status and privilege of a person, or that no technological effort will be spared in the prolongation of a patient's life. Your agreement or disagreement with these expectations is most likely a product of your own culture and thus serves to demonstrate the concept.

Cultural frameworks can crosscut in an individual. Thus, it would not be altogether surprising to find that the world view of a Western-trained Vietnamese physician was more like that of a U.S.-born physician than of a fellow refugee who had been a farmer in Vietnam. Furthermore, it is important to distinguish the influence of culture from idiosyncratic differences in opinion; culture is shared by and taught to members of a group, however loosely identified. Thus, in this discussion of culture and ethics, we would be less interested in, say, a Vietnamese physician's personal fear of death than in his or her orientation toward a "technological imperative"[2] derived from medical training. Also, it must be remembered that culture refers to a *tendency* in shared behavior, thought, feeling, or mores; it is not necessarily predictive for any one individual or a permanent absolute in its expression. Often, as we will see in the discussion of the allocation of medical resources in the United States, values can compete and some can prevail over others when put into actual practice.

No one culture expresses universal "truth"; there are many cultural truths. The three examples mentioned above can illustrate this point: the members of some cultures may abhor the practice of telling patients that they will die, whereas such disclosure may be "normal" in another culture; one cultural group might believe that a fetus is a person only after birth, or even after several days following birth, whereas another cultural belief might assume that personhood begins at the moment of conception; one cultural framework can easily justify what another might define as euthanasia. Evidence, rational argument, and other forms of persuasion can be brought to defend a cultural truth or its converse.

The term *ethical relativism* refers to the idea that, as cultural products, ethics are derived from and reflect different cultural contexts. This means that prohibitions and advice about what is or is not to be approved, rewarded, desired, or considered virtuous and right will vary according to the cultural framework in which they cohere. These rules and value judgments are taught and reinforced through rewards and punishments that have value within a cultural context. It is conceivable that even what is considered within the domain of ethical inquiry may vary from culture to culture. For instance, members of one culture may consider giving gifts to health practitioners to be an ethical problem, whereas people in another culture would see this as "natural," expected, and kind. If many people around you are doing something that has been done this way for years, and not doing it will bring moral censure, it will probably make cultural sense for you to do it, too.

Ethical relativism is troubling because it leaves little basis for judging something to be wrong or harmful if it is to be considered only in the context in which it "makes sense." If we are to be hindered from judging another culture on the basis of our own culturally informed ethics, then would we have to stop short of criticizing the dehumanization required for Nazi experimentation on Jews during World War II? I would hope not. Furthermore, ethical relativism has been criticized because of its use in justifying support for a status quo that serves only the interests of those in power. For example, a policy of relativism toward indigenous social structures may well have served French colonial interests by condoning the continuation of "traditional" subordination of groups of people.

On the other hand, much damage has been done to the integrity and health of entire populations when, in the name of moral righteousness, the ethical framework of one culture has been used to dominate, intimidate, or regulate the behavior and values of another group. For instance, this kind of ethical imperialism has influenced birth control campaigns: both the withholding of contraceptive information and devices and—at the other extreme—the wholesale sterilization of women, each with a detrimental effect.

In this chapter I discuss a number of different cultural practices and beliefs found in the United States and abroad as they bear upon clinical decisions about death and policy debates about medical resources. A relativistic stance is taken until the conclusion, where I discuss the limits and merits of such an approach in the context of medical care in the United States. There I return to such questions as: Whose reasoning should decide the "best" course of action? Is ethical consensus desirable, or even possible, at the bedside or in the policy agenda? Inevitably these questions pivot on issues of power as well as morality and so pose important and complex problems. First let us examine some of the ways in which culture gives meaning to quite divergent responses to death in clinical settings.

Death

New technologies that can detect, measure, and prolong life have confounded old truths about death in the United States. Respirators can now continue the body's capacity to breathe and defibrillators can shock a recalcitrant heart into beating again, thus obscuring traditional indicators of death. What then defines death in this age of technological assists? Pernick's historical review of the controversy over defining and diagnosing death makes it abundantly clear that we are far from close to an "objective" definition of death in the United States.[3] The technologies we use to assess brain death, for instance, can provide measurable data that are correlated to a physical phenomenon, but the meaning of these data is subject to different interpretation, much of it based in culture. The trail of court cases, special commissions, and publications that have dealt with the question of how to tell whether someone is dead provides eloquent testimony to the wide range of possible meanings given to these objective data about death.[4] Zaner asserts that the criteria for determining death must first be culturally based in the conceptions of personhood or personal identity and that the United States has failed to reach consensus in this regard.[5] In culturally pluralistic countries such as the United States, it may be impossible to reach agreement about such fundamental cultural ideas.

Lock and Honde contrast the scientific attempts to define death in the United States with the experience of the relatively homogeneous nation of Japan in order to explain the lack of acceptance of organ transplantation in that country. These authors identify several factors that have contributed to what they term the "cultural construction of death"[6] in Japan and the United States. Many people in the United States would agree that the personal expression of self is dependent on brain function. However, in Japan it is much harder to find an expression of the person outside of the social context, much less isolated in a body organ. The researchers do identify " 'kokoro,' located somewhere in the chest or thorax,"[7] which is believed in Japan to be associated with what is most unique about an individual. This difference in belief about which organ best reflects personhood might explain why heartbeat is a more accepted indicator of death than brain wave in Japan and why brain death has more likelihood of acceptance in the United States than in Japan.

Definition of death becomes crucial in organ transplantation because (both in the United States and Japan) what has been called "harvesting," the taking of organs, would be called murder if the liver or heart donor is considered to be alive. Many Japanese believe that the spirits of their dead relatives continue to interact with the living; spirits can influence the living and vice versa. Therefore, ritual observances can influence the dead. Lock and Honde report that Japanese ancestor beliefs dictate that "a corpse should be complete (gotai manzoku) otherwise the spirit will suffer and is potentially able to cause bad luck for the living."[8] The authors report that respect for this belief is widespread even among Japanese who are not religious.

The meaning of death varies cross-culturally and will justify different decisions about treatment of the dying. Lock and Honde argue that attempts to modernize definitions of death in the United States through "the establishment of universal, scientific criteria"[9] are reflections of medical practitioners' emotional discomfort with death. The tremendous sense of responsibility felt by practitioners who believe that death is the end of a person or that death is a "technical failure"[10] leads them to seek certainty in what Kundstader calls the "technocratic culture of practitioners." He is referring to the dominant influence technology has had in shaping the ideology, socialization, and organization of Western medical practice.[11] Within this cultural framework it makes sense that technological imperatives and measurable responses are sought to provide safe haven in storms of emotional and legal uncertainties. Within a different cultural system of belief, other factors are more compelling. For instance, Lock and Honde explain that despite the acceptance of eternal life for ancestors, many Japanese physicians may feel ambivalence about their decisions to terminate life-support technologies (even when pain killers have been used to accelerate the process of dying) because of the Buddhist prohibition against killing. Similarly, within the United States, compelling values come out of religious cultures. For example, I have observed that some members of an ethics committee in a Catholic hospital will speak as much from their religious beliefs as their medical training when making recommendations about withdrawing life supports.

Because ethics is embedded in cultural traditions and circumstances, it is not surprising that different arguments for terminating treatment are salient in different cultural settings. Illustrating this point further, Lieban has contrasted decisions about terminating treatment for infants in Israel and Sri Lanka, using studies by Eidelman[12] and Subramanian.[13] Factors such as "religious beliefs about the sanctity of life, the experience of the Holocaust . . ., government spending (priorities) . . ., and concern of Jews that they will be outnumbered by the increasing Arab population"[14] all seem to figure in Israeli practitioners' decisions. In Sri Lanka, it seems that the ability of a family to pay for treatment and aftercare is a stronger determinant of treatment for infants. These "quality of life" considerations in Sri Lanka are supported by the Hindu cultural belief in rebirth.

Prakash Desai explains that in India, also, Hindu clinicians and patients may believe that "death is not the opposite of life — it is the opposite of birth"[15] and that death is a passage to another, possibly better life. However, this does not mean that Indian clinicians are likely to hurry someone along to that new life. Actually, in India there is a strong prohibition against telling dying patients of their prognoses for fear that this may cause demoralization and bring death prematurely. Desai writes, "The impending death is not explicitly pronounced because words have power, the naming of death may invite death quickly."[16]

The belief that speaking of death can hasten it influences medical practice in many places around the world. Full and frank disclosure of a terminal prognosis by clinicians is a relatively recent development even in the United States,[17] and certainly it is not the predominant practice worldwide. Problems can arise when patients, families, and clinical staff do not share expectations for how to talk about such matters. Meleis and Jonsen's discussion of a case of miscommunication between the family of an Egyptian patient and the staff of a hospital in the United States illustrates the potential for problems when cultural expectations collide. The patient, diagnosed with Hodgkin's disease, choked on some soup the day after his admission; he suffered five to seven minutes of anoxia before a tracheotomy tube was placed. The authors detail a subsequent series of tragic misunderstandings that crescendoed in one horrible incident of mutual distrust when the staff conscientiously gave news of the patient's irreversible brain damage and imminent death. The family's reaction was stunning: they set up a full-time guard rotation to protect their relative from what they believed to be the murderous intentions of his health care providers.[18]

This case also serves to illustrate another potential cultural difference in our range of ethical responses to death, namely, the role of the family and community in death. Folk expressions such as "just as we come into the world alone, we will die alone," and folk songs with lines such as "that long, lonesome highway that I'll travel all by myself" key us into how the predominant view of person-as-individual figures in death in the United States. In this conception, each person is regarded as his or her own person, existentially separated from others throughout life, and most symbolically at its beginning and end. This belief holds firm even though in actual fact most births and deaths are attended and interpreted by numerous others in varying social roles, including (at minimum) relatives and medical personnel. Signed consents that permit ordering that medical personnel do not resuscitate and the new "advance directives" regarding the termination of life supports are bureaucratic responses derived from this cultural celebration of the autonomous person. In the dominant culture of the United States it makes perfect sense to act on the expressed wishes of the individual who will be most affected by medical decisions at the end of life, that is, the patient. It seems ridiculous, immoral, and even suspicious to constrain an individual's choice in such a matter.

However, it should not surprise the reader to learn that people from more communitarian cultures might find this a strange and lonely picture of death and far from what they feel is an appropriate description of their feelings, expectations, or observations. The legalistic or moral conundrums that surround the use of "proxies" and "substituted judgment" in health care institutions here[19] would not have meaning in much of the world and in marginalized cultural groups in this country (for example, African-Americans, rural farm residents[20]), in which more emphasis is given to the network of social relations that make up the community, whether that be the extended family, village, or nation. Within the framework of these more communitarian cultures, a person is more likely to be defined as a part of a group, not as separate from that group, and, ideally, one's fate is negotiated through a network of relations held together with mutual obligations. More often than not, patients in these more communitarian cultures might not even be aware of the medical decisions that were being made on their behalf by those who would "naturally" be expected to bear such responsibilities. For example, in the People's Republic of China members of a patient's family, representatives from the patient's work unit, and the hospital staff meet to decide the progress of dying patients. The absence of the patients themselves from such discussions is not remarkable; on the contrary, their presence would be.[21]

The possibility of different interpretations for family responsibility at the time of death was poignantly illustrated by a conversation I had once with a Chinese-American medical student. In class, the lecturer had defended his strong reaction against "mercy killing." His arguments pivoted on the Western moral claim that individuals have intrinsic worth and thus physicians have a professional and legal obligation to not harm individual patients.

Afterward, the student approached me about his confusion with such a position. He explained that his mother had asked him explicitly, as oldest son, to use his medical knowledge if she ever became a "vegetable" so that she would die swiftly and painlessly.[22] Although he could understand the moral arguments about individual worth that supported the lecturer's position, he also knew that he would have to respect his mother's wishes, not in support of her autonomy, but to comply with his filial duties. These duties, he said, would take precedence over the possibility of a murder arrest or the loss of his medical license. Furthermore, he feared that if he did *not* thus respect his mother's request, his relatives would think less of him for bringing shame to the whole family. His connection to these significant family relationships was still more important to him than his relationships with his peers and what he was learning of the profession's value system.

As these examples suggest, cultural frameworks create, support, and influence the definition of death, the meaning of death, decisions about when to terminate treatment for a dying patient, rules for disclosure of terminal prognoses, and expectations about who should be involved in decisions concerning a patient's death. I do not believe that these cultural differences necessarily mean that one group cares more or less for the dying; rather, they mean that we tend to express our care for these patients in different ways.

Allocation of Health Care Resources

Cultural values also influence health policy, including the reasoning behind decisions about who will receive health and medical care. In this section I explore some of the beliefs and practices that influence the ways in which health and medical resources are distributed in different cultural contexts, in the United States and abroad. Generally, these resources are in real or perceived short supply,[23] making necessary some kind of judgment about how to distribute them among those in need. In a system of scarcity, not everyone can receive all that medical science has to offer; thus, culture provides the rationale for deciding who can and who should receive these scarce benefits. The criteria and reasoning for selection prioritize certain qualities above others and are thus subject to ethical inquiry. What is interesting from a cross-cultural perspective is the wide variation in which priorities are acceptable and why.

Take India for instance. This year's census in India again reports that there are fewer women than men in the population. Many Indians believe that boys are of more value than girls.[24] This culturally informed gender difference translates into the observation that girls are more likely to fare poorly in terms of their nutrition and health care, and thus in morbidity and mortality.[25] Similar patterns have been observed in Bangladesh by Koenig and D'Souza. They noticed that a strong cultural advantage for boys begins early, when families decide whether food will be purchased to supplement breastfeeding and whether to seek medical care if the child becomes ill. When breastfeeding can no longer provide the nutrients necessary for growth, girls who are not receiving food supplements are likely to fall into a downward spiral of poor health, limited access to medical care, and possibly

death.[26] Fox reports a case that reflects a similar gender bias in China. The parents of a girl in acute renal failure refused dialysis; Fox was later told that these parents would have probably agreed to therapy had the child been a son.[27]

As Lieban explains, such bias makes sense in these cultural frameworks, where economic and spiritual traditions reinforce such practices. In India, Bangladesh, and China the productive labor of sons provides security to aging parents, whereas daughters traditionally marry into other families and leave their parents. These filial obligations are supported by the belief that family ancestors are linked to the future "line" of progeny through sons, not daughters.[28] Boys and girls in such cultures have relative value not so much for their intrinsic, individual existence, but more for the role they can play in the thick network of past, present, and future relationships in their extended family and community.

The Akamba of Kenya give similar weight to the importance of interpersonal relationships when deciding on how scarce medical resources will be distributed. In a fascinating study by Kilner, traditional healers and Western-trained health workers were given the hypothetical choice between two male patients (one old, the other young; one with children, the other without; one who is of service to many people, the other who is not) and asked who should be saved if there were only a limited supply of medicine. Most of the respondents without formal education preferred not to choose between the patients or chose to give half dosages to each, even with the knowledge that this would be ineffective for both. The meaning and significance of their notions of equality are expressed in a proverb that says, "No matter how many Akamba are gathered, the mbilivili (a small bird) will be shared."[29]

When pushed to respond to the dilemma of allocation, these respondents clearly gave weight to the patients' place in the social web of family and community. For instance, it was explained that the older patient would be chosen for treatment because as one becomes older, connections with others become stronger and more complex, and thus the loss of an elder would be more damaging to the group. Likewise, the man without children would be saved so that he could live to "raise up a name"[30] and thus perpetuate his strand in the past and future social fabric of Akamba life. Kilner explains, "The self, for the Akamba, is not solely an individual, mortal life in the present; it is also a vital link in a chain that reaches through time."[31]

The matrix of "modernization," with its double-edged gifts of education in Western values and knowledge, increased economic mobility for women and men, and an emphasis on individual competition and reward, has strained the traditional communal orientations among the Akamba and other cultures around the world. Kilner observed that when responding to the hypothetical triage question, the Akamba health workers who had attended school were more likely to consider the patients in isolation from their social connections. This transition to a more individualized assessment of need is not always comfortable for people who have been raised in a more communitarian culture and who then work in a "modern" institutional setting. They must straddle the fence between two cultural value systems: one that reinforces the coherence of interpersonal relationships and another that is founded on more individualized notions of justice.

A Sierra Leonean physician who trained in the United States told me about the weekly dilemma he faces because he chose to return to his home town to practice medicine. There he must juggle his limited funds and medicines between his many relatives who call upon his services and patients who are not kin. One side of him feels that he is often "taken advantage of" by his relatives, who expect preferential treatment; his other side knows that their expectation is only right and just and that to do otherwise would mean that he had become callous and "too American."

Is it possible to identify "American" priorities for health and medical resource allocation? The previous examples from other countries may serve to identify what mainstream U.S. priorities are not. For instance, some readers raised in the United States might have felt alarm that gender would be considered so explicitly in distributive equations in India and Bangladesh. Or perhaps the reasoning behind the decision to save the older Akamba patient was surprising. Such feelings—abhorrence, shock, anger, fear, astonishment, or confusion—when they arise, can serve as a litmus test for identifying cultural differences. From these feelings it is an easy step into judgment about the morality and fairness of particular schema of distribution. But before we address the important issue of whether and how judgments can be made about the relative merit of different criteria and reasoning, let us consider the dominant cultural values that influence how medical services and personnel are distributed in the United States.

Depending on whether the focus is on "ideal" or "real" cultural values, it is possible to describe quite different justifications for the way medical resources are allocated in the United States. Ideally, given the compelling cultural appeal to the equality of each individual in the United States, one important measure of a just system of allocation would be equal access to health and medical services. This position is built upon the notion that individual persons, quite removed from their extrinsic relations to others, to their productivity, or their wealth, have the right to such services. Although such a framework stresses the importance of individual rights, the ultimate goal is quite communitarian in that realizing what is good for individuals is believed to result in the good of the overall community.

Contrary to this goal, as the reader knows, tension between competing values in the United States tends to obscure the ideal of equality when it comes to access to health and medical services. As Victor Fuchs explains, "On the one hand, we believe that all people should be treated as equals, especially in matters of life or death. Against this we have what Raymond Aron calls the imperative 'to produce as much as possible through mastery of the forces of nature,'[32] a venture requiring differentiation, hierarchy, and inevitably unequal treatment."[33] This imperative and the resulting social stratification are cultural, as we know, and thus neither inevitable nor celebrated by everyone. But this cultural imperative forms a dominant quality in the United States and colors much of what might seem "natural" in the order of things. We see its influence in the fact that priority access to medical services in the United States is actually given to groups that succeed in and are rewarded for this kind of social mastery—generally those who have money (or insurance coverage)[34] and/or are racially "white."[35]

The cultural reasons supporting the primacy given to the interrelated criteria of wealth and race are probably more related to political and economic dominance in the United States[36] than to spiritual beliefs. However, Weber's thesis linking the growth of capitalism with the Protestant idea that material success came from following God's will[37] might go far in explaining some of the disdain so often felt by more wealthy citizens toward the "undeserving" welfare poor in the United States. I am always struck by the level of animosity expressed by some medical students, for instance, toward poor mothers on Medicaid who use the emergency room for their routine medical care. These students have no sense of the cultural and socioeconomic reasons for such choices and resent these women as if they were personal affronts to the students' own ambitious professional goals, which they think they will reach from individual effort alone. Perhaps the students' feelings of righteousness and self-pride are the hubris born in some latent pact with their God?

Boundaries of Tolerance

The above somewhat facetious question leads to an examination of the limits and merits of ethical relativism in U.S. medical care and policy. If it were true that the medical students' assumptions about "poor people" were indeed based in culture—learned through the informal channels and rituals of medical training, shared by many of their colleagues, reinforced by their mentors, and supported by institutional practices—would we then, as relativists, be compelled to tolerate their views? Should such attitudes then be understood as ethically acceptable?

I have presented some examples of significant cultural difference regarding death and the allocation of medical resources. Many of these examples are drawn from around the world, but it is realistic to suppose that a health professional working in the United States will have ample opportunity to meet not only representatives from these international cultures, but also people from a diverse range of indigenous cultural groups of different ethnic, occupational, regional, economic, gender, or religious backgrounds. These cultural groups will not always share the ethical reasoning that informs clinicians' decisions about death. Nor will they necessarily agree with the policy decisions regarding access to medical resources.

Given the inevitability of disagreement about such issues, how far should the health professional go in tolerating difference? I say very far for a number of reasons, especially when disagreement occurs in a clinical context. First, there is the argument that there will be greater likelihood of one's own cultural views finding respect in an environment that tolerates differences. Support of intolerance never guarantees that one's own cultural framework would be the standard by which others are judged. So, cultural self-interest (if there is such a thing) would encourage an argument for this "good neighbor" brand of tolerance.

A more complex response rests on the metaphor of a "mosaic" rather than a "melting pot" for our image of ourselves as a nation. We need not strive toward some homogenization of nationhood, for this is bound to silence the less powerful. And in so doing we could lose the opportunity to enrich our perspectives about and expand the possible range of responses to the medical dilemmas that we all face. In the image of the mosaic, where cultural groups are arranged side by side, there will be tension. But why shy away from that tension? Instead, we can learn to converse about our differences, even where a negotiated consensus is impossible. Within such a dialogue lie solutions that we have not yet even considered and the possibility of self-knowledge that would otherwise remain obscured to our vision.

So we have reasons to beware of the efforts to impose consensus upon moral divergences in medical care that come from the law or bureaucratic routine. The law, if based on majority rulings, tends to reflect the morality of the more dominant voices in the society; bureaucracies, in the interest of efficiency, either run roughshod over, or forget entirely, those with different moral priorities. Instead, we need to ensure that institutional "room" is given for disagreement over and exploration and arbitration of cultural differences and similarities among staff and patients regarding clinical decisions. Often ethics committees can supply such a place, especially when informal efforts have failed to bring satisfactory solutions. The reflectivity awakened through such conversations with others who do not share cultural frameworks allows cul-

ture to change and adapt and thus become better prepared to deal with challenges that may affect even our very survival as a species.

But what about those troubling medical students and the other, more disturbing cultural practices I describe here, such as gender-based favoritism? To answer this question I turn to my own experience, because I think that we will each find our own (no doubt culturally informed) ways to respond. I agree that it is important to wander in what Keesing calls the "desert of relativism . . . in search of a clearer vision"[38] of our own cultural backyards. However, I inevitably face the limits of the perspective when I return from such quests. There are times when it is not only hard to work with another cultural point of view, but also when to do so would compromise too much my sense of right and wrong. If this occurs on a one-to-one basis, say, at the bedside, then I think that it is better to find someone else who can work with the differences at hand. There is precedent for this in health care when, for instance, a staff person does not feel ethically comfortable participating in an abortion. In my own case, it would be very difficult to support an abortion done for purposes of sex selection, and I probably would decline to be involved.

There are other times when it has been important for me to take an active stand against certain cultural expressions that may make sense from within the culture but that create harms to people. These harms would include control through dominance, intolerance of differences, discrimination, the commercialization of relationships, and greed. When these "wrongs" are expressed in faraway places, it is harder for me to justify taking action against them, but when they occur within the U.S. health care environment, we are on my own turf and my assault can be less ambivalent. Usually, as in the case of the medical students, what I find objectionable is not the whole cultural framework, but rather the particular way in which one component of the framework is being expressed. Thus it is possible to appeal to other values from within the culture to make my point; I may remind the medical students of the ethic of service and the sanctions against discrimination that run strong in their profession. Then my work is to reinforce these values within the structure of medical education and practice.

Each of us will have some line, some position, some belief that forms the boundaries of our tolerance. I believe that this is right and good in a moral sense, because such positions can provide an internal sense of integrity and commitment to things larger than ourselves. Only when they remain unexamined and unquestioned do such views become rigid and thus may cause harm where none was intended. It remains helpful for me to "step in another's shoes" for a while on the journey toward finding what values really make sense to me. Experiences with patients and professionals who do not share similar ideas about such important aspects of our humanity as death and health care access inevitably lead to an expansion and clarification of my own ideas. And so far, despite the inevitable frustrations, this reward seems to merit the effort.

Notes

1. Lynaugh, J., and Bates, B. The two languages of nursing and medicine. In: N. Klein, editor. *Culture, Curers, and Contagion.* Novato, CA: Chandler and Sharp Publishers, 1979, pp. 129–37.

2. Koenig, B. The technological imperative in medical practice: The social creation of a "routine" treatment. In: M. Lock and D. Gordon, editors. *Biomedicine Examined.* Dordrecht, Holland: Kluwer Academic Publishers, 1988, pp. 465–96.

3. Pernick, M. Back from the grave: recurring controversies over defining and diagnosing death in history. In: R. Zaner, editor. *Death: Beyond Whole-Brain Criteria.* Dortrecht, Holland: Klumer Academic Publishers, 1988, pp. 17–74.

4. The following are examples:

   Ad Hoc Committee of the Harvard Medical School to Examine the Definition of Death. A definition of irreversible coma. *Journal of the American Medical Association* 205(6):337–40, Feb. 1968.

   President's Commission for the Study of Ethical Problems in Medicine and Biomedical and Behavioral Research. *Defining Death: A Report on the Medical, Legal, and Ethical Issues in the Determination of Death.* Washington, DC: U.S. Government Printing Office, 1981.

5. Zaner, R., editor. *Death: Beyond Whole-Brain Criteria.* Dordrecht, Holland: Kluwer Academic Publishers, 1988, p. 5.

6. Lock, M., and Honde, C. Reaching consensus about death: heart transplants and cultural identity in Japan. In: G. Weisz, editor. *Social Science Perspectives on Medical Ethics.* Philadelphia: University of Pennsylvania Press, 1990, p. 109.

7. Lock and Honde, p. 109.

8. Lock and Honde, p. 110.

9. Lock and Honde, p. 103.

10. Foster, G., and Anderson, B. *Medical Anthropology.* New York City: Alfred A. Knopf, 1978.

11. Kundstader, P. 19 Medical ethics in cross-cultural perspective. *Social Science and Medicine* 14B:290, 1980.

12. Eidelman, A. In Israel people look to two messengers of God. *Hastings Center Report* 16(4):18–19, Aug. 1986. Cited by Lieban, R. Medical anthropology and the comparative study of medical ethics. In: Weisz, G., editor. *Social Science Perspectives on Medical Ethics.* Philadelphia: University of Pennsylvania, 1990, pp. 221–39.

13. Subramanian, K. N. S. In India, Nepal, and Sri Lanka, quality of life weighs heavily. *Hastings Center Report* 16(4):20–22, 1986. Cited by Lieban, R. Medical anthropology and the comparative study of medical ethics. In: G. Weisz, editor. *Social Science Perspectives on Medical Ethics.* Philadelphia: University of Pennsylvania, 1990,

14. Lieban, R. Medical anthropology and the comparative study of medical ethics. In: G. Weisz, editor. *Social Science Perspectives on Medical Ethics.* Philadelphia: University of Pennsylvania, 1990, p. 231.

15. Desai, P. Medical ethics in India. *Journal of Medicine and Philosophy* 13(3):251, 1988.

16. Desai, p. 252.

17. Oken, D. What to tell cancer patients: A study of medical attitudes. *JAMA* 175(2):86–94, Jan. 14, 1961. Novack, D., et al. Changes in physicians' attitudes toward telling the cancer patient. *JAMA* 241(9):897–900, Mar. 2, 1979.

18. Meleis, A., and Jonsen, A. Ethical crises and cultural differences. *The Western Journal of Medicine* 138(6):889–93, June 1983.

19. Meizel, A. *The Right to Die.* New York City: John Wiley, 1989.

20. Dula, A. Is there an African American bioethics? In: E. Pellegrino and H. Flack, editors. African American Bioethics. Washington, DC: Georgetown University Press. In Press. Brown, K. Connected independence: A paradox of rural health. *Journal of Rural Community Psychology* 11(1):51–64, 1990.

21. Personal communication with Yunfee Kuang, M.D., medical director of the Yangzhou Hospital, Yangzhou, People's Republic of China, Oct. 1989.

22. The reader may be interested in an article that outlines the current debate about euthanasia in the People's Republic of China. Shi Da Pu. Euthanasia in China: A report. *Journal of Medicine and Philosophy* 16(2):131–38, Apr. 1991.

23. Some measures of scarcity are objective. For example, there is a limited number of livers available from donors for transplantation purposes. But economic scarcity is actually a relative measure. The scarcity that is talked about in the U.S. medical system is largely the result of distributive practices that deny access to those who are poor and/or rural; in the overall "system," there is surplus (e.g., hospital beds, specialists in urban centers, etc.). But because we are unlikely to see these surpluses shifted to respond to need, it is realistic to speak of scarcity even here in the United States, where (objectively) $600 billion is spent on health care every year.

24. Just as in the United States, it is important to appreciate that there are many different cultural frameworks in India. For instance, there are over 100 different language groups in that country. Certainly religious and social classes differ in their orientations to the world. There are regional and urban/rural cultural differences, too. Here, and later when discussing cultural trends in Bangladesh, note is made of the dominant cultural framework in each country.

25. India finishes census; figures are alarming. *Los Angeles Times,* May 5, 1991.

26. Koenig, M., and D'Souza, S. Sex differences in childhood mortality in rural Bangladesh. *Social Science and Medicine* 22(1):15–22, Jan. 1986.

27. Fox, S. China: Diary of a barefoot bioethicist. *The Hastings Center Report* 14(7):18–20, Dec. 1984.

28. Lieban, p. 221–239.

29. Kilner, J. Who shall be saved? An African answer. *The Hastings Center Report* 14(3)18–22, p. 19, June, 1984.

30. Kilner, p. 19.

31. Kilner, p. 19.

32. Aron, R. *Progress and Disillusion.* New York City: Prae-ger, 1968, p. 3. Cited by Fuchs, V. *Who Shall Live? Health, Economics, and Social Choice.* New York City: Basic Books, 1974, p. 25.

33. Fuchs, p. 25.

34. Dougherty, C. *American Health Care Realities, Rights, and Reforms.* New York City: Oxford University Press, 1988.

35. Jones, W., and Rice, M., editors. *Black Health Care Issues in Black America: Policies, Problems, and Prospects.* New York City: Greenwood Press, 1987.

36. Navarro, V. *Crisis, Health, and Medicine.* New York City: Tavistock Publications, 1986.

37. Weber, M. *The Protestant Ethic and the Spirit of Capital-ism.* New York City: Charles Scribner's Sons, 1958.

38. Keesing, R. *Cultural Anthropology: A Contemporary Per-spective.* New York City: Holt, Rinehart, and Winston, 1976, p. 179.

Part IV

Ethics and the Health Care Professional

Bioethics, like any other discipline, has its cycles and phases. At one time, the focus of professional bioethics in health care was on fairly narrow issues, such as whether physicians should advertise. In more recent times, the scope of professional bioethics has expanded to other issues, most notably the debate over whether patients in a persistent vegetative state should receive life-sustaining (or existence-prolonging) technological support. However, most discussion of professional ethics still focuses on the profession of medicine.

The literature is now expanding to include other health care professions. In this section, two essays focus on nursing: Donald F. Phillips examines a remarkable survey of the sources of nurses' moral distress, and Andrew Jameton, Ph.D., discusses some of the key ethics dilemmas and moral conflicts faced by nurses today. Emily Friedman provides guidelines for creating an ethics-sensitive environment throughout a health care organization, including the administrative leadership. In a separate essay, she discusses the moral implications of health care organizations' profits and the uses to which they are put, with particular emphasis on trustee responsibilities. Finally, Ralph Crawshaw, M.D., in telling a very personal story, provides a lesson that too many providers forget: that the most caring of practitioners can fall victim to fear and hard-heartedness, despite the best of intentions.

Chapter 15

Moral Distress in Nursing

Donald F. Phillips

Donald F. Phillips is the editor of Hospital Ethics, *publilshed by the American Hospital Association, Chicago.*

National attention is currently focused on the nursing shortage, and the same issues and problems seem to be at the center of discussion as they were eight years ago when the National Commission on Nursing was formed to deal with an anticipated shortage. Thus, the reasons given then, which are just as current now, include dissatisfaction with working conditions (staffing patterns, career advancement programs, and recognition), insufficient salaries and benefits, inadequate recruitment and retention programs, lack of leadership, and the poor image of nursing.

But to what extent are moral problems a factor? In his book, *Nursing Practice: The Ethical Issues* (1984, Englewood Cliffs, NJ: Prentice-Hall, Inc.), Andrew Jameton sorts moral problems in the hospital into three different categories:

- Moral uncertainty—when one is unsure of what principles or values apply, or even what the moral problem is
- Moral dilemmas—when two (or more) clear moral principles apply, but they support mutually inconsistent courses of action
- Moral distress—when one knows the right thing to do, but institutional constraints make it nearly impossible to pursue the right course of action

The problems are all similar in their effect, in terms of the psychological suffering that results, but they are different as to cause. Moral uncertainty and moral dilemma produce negative feelings because of the nurses' inability to decide what is right. Moral distress, on the other hand, produces negative feelings because nurses are prevented from *doing* what they have decided is right.

Moral Distress Often Cited

Judith M. Wilkinson, R.N., for her master's thesis at the University of Missouri, Kansas City, examined nurses' perceptions of (1) the kinds of patient-care situations that produce moral distress, (2) the contextual constraints that limit their freedom to implement moral decisions, (3) the effect of moral distress on their personal wholeness, and (4) the effect of moral distress on their patient care.

Because nurses' actions are constrained by many conflicting loyalties and responsibilities (to licensing bodies, employing institutions, physicians, other nurses, patients and families), Wilkinson found that nurses frequently encounter moral distress in the course of their work. "All health care workers probably experience moral uncertainty and moral dilemma with equal frequency," Wilkinson said, "but because of their peculiar position in the health-care power structure and because of their conflicting loyalties, nurses are especially prone to suffer moral distress."

Wilkinson mailed letters to 382 nurses in the Kansas City area, asking those who had experienced moral distress if they would participate in a face-to-face interview that would be tape-recorded as a means of collecting data for her study. She received 26 responses and completed 24 interviews. The various types of situations that produced moral distress, as well as the total number of nurses and cases for each situation, are shown in the table.

Wilkinson notes that moral distress begins with the existence of a case involving a moral issue, where certain conditions of feeling and cognition are present in the nurse, and where the nurse makes a decision as to what his or her own action should be in the case. Those issues most often involved were harm to the patient (pain and suffering), and treating the patient as an object (dehumanizing). Other moral principles involved the use of scarce resources, killing, patient autonomy, lying, and failure to benefit the patient.

"The nurses' moral frameworks were more often based on consequences than on rules," she noted, "except in those cases involving lying to patients. The rule 'Do not lie' seemed to be the basic principle, and nurses did not speculate whether or why lying is wrong or what effects it might have.

"Moral distress does not automatically occur just because a certain type of case exists," Wilkinson said. "It requires the case plus the nurse's belief system. For instance, in cases of Code Blue, some nurses would suffer moral distress if resuscitation *was* done, while others would suffer moral distress if resuscitation was *not* done, depending on their beliefs about quality of life, killing, and letting die."

Wilkinson found that the nurses were clear about what or who they perceived as the source of the constraints involved in the situations, although they were somewhat less clear about what the nature of the sanctions would or could be. Physicians, law/lawsuits, nursing administration, hospital policy and administration, peers, patients

and families, and the immediate situation in terms of time and workload were mentioned as external constraints, whereas the most frequently mentioned internal constraints were nurses' background and experiences (socialization), lack of initiative because of the futility of past actions, and the value they placed on the job, or the fear of losing it.

"It is interesting to note that the nurses perceived their work environments as more threatening than supportive," she said. "They reported a number of serious sanctions that could be brought to bear upon a nurse, and an almost total lack of support. Only 3 of the 24 nurses mentioned that they had some support in a situation."

"It seems clear that contextual constraints do exist and pose a real threat to nurses who presume to oppose sources of power within the hospital," Wilkinson said. "It also appears that the nurse's 'real' perception of the constraint is more important than whether the constraint is actually 'real.' Nurses seem to fear severe, but unlikely, consequences (such as loss of license to practice) equally as much as they do the more likely, but less severe, consequences (such as a physician's anger)."

The nurses reported feeling anger for those controlling the situation (such as physicians, hospitals, or laws), guilt for their part in the situation, frustration at their inability to change the situation, sadness and pity for the patient, anger in Code Blue cases, and many other negative feelings, such as nervousness and tension, worry and fear, disgust (with others/for self), sickness, helplessness, discomfort, self-doubt, emptiness, and inadequacy.

Nurses who perceived the physician as "the decision-maker" and the nurse as "order-follower" experienced less

Table. Classification of Cases of Moral Distress

Type of situation	Number of Nurses Describing Such a Case	Total Number of Cases Described*
1. Coding patients who are dying (or "not salvageable")	12	12
2. Performing unnecessary tests and/or treatment on patients—for profit or to protect from malpractice	10	12
3. Lying to patients; withholding information from patients	9	12
4. Witnessing incompetent or inadequate treatment by a physician	6	9*
5. Performing tests/treatment without informed consent (or with no consent)	5	8
6. Observing work conditions that risk patient safety	4	5
7. "Practicing" procedures on patients	4	4
8. "Pulling the plug" or "no code" orders	3	4*
9. Giving chemotherapy to dying patients	3	3
10. Discontinuing treatment because patient can no longer pay	3	3
11. Prolonging life (e.g., dialysis, ventilators) when there is no hope for meaningful life	3	3
12. Not respecting patient's dignity	2	2
		72

*Some nurses described more than one incident of the same type of case.

guilt than those with a strong feeling for nursing autonomy and personal moral responsibility.

"Four patterns of nursing care behavior emerged," Wilkinson said. "Subjects reported behaviors that could be classified as avoiding the patient, compensating the patient, changes in emotional state, or neutral (no effect, don't know). The strongest patterns were those of avoiding or compensating. Subjects who avoided patients because of their own psychic pain reported their care had suffered in quality. Subjects who reported compensating behaviors believed their patient care had improved."

Coping Mechanisms

Nurses tried to resolve their painful feelings in a variety of ways, both conscious and unconscious, Wilkinson said. Unconsciously, they may have (1) focused on the immoral actions of others, (2) focused on the powerful constraints that prevented them from acting morally, or (3) become unable to perceive negative changes in their patient care. One of the most common, but less successful, coping behaviors was avoidance, either of patients or of situations. The most common successful coping behaviors were to (1) deny responsibility for either the situation or their own immoral action and/or (2) believe they were able to have some control and effect upon patient situations.

"Most nurses did not cope successfully with moral distress by staying and dealing with it," Wilkinson said, "instead, they changed jobs or left nursing." Those who coped successfully tended to (1) believe they could have some control/effect on patient situations, (2) believe their patient care was good, and (3) compensate rather than avoid patients.

Implications

Wilkinson believes that nursing is a moral endeavor and that nurses are morally autonomous and are, therefore, responsible for recognizing moral issues in patient-care situations and for their own actions in these cases, despite contextual constraints.

"If nursing is to be approached holistically," she said, "nursing diagnoses must include moral aspects of the patient situation as well as biopsychosocial aspects. In addition to responsibility for their own moral actions, nurses are responsible for supporting patients and families who are making moral decisions, and for serving as advocates for patients when moral decisions are being made either for them or about them. This requires that nurses be active decision-makers rather than passive rule-followers — a role that is difficult, at best, within the constraints of hospital bureaucracies."

In the last section of her thesis, Wilkinson outlines some implications of her research for nursing practice, education, and research. Nursing administrators, she contends, need to clearly define for themselves what kind of nurse they wish to have at the bedside. Do they want nurses with a strong sense of responsibility, or do they actually prefer those who are content to relegate the thinking to others and function simply as rule-followers?

"The nurses who are unable to cope with moral distress and who leave bedside nursing entirely seem to be those who are most aware of and sensitive to moral issues, and who feel a strong sense of responsibility to patients and for their own actions," Wilkinson said. "These are the very qualities that are found in the caring kind of nurse that *should* remain at the bedside if patient care is to be humane instead of mechanical and routine."

To aid in the retention of the most caring, sensitive, and responsible nurses, Wilkinson advises efforts to help them cope with their feelings. The services of an ethicist and/or a mental health nurse could be utilized, and time should be given, and even required, for support groups to discuss moral issues.

For those nurses who stay at the bedside and are unable to recognize moral issues or to sense their own responsibilities in such cases, she advises in-service programs to increase awareness of moral issues and to give nurses tools to cope with the feelings that develop from such awareness.

Wilkinson believes that moral distress is probably one of the sources of psychological discomfort that leads to burnout. Therefore, she suggests that moral issues should be included in orientations and internships to lessen the contribution of moral distress to reality shock and burnout.

At present, she said, such programs do not address ethical issues because the people who plan the programs have not been sensitized or educated about them. Continuing education in nursing ethics should be required for hospital in-service educators, and it should aim to keep nurses informed of laws and hospital policies and procedures in order that contextual constraints to moral action will be perceived realistically.

Wilkinson notes that moral distress occurs in every type of patient care setting, but that it is probably more intense on units, such as ICU and labor and delivery, where nurses have a high degree of autonomy. She argues that nurses who exercise their judgment in other aspects of patient care are especially frustrated when they cannot do so with regard to moral aspects. These nurses, especially, need support in coping with moral distress.

"Nursing administrators should be aware that staff nurses view them more as a part of the contextual constraints than as a part of their support system in moral matters," Wilkinson said. "If this is not a realistic perception, then better communication is needed between nursing administrators and staff nurses in this regard.

"Efforts should be made to support nurses who are being sanctioned in moral distress cases. Nursing administrators should attempt to have ethics committees established in their hospitals to assure that nurses have input in moral matters," Wilkinson said. "Such committees may be helpful in differentiating between medical and moral decisions for both nurses and physicians, and in removing some constraints and sanctions in some cases."

With regard to nursing education, Wilkinson argues that if the profession is to give other than lip service to holistic medicine, then nursing ethics must be included in the nursing curriculum. "Presently," she said, "nurs-

---

Shortly after completing her master's thesis, Judith Wilkinson, R.N., left the field of nursing. Her work has never been published.—Editor

ing ethics is included in very few nursing programs in a planned, structured manner. It is usually hit-or-miss, and few faculty members are actually prepared to teach the content."

Additional Resource

The Nursing Shortage: Facts, Figures, and Feelings is the title of a new research report, recently published by the AHA, that provides detailed and candid insight into how student and practicing nurses, nurse executives, and hospital administrators view the nursing shortage and what steps they would take to diffuse the crisis.

Attention is given to suggested strategies for stemming the drop in enrollment in nurse programs and countering the frustrations of practicing nurses. A major thrust of the book is to give hospitals help in designing and implementing their nurse recruitment programs.

Chapter 16

Nursing Ethics and the Moral Situation of the Nurse

Andrew Jameton, Ph.D.

Andrew Jameton, Ph.D., is an associate professor in the Department of Preventive and Societal Medicine, University of Nebraska Medical Center, Omaha.

L ike the professions of medicine, law, and engineering, the nursing profession has created a tradition of ethical codes, teaching, and analysis. Work on nursing ethics began to be published soon after schools of nursing were founded in the late 19th century and as the nursing organizations and journals developed. Nursing ethics textbooks have been used in nursing courses since the end of the 19th century, the most prominent of the early texts being Isabel Hampton Robb's *Nursing Ethics* (1901).[1] A number of texts have been published during the 20th century, and the *American Journal of Nursing* published a column of ethical advice during various periods in the first half of the century.[2] The American Nurses' Association (ANA) first published a code of ethics in 1950, and the ANA Code for Nurses has undergone a series of revisions since then. A number of nursing subspecialty groups also publish codes of ethics and standards of conduct. The bioethics renaissance since the 1970s has fostered a rapid increase in the publication of texts, magazine articles, and journal research on nursing ethics.

As the ethical analysis of day-to-day decisions by individual professionals functions partly to set these actions in a globally coherent context, nursing ethics shares its most important features with issues discussed in medical ethics, bioethics, and ethics generally. Nurses are concerned with their responsibilities toward patients,

the values inherent in the goals of therapy, appropriate decisions about the care of patients, the ethics of relations among professionals, and the social responsibilities of the nursing profession. Nursing ethics nevertheless has its own unique features and particular concerns.

The special flavor of nursing ethics arises from the *moral situation* of nurses, that is, the typical ethical concerns that arise from the daily decisions and circumstances of nurses. One important aspect of the daily work of nurses is the care of patients and the commitment to caring for patients. Thus, ethics in nursing is distinguished by a strong focus on care. Caring is a difficult concept, and its function as an ethical concept is only recently beginning to be appreciated by ethicists. At the same time, health care institutions have shown ambivalence toward caring, and more concrete and technologically exciting procedures have drawn attention toward the technical side of health care and away from the emotional side.

A second focus of nursing ethics, which relates closely to the first, is communication with patients. Dialogue and exchanges of information must be woven among nursing tasks and considered in the shifting participation of staff, family, and patient. Truth telling is a delicate issue for nurses in their work settings, where differing interpretations of the patient's condition compete against a background of sickness and uncertainty.

A third focus of nursing ethics is the authority of the nurse in relation to other health professionals. Although medical ethics focuses heavily on the two-person physician–patient relationship, nursing ethics looks broadly at the nurses' role in a complex situation involving patient, family, supervisory nurses, physicians, and the hospital or other health care institution. Choices often need to be made as to how to relate to and negotiate among these various parties. When things get tense, nurses sometimes speak of the problem of being "the nurse in the middle." The nurse typically works at a midlevel in highly stratified institutions. Because nurses have are responsible for the welfare of patients but have limited authority, delicate issues of conscience arise in balancing the needs of the patient against the limitations of the institution.

A fourth focus of nursing ethics — justice — considers issues affecting the access of patients to care and the allocation of scarce nursing resources to patients already receiving care. An example of this is deciding, on a busy service, which patient requests to attend to first. Issues of justice also affect the relationship of nurses to patients, to each other, and to other health professionals. The most prominent question regarding the justice of nurses' relations to others is whether nurses receive adequate rewards in relation to their contribution to others.

Caring and Emotional Labor

The concept of caring plays an important role in nursing ethics. "Caring" identifies a primary obligation and contribution of nurses to patients. It combines two different concepts: (1) performing the various specific tasks done by nurses to and for patients, such as administering medications, observing physical signs and symptoms, teaching self-care skills, and so forth, and (2) maintaining a personal commitment to the welfare of the patient, that is, communicating empathetically, displaying compassion, engaging with the patient's concerns, and providing emotional support. Crucial to meaningful nursing practice is the ability to provide care in the first sense, or daily "cares" as these activities are sometimes called, along with care in the second sense. This commitment to "emotional labor," to use sociologist Arlie Hochschild's term,[3] distinguishes nursing ethics from medical ethics, which traditionally maintains an emotive posture of "detached concern,"[4] and from bioethics, which currently draws primarily from the Kantian tradition of nonemotional rationality.

This central commitment to caring in its second sense has posed problems for the status of nursing. Emotional labor, although widely recognized as a teachable and marketable skill, is usually of only moderate value economically; indeed, it has often been a mark of serving occupations, such as flight attendant and waiter. To emphasize emotional labor is also to associate nursing with traditional "women's work" at a time when ethical analysis is striving for gender neutrality in its conceptions of humanity. Moreover, the skills of emotional labor are not teachable in an obvious, concrete way that is easily described and measured. Thus, these skills are not univer-

sally recognized as warranting professional standing. Lastly, emotional labor is a personal human skill not easily enhanced by technology. It is easy to imagine computers assisting diagnosis and robots providing "cares," but an empathetic and emotionally supportive robot is far beyond our present understanding of the difference between humanity and machinery. Unfortunately for practitioners of emotional labor, current conceptions of progress and economic rewards in health care are products of technological development, not increasing skill in caring — indeed, time for care, empathy, and support is rarely budgeted as a hospital service.

Despite these obstacles, it is clear that emotional labor is an essential and developing aspect of health care. To see that it is essential, one need only imagine an acute care hospital employing only robots or distant, unempathetic technicians. For the patient, serious illness is an emotional roller coaster of fear, pain, joy, relief, horror, nausea, grief, hope, and the like. Indeed, as the severity of illness of hospitalized patients continues to increase, so does the difficulty of emotions experienced by patients and families. Few patients could survive the ordeal of hospitalization psychologically or physically without substantial empathy and support from caregivers.

The development of counseling and the human potential movement of the past three decades also supports the importance of skills in caring, as exemplified by nursing courses with titles such as "Therapeutic Communication." Moreover, the bioethics literature increasingly is recognizing the value of ethical concepts developed in feminist literature, such as community, connection, context, responsibility, and caring.[5] Finally, it is obvious that ethics cannot reflect the full range of human experience without being sensitive to human feelings as well as to the capacity for reason; as Sidney Callahan put it, emotion and reason are both "tutors" of ethical decisions.[6]

For the nurse committed to skilled, professional emotional labor, a number of subtle ethical questions arise:

1. *How should the nurse balance emotive and technical skills in the routine of patient care?* When efficiency demands speed and patients in critical care units communicate with difficulty and meet the caregiver through a screen of tubes and monitors, how strenuously should the nurse press to connect with the patient?
2. *How should the nurse balance professionalism and friendship with the patient?* Sharing family communication, gifts, toasts, touch, funerals, and favors are partly the vocabulary of friendship and partly of professional support. Is the relationship always well defined, and should it always be well defined? Perhaps the ability to give an appearance of friendship is one of the skills needed to

provide support, and if so, when is an appearance of friendship dishonest?

3. *When are the nurse's ethical uncertainties about patient care professional questions and when are they personal questions?* Because emotional labor is not well defined as part of the nursing job, a nurse who feels that a patient is unhappy, suffering, or dissatisfied may experience opposition from other staff if he or she pursues this concern forcefully. Or the nurse may mistakenly define a professional ethical concern as a "merely personal" moral concern and fail to initiate a remedy.

4. *How should a nurse balance his or her personal emotional needs in relation to the patient?* Is there a point in the day when a nurse has seen too much suffering and should stop work? When is it appropriate to cry with patients, to show anger or disgust toward them? And if clinicians are expected to suppress their own strong feelings, what institutional mechanisms should be available to them for relief from their emotional burdens?

This set of concerns poses important questions about the nature of professionalism. The questions lack immediate answers and need more exposition in the literature. The first question, about balancing emotive and technical skills, requires careful discussion by nursing and medical ethics committees, public discussion of health care priorities, and a careful look at how nurses communicate compassion and empathy to patients while accomplishing concrete care tasks. The second question, about friendship and professionalism, can be addressed in teaching by distinguishing the elements of friendship that enhance professionalism from those that do not, by characterizing codependency and under- and overcommitment, and by testing the thesis that the nurse should be equally committed to all patients. The third question, about the line between the professional and the personal, is implicit in the bioethical literature, which attempts to relate professional ethics to larger moral questions. Thus, the nurse on the scene is both moral agent and professional and should not do what he or she regards as immoral even if professionalism seems to demand it. The fourth question, about the emotional burdens of caregiving, requires separate analysis of specific feelings and a better understanding of how clinical staff experience them. The role of clinical humor is, for instance, controversial and in need of careful analysis in an ethics context.

Communication with Patients

Emotional labor is one aspect of nursing communication with patients. Nurses also have substantial responsibility for educating patients, instructing them about hospital procedures, informing them about their condition, and listening to and acting upon their concerns. The term *advocacy* has been used often by nursing ethicists to articulate the nurse's responsibility in communicating with patients.[7] Advocacy combines the nurse's responsibility for (1) protecting the patient and (2) acting as the patient's agent. The word *advocacy* also suggests that the patient is on trial, perhaps with the disease as punishment and the physician or hospital as judge. Nurses face important ethical questions about how strenuous their advocacy of patients' interests should be and how extensive and honest their communication with patients should be. In their efforts to speak for patients' interests, nurses risk communicative paternalism by overinterpreting patients' wishes, perhaps in the patients' interests, but perhaps in the nurses' or institutions' interests. Moreover, institutional concerns may limit the ability of nurses to be effective advocates for patients. For instance, telling the patient his or her diagnosis is still widely regarded as the privilege and responsibility of the physician. But what if the physician has not met this responsibility in a timely or effective way? Is it appropriate for the nurse to step in and act as an advocate by disclosing a diagnosis? Tradition may say "no," but there surely are cases in which the diagnosis is clear and the physician so unavailable that simple respect for the patient requires the nurse to speak.

It is common for nurses to feel that patients do not know enough about their prognosis and therapy. For instance, intensive care unit nurses may feel that patients should be made aware of possible complications of care in the unit. At the same time, they do not wish to burden patients with frightening explanations. Because some of the things that can happen to patients in intensive care are frightening, it is difficult for nurses to balance the commitment to disclosure with the commitment to support the patient emotionally. Although the nurse will want to be the patient's advocate, in this circumstance it is unclear how much disclosure best protects and represents the patient.

Communication with the families and friends of patients presents complex ethical issues. Nurses often maintain the bulk of hospital communication with families. Decision making within families can be an intricate matter as longstanding familial concerns become involved in the clinical decision at hand. Also, clinical staff may disagree on how involved the family should be in the care and on who constitutes the family. The nurse may be actively involved in supporting family members who hold what seems to the clinical team to be the soundest point of view. Keeping family members up-to-date, correcting misunderstandings, maintaining the family's support for the therapy, helping family members to feel included in decisions, teaching the family how to care for the patient, and negotiating the borderline between nursing and family services all require careful ethical and psychological analysis.

Because nurses are aware of working in a complex institutional context, some communication issues are awkward. For instance, a patient may ask a nurse for his or her opinion of a physician, the hospital, or another nurse. Patient advocacy would require a knowledgable nurse to render an opinion, but loyalty to the health care team supports avoiding a direct answer. A similar issue arises when the patient tells the nurse a secret and asks the nurse to keep it from the rest of the health care team. What is the nurse's responsibility when the information is needed for effective care of the patient? Although it is clear that team loyalty should serve the aim of the best patient care, it is not immediately clear how and when a particular patient's interests should be balanced in relation to the team's long-term efficacy, which depends on loyalty and trust among team members.

Authority, Responsibility, and Interprofessional Relations

Although nurses have authority to determine many aspects of the patient care plan, this work needs to be coordinated with and sometimes subordinated to the medical care plan. Because only physicians can write medical orders, nurses must work through physicians when they judge that a problem exists with the medical care plan. When nurse and physician disagree about the care plan, the nurse's main recourse is to persuade or influence the physician. But the physician has no well-defined responsibility to listen to the nurse, and the physician's special expertise creates a presumption in the physician's favor. Yet, it is not difficult to find circumstances in which the nurse could reasonably disagree with a medical order. He or she may have observed something about the patient that the physician missed, or the physician may have overlooked a possible complication or miscalculated a dosage. Where the medication order is unquestionably wrong or even dangerous, the nurse has a clear legal and moral responsibility to have the order changed. Where the issue is more subtle, where the order constitutes standard care but is otherwise suboptimal, or where the nurse feels that the patient's values have been insufficiently considered, the courses of action open to the nurse are less obvious.

If the physician fails to talk with the nurse or neglects to take his or her concerns into account, the nurse usually has no direct course of action. Because the physician (unless a medical resident) does not usually have a clearly defined supervisor, the nurse must either do nothing or fish for assistance among consulting specialties and on-call physicians. This can be a time-consuming nightmare for nurses and physicians alike. The nurse also can choose to express his or her concerns to the patient or family in the hope that they will act on them, but then the nurse risks the appearance of breaching loyalty to the team. The paradigm experience of being "in the middle" arises when the nurse attempts to communicate his or her concerns to the family inobtrusively, the family does not take the hint, and problematic care continues. A staff nurse can take the problem to a nursing supervisor, but the nursing supervisor also must work within the complex network of medical consulting and specialty relationships.

Thus, nurses sometimes find themselves in the position of moral witness. They see things going on in the hospital that they regard as morally reprehensible but feel powerless to stop. A nurse may witness a medical student causing a patient pain while practicing a venipuncture, a procedure that the nurse could do less painfully. Although the institution may support balancing the patient's interests with the needs of medical education, the nurse, with a less compromised dedication to the patient's welfare, need not accept this balance. Although the institution may allow the nurse to step in when the student has gone too far, the nurse has not been given a defined authority in the area and so may feel unsure about speaking out except in the most offensive cases.

Nurses may also be expected to perform procedures they feel are unwise or unethical. A few institutions have "conscience clauses" permitting nurses to refuse to assist with or to perform procedures, such as abortions, that they feel are unethical. Such clauses, however, usually require the nurse to assist if no substitute can be found. Moreover, the institution may impose formal and informal personal costs on an employee who does not cooperate. Some nurses exaggerate this cost and relate stories, many of them true, about nurses who suffered for raising moral questions about procedures. However, for each story of moral tragedy there are many more stories of nurses who objected reasonably to problematic practices and whose point of view was heard and acted upon. As players of middle standing in hospitals, nurses focus much of their ethical thinking on the finesse needed to adjust moral ideals in relation to institutional realities.

The nurse–physician relationship, although in many respects highly cooperative, can be difficult. The status of the two professions is very different. For instance, pay for registered nurses ranges from an average starting salary of about $24,000 to an average maximum of about $35,000.[8] Physicians' net salaries average about $144,700, with specialty averages ranging from about $85,000 to $180,000.[9] The focus of interest in hospital acute care also is often different, with the nurse focused on care, comfort, and the patient's overall sense of well-being and the physician focused on specific goals of therapy and particular, measurable aspects of the patient's condition. Nurses and physicians also do not understand each other's jobs very clearly. Physicians may overemphasize the physician-related aspects of the nurse's job (such as administering medications or reporting observations to the physician), whereas the nurse may fail to appreciate the great uncertainty with which the physician must work or react too quickly against a physician's carefully thought-out decision to deviate from a standard medical procedure.[10]

These conflicts would not be so sharp if the two professions had not inherited the power relationship that existed when nursing was born as a profession in the late 19th century. Even though nursing and medicine have made tremendous progress toward accommodation and women in medicine have increased in number,[11] some of the imbalance of the two complementary roles has been preserved, though stripped of its gender associations. If it were not for this historical imbalance, it would be easy to establish a more cooperative nurse–physician relationship. For instance, the staff decision-making unit for patient care could be a nurse–physician team, or the physician could provide diagnostic information to the nurse, who would then formulate an overall care plan. There have been some efforts along these lines.[12] Physicians and nurses could both be required to start their careers as nursing aides and with education and experience work themselves into their respective professional specialties. Nurses and physicians could share more classes in medical and nursing school. Nurses at teaching hospitals who teach clinical skills to medical students could be given formal recognition and rewards for this sometimes unrecognized work. It is clear that there is an imbalance in nurse–physician relationships, because nursing ethics discussions often involve consideration of the physician, but medical ethics discussions rarely take the nurse's participation into consideration.

Justice and Nursing

In nursing ethics, the concept of justice applies both to fairness for nurses and fairness for patients. We have already touched on inequities in the nurse–physician relationship. In general, the choice to do bedside service and emotional labor puts nurses at risk for exploitation. Advocacy by nurses for the needs of suffering patients makes nurses vulnerable to excessive claims on their labor by those who are more distant from patients or more concerned with the institution's financial bottom line. Indeed, the history of nursing ethics literature is full of exhortations for self-sacrifice and high levels of dedication to the calling. But justice requires that the needs of both nurses and patients be considered; nurses need to be able to provide adequate support to patients and receive appropriate rewards without excessive sacrifice.

One of the most important concerns around which to articulate justice for nurses is the elimination of abuse and sexual harassment. The surgeon who throws instruments at nurses during surgery, the physician who yells at nurses in the hallway, and the resident who pinches nurses all need restraint and reeducation (these phenomena are widespread according to nursing lore and are well documented by studies).[13] Successfully countering these very public examples of harassment can do much to improve an atmosphere that now too easily permits abuse of nurses.

An interesting and difficult ethical problem of justice is finding the balance between the personal risks nurses can be expected to take in the care of patients and their responsibility to provide patient care. Violent or contagious patients pose risks for nurses and schedules can sometimes be arranged to keep pregnant nurses from contact with such patients. In general, nurses have a right and obligation to protect themselves from harm while doing their work. If the risks of violence are high, nurses can justifiably call security or the police to subdue patients.

AIDS patients pose an interesting problem of justice. Physicians have generally articulated a responsibility to care for AIDS patients; however, this principle has been strongly questioned by surgeons, who undergo the greatest exposure to patients' blood. Like surgeons, nurses come into more contact with patients' blood and body fluids than do most physicians. Should nurses accept the same responsibility as physicians to care for AIDS patients? Understanding that the risk of contagion from HIV is extremely small and using universal precautions (not always practiced by nurses, partly because gowns and gloves hinder emotional labor) should resolve the conflict. However, conversations with nursing students and a recent study seem to indicate that reluctance to work with AIDS patients is common among nurses, perhaps because of a degree of homophobia.[14] The ethical question for analysis is: Why would it be justifiable for a nurse to refuse to work with a patient because of danger to himself or herself and not justifiable to refuse to work with a patient because he is gay? A reasonable initial response is that the first decision rests on a moral principle (the right and responsibility of self-protection), whereas the second rests on mere prejudice. But what if the nurse claims that his or her view of homosexuality is based on a moral principle and not prejudice? One would not want to argue initially that, contrary to his or her assertions, the nurse is actually morally unprincipled, but if the nurse really takes this position out of principle, it may not be difficult to argue that the nurse is mistaken.

One could counter the second view with the ANA Code for Nurses nondiscrimination clause:

> The nurse provides services with respect for human dignity and the uniqueness of the client, unrestricted by considerations of social or economic status, personal attributes, or the nature of health problems.[15]

The ANA commentary on this point refers specifically to "sexual differences," although it is unclear whether this phrase is intended to refer to gender differences, sexual preferences, or both. Because of its support for non-discrimination, the clause forces nurses who would discriminate as a matter of principle to distinguish between the claims of their profession and their own personal moral view. The commitment to nondiscrimination by the profession weighs heavily against these nurses' personal view. It should be distinguishable from other ethics cases, such as abortion, where the profession has not yet reached a consensus and about which the profession can thus permit practice based on a range of personal opinions.

One might also distinguish between procedure-oriented objections, such as objections to abortion, and patient-oriented objections. Indeed, most nurses would hold that the perceived social worth of the patient is not an appropriate attribute to consider in deciding which patients to treat, so that even if a nurse held that sexual orientation spoke in some way to moral worthiness, and thus the social worth of the patient, this factor should not be considered in allocating care.

Some nurses will argue that they are emotionally unable to give respectful care to certain patients (for example, child abusers, rapists, racists) because of their strong feelings about them. This line of analysis returns us to our initial concerns about emotional labor and raises the question of whether there are emotional burdens nurses should or should not in fairness be obligated to undertake. Given that a dislike of gays is usually based on ignorance and fear of the unknown, homophobic nurses would be expected to benefit from working with gays, and so there would be no conflict in asking a nurse to overcome or repress such feelings. This position, however, displays a touch of paternalism with regard to the nurse, which may be appropriate in nursing education but is not respectful of a mature nurse who holds a well-conceived, albeit professionally deviant, position.

Underlying this discussion is a general question about the moral authority of the individual nurse with regard to the moral rules of nursing and other health professions. The moral authority of individual nurses tends to be limited, to a degree, by the general institutional limitations on nurses' decision-making authority. For instance, unlike most physicians, most nurses are expected to treat any patients the institution admits, and unlike the American Medical Association, the ANA has not included a provision in its ethics code supporting the right of nurses to select which patients they treat.

Issues of distributive justice for nurses in relation to patients are complex and little discussed in the bioethics literature. For a staff nurse, these involve frequent decisions during the day as to how best to allocate his or her labor on the basis of many factors—the legitimacy and persistence of patients' requests, the comparative urgency of patient care tasks, the patient's compliance, the patient's need for supportive communication, and the like. Although many ethical concepts are involved in allocating these activities—such as maximizing the overall welfare of patients or, alternatively, the approval of administrators—justice certainly applies and is seen by nurses to apply. Nursing time is scarce and nurses want to allocate their time fairly. Nurses also are frequently involved in, or are primarily responsible for, triage decisions in allocating bed space and determining emergency department queues. Because an intensive care bed may not be available to every patient who could benefit from one, nurses and physicians must decide which patients should be admitted to or maintained in the intensive care unit and which patients must be cared for on the floor. Nurses also make decisions about overtime schedules, float assignments, assignment of nurses with appropriate capacities or congeniality to match the needs of particular patients, and special services to VIP patients. Many of the controversies over fairness among hospital nurses focus on decisions about such matters.

Like most health professionals, nurses generally believe that health care should be available to all who need it. And, like most health professionals, nurses hold a wide range of political and economic views as to how this might best be achieved. Much attention is paid in the health services literature to getting the patient to the physician, but less is said about getting the patient to the nurse, although nursing represents the major portion of labor to which patients need access. This is regrettable. Nurses have significant interest and expertise relevant to planning for health care systems and should be amply consulted. In the event that a more universal but sparer health care system is established, nurses could undertake some of the responsibility as gatekeepers in rationing health care. Nurses have views about which nursing services should have priority over others, and thus can play an important role in articulating criteria for rationing. Finally, if health care is to be made more efficient, some thought needs to be given to which health care services could be made more accessible by relying on nurses and other allied health practitioners rather than on more expensive physicians. Many nursing professional societies are studying these issues and making alternative proposals for funding and delivery of health care.[16]

Pitfalls and Cautions

As nursing ethics continues to develop as a field of study, work in certain areas needs to continue. First, although too much discussion in nursing focuses on the nurse's relation to the physician, this reflects a reality of the professional situation of many nurses. Until physicians are more prepared for dialogue, energy could be better spent on what nurses can control. For instance, nurses often speak informally of nurse–nurse abuse; yet the nature, causes, and reduction of intraprofessional nursing difficulties seldom receive ethical analysis.

Second, like most people, nurses tend for good reasons to focus much of their attention on those above them in status. Yet there is much to be said about the nurse–aide relationship and the nursing–environmental services relationship, to say nothing of relations with materials services workers, unit clerks, social workers, and technologists — those whose status is similar to or less than that of nurses and whose work is often greatly influenced by nurses. The triad of patient–nurse–physician is only part of a much larger structure that has many active and potentially active players who have important values that bear on patient care.

Third, nursing ethics tends to focus too much on the hospital (the author admits to this fault) at a time when we can expect an increasing need for ethical analysis of other areas of nursing practice. A few nursing ethicists are beginning to work on special areas of nursing ethics, and more work is needed in such areas as:

- *Home care:* Relations with the family, the safety of the nurse, observations of other health problems in the home, relations with physician and pharmacy, nonnursing assistance to the patient, reporting of illegal activities, financial problems, and so forth[17]
- *Long-term care:* Chronic illness, nursing home as home *versus* as health care institution, relations with nursing aides and assistants, falls, restraints, mental competence and consent of patients, scarce resources, and so forth[18]
- *Administration:* Creation of an ethical environment, ethics committees, policies with ethical implications, ethics of supervision, quality assurance, institutional responsibility, business ethics, and so forth[19]
- *Utilization review:* Priorities for review, fairness to practitioners with differing practices, balance of a documentation focus with meeting patients' needs, discretion and flexibility in following rules, destination of one's primary client, and so forth
- *Nursing subspecialties:* Nurse practitioners, nurse midwives, quality review, public health, intensive care, emergency department, surgery and recovery, newborn intensive care, pediatrics, psychiatry, and so forth[20]

Fourth, nursing ethics writing in the journals tends to be somewhat derivative; this may arise from a wish to connect writing on nursing ethics with other well-established areas, as well as from the unjustifiable lack of interest by philosophers in nursing ethics. However, nursing ethics writers need to find their own voice in addressing ethical issues. An abundance of new material on ethics has appeared since the advent of feminist ethics writing; the growth of the sociological, anthropological, and psychological study of ethics; and the great expansion of applied ethics. Nursing's unique point of view needs to be heard in order to educate the bioethicists, who for the most part follow older and decreasingly viable traditions.

Fifth, trained by years of invisibility, nurses tend to be too cautious and covert in their statements of issues and solutions. For example, it is clear that one objective of emotional labor is to control the patient to ensure his or her safety and compliance to regimen; there is otherwise little reason to admit the patient to the hospital. Yet few nursing ethicists clearly address the nurse's role in controlling and manipulating patients. This is partly because the bioethics literature is currently so strong in articulating patient autonomy that it is difficult to defend a legitimate role for manipulation. Yet this "dark side" of nursing ethics needs to be acknowledged. Moreover, nurses who make strong moral judgments about care sometimes temper their statements of concern by expressing their judgments as questions or dilemmas when outcry is called for. If we are to fully appreciate the depth and interest of nursing ethics, nurses need to address ethical concerns as forthrightly as possible.

Last Words

Although the number of texts and articles in nursing ethics is increasing, the field is far outpaced by work in medical ethics. This displays a regrettable lack of attention by ethicists to the most complex and interesting problems of bioethics. The phenomenon of the focus of bioethics on medicine and law highlights the relationship of ethics to power — the ethics of the most powerful professions in our society appears to interest us the most. Indeed, writing about ethics carries the risk of articulating theories and views that serve the continuing influence of the powerful. But one quite wonderful thing about the field of ethics is that moral language can be used not only by the powerful, but also by the less powerful who seek to defend and empower themselves. For ethics to be honestly handled, ethicists must address the concerns of the less powerful and find ways to teach those in power how to serve the good rather than allow conceptions of the good to serve the powerful.

For those interested in the full range of ethics, nursing ethics is an important area for study. Indeed, its attention to interprofessional relations is one of its great virtues. It is plausible that the moral quality of patient care depends much more on the moral quality of interprofessional relations than it does on what we might say about the ethics of patient care.[21] Historically, professional codes of ethics have been developed primarily to improve relations within a profession, even though much of the language of the code addresses issues in patient care. By addressing patient care, a code draws the attention of professionals in conflict to their major goals and obtains mutual cooperation through idealism. However, in the complex world of the health professions, ethics needs to address more explicitly the issue of interprofessional relations. Nursing ethicists may be able to engage those working in other professions to analyze these issues. Meanwhile, nursing ethics continues to contribute its own significant voice to the dialogue.

Notes

1. Robb, I. H. *Nursing Ethics: For Hospital and Private Use.* Cleveland: J. B. Savage, 1901.
2. For example: Aikens, C. A. *Studies in Ethics for Nurses.* 5th ed. Philadelphia: W. B. Saunders, 1943. Densford, K. J., and Everett, M. S. *Ethics for Modern Nurses: Professional Adjustments I.* Philadelphia: W. B. Saunders, 1947. Benjamin, M., and Curtis, J. *Ethics in Nursing.* 2nd ed. New York City: Oxford University Press, 1986. Davis, A. J., and Aroskar, M. A. *Ethical Dilemmas and Nursing Practice.* 3rd ed. Norwalk, CT: Appleton & Lange, 1991. At least 78 ethics columns appeared in *American Journal of Nursing* between 1926 and 1934.
3. Hochschild, A. R. *The Managed Heart: Commercialization of Human Feeling.* Berkeley, CA: University of California Press, 1983.
4. Fox, R. C. *Experiment Perilous: Physicians and Patients Facing the Unknown.* Glencoe, IL: Free Press, 1959.
5. Watson, J. *Nursing: The Philosophy and Science of Caring.* Boston: Little, Brown, 1979. Noddings, N. *Caring: A Feminine Approach to Ethics and Moral Education.* Berkeley, CA: University of California Press, 1984. Ruddick, S. *Maternal Thinking: Toward a Politics of Peace.* Boston: Beacon Press, 1989. Chinn, P. L., editor. *Anthology on Caring.* New York City: National League for Nursing, 1991. Benner, P. E., and Wrubel, J. *The Primacy of Caring: Stress and Coping in Health and Illness.* Menlo Park, CA: Addison-Wesley, 1989. Neil, R. M., and Watts, R., editors. *Caring and Nursing: Explorations in Feminist Perspectives.* New York City: Center for Human Caring, National League for Nursing, 1991. Muff, J., editor. *Socialization, Sexism, and Stereotyping: Women's Issues in Nursing.* Prospect Heights, IL: Waveland Press, 1982.
6. Callahan, S. The role of emotion in ethical decisionmaking. *Hastings Center Report* 18(3):9–14, June–July 1988.
7. Kohnke, M. F. *Advocacy: Risk and Reality.* St. Louis: C. V. Mosby Co., 1982. Winslow, G. R. From loyalty to advocacy: A new metaphor for nursing. *Hastings Center Report* 14(3):32–40, June 1984. Gadow, S. Existential advocacy: philosophical foundation of nursing. In: S. F. Spicker and S. Gadow, editors. *Nursing: Images and Ideals: Open Dialogue with the Humanities.* New York City: Springer Publishing Co., 1980, pp. 79–101. Curtin, L. L. The nurse as advocate: A philosophical foundation for nursing. *Advances in Nursing Science* 1:1–10, April 1979.
8. *Facts about Nursing 86–87.* New York City: Nursing Information Bureau, American Nurses' Association, p. 162.
9. Gonzalez, M. L., and Emmons, D. W., editors. *Socioeconomic Characteristics of Medical Practice, 1989.* Chicago: American Medical Association Center for Health Policy Research, 1989.
10. Kalisch, B. J., and Kalisch, P. A. An analysis of the sources of physician-nurse conflict. In: J. Muff, editor. *Socialization, Sexism, and Stereotyping.* St. Louis: C. V. Mosby, 1982, pp. 221–33.
11. Because there are so many more nurses than physicians, the *number* of men in nursing is high even though the *percentage* of men in nursing is low. Indeed, if one counts both RNs and LPNs, there are more men in nursing than there are women in medicine.
12. Friedman, E. Nursing: Breaking the bonds? *JAMA* 264(24):3117–22, Dec. 26, 1990. Mechanic, D., and Aiken, L. H. A cooperative agenda for medicine and nursing. *The New England Journal of Medicine* 307:747–50, 1982. Stein, L. I., Watts, D. T., and Howell, T., The doctor-nurse game revisited. *The New England Journal of Medicine* 322:546–49, 1990.
13. Braun, K., Christle, D., Walker, D., and Tiwanak, G. Verbal abuse of nurses and non-nurses. *Nursing Management* 22(3):72–76, March 1991. Cox, H. Verbal abuse nationwide, part II: Impact and modifications. *Nursing Management* 22(3):66–69, March 1991.
14. Young, M., Henderson, M. M., and Marx, D. Attitudes of nursing students toward patients with AIDS. *Psychological Reports* 67:491–97, 1990.
15. American Nurses' Association. *Code for Nurses with Interpretive Statements.* Kansas City, MO: American Nurses' Association, 1976, 1985.
16. American Nurses' Association and 42 nursing specialty associations. Nursing's agenda for health care reform. *The American Nurse,* suppl., 1991.
17. Haddad, A. M., and Kapp, M. B. *Ethical and Legal Issues in Home Health Care: Case Studies and Analyses.* Norwalk, CT: Appleton & Lange, 1991.
18. Kane, R. A., and Caplan, A. L., editors. *Everyday Ethics: Resolving Dilemmas in Nursing Home Life.* New York City: Springer Publishing Co., 1990. Schmit Kayser-Jones, J. *Old, Alone, and Neglected: Care of the Aged in the United States and Scotland.* Berkeley, CA: University of California Press, 1981, 1990.
19. Levine-Ariff, J., and Groh, D. H. *Creating an Ethical Environment.* Nurse Managers' Bookshelf, vol. 2, no. 1. Baltimore: Williams & Wilkins, 1990.
20. For example: Fowler, M. D. M., and Levine-Ariff, J., editors. *Ethics at the Bedside: A Source Book for the Critical Care Nurse.* Philadelphia: J. B. Lippincott, 1987.
21. Waddington, I. The development of medical ethics: A sociological analysis. *Medical History* 19(1):36–53, Jan. 1975.

Basic Works in Nursing Ethics

Aikens, C. A. *Studies in Ethics for Nurses.* 5th ed. Philadelphia: W. B. Saunders, 1943.

Ashley, J. A. *Hospitals, Paternalism, and the Role of the Nurse.* New York City: Teachers College Press, 1976.

Bandman, E. L., and Bandman, B. *Nursing Ethics through the Life Span.* 2nd ed. Norwalk, CT: Appleton & Lange, 1990.

Benjamin, M., and Curtis, J., *Ethics in Nursing.* 2nd ed. New York City: Oxford University Press, 1986.

Bishop, A. H., and Scudder, J. R., editors. *Caring, Curing, Coping: Nurse, Physician, Patient Relationships.* Tuscaloosa, AL: University of Alabama Press, 1985.

Davis, A. J., and Aroskar, M. A. *Ethical Dilemmas and Nursing Practice.* 3rd ed. Norwalk, CT: Appleton & Lange, 1991.

Fromer, M. J. *Ethical Issues in Health Care.* St. Louis: C. V. Mosby, 1981.

Husted, G. L., and Husted, J. H. *Ethical Decision Making in Nursing.* St. Louis: Mosby-Year Book, 1991.

Jameton, A. *Nursing Practice: The Ethical Issues.* Englewood Cliffs, NJ: Prentice-Hall, 1984.

Jones, A. H., editor. *Images of Nurses: Perspectives from History, Art, and Literature.* Philadelphia: University of Pennsylvania Press, 1988.

Ketefian, S., and Ormond, I. *Moral Reasoning and Ethical Practice in Nursing: An Integrative Review.* New York City: National League for Nursing, 1988.

Moore, J. *A Zeal for Responsibility: The Struggle for Professional Nursing in Victorian England, 1868–1883.* Athens, GA: University of Georgia Press, 1988.

Murphy, C. P., and Hunter, H., editors. *Ethical Problems in the Nurse-Patient Relationship.* Boston: Allyn and Bacon, 1983.

Muyskens, J. L. *Moral Problems in Nursing: A Philosophical Investigation.* Totowa, NJ: Rowman and Littlefield, 1982.

Pence, T., and Cantrall, J., editors. *Ethics in Nursing: An Anthology.* New York City: National League for Nursing, 1990.

Quinn, C. A., and Smith, M. D. *The Professional Commitment: Issues and Ethics in Nursing.* Philadelphia: W. B. Saunders, 1987.

Reverby, S. M. *Ordered to Care: The Dilemma of American Nursing, 1850–1945.* Cambridge: Cambridge University Press, 1987.

Steele, S., and Harmon, V. M. *Values Clarification in Nursing.* 2nd ed. Norwalk, CT: Appleton-Century-Crofts, 1983.

Thompson, I. E., Melia, K. M., and Boyd, K. M. *Nursing Ethics.* Edinburgh: Churchill Livingstone, 1983.

Thompson, J. E., and Thompson, H. O. *Bioethical Decision Making for Nurses.* Norwalk, CT: Appleton-Century-Crofts, 1985.

Veatch, R. M., and Fry, S. T. *Case Studies in Nursing Ethics.* Philadelphia: J. B. Lippincott, 1987.

Chapter 17

Ethics and Corporate Culture: Finding a Fit

Emily Friedman

Reprinted, with permission, from *Healthcare Executive,* March/April 1990, pp. 18–20. Published by the American College of Healthcare Executives, copyright ©1990.

Emily Friedman is a writer, lecturer, and health policy analyst based in Chicago. She writes for several leading health and business publications. In 1987–88 she was Rockefeller Fellow in Ethics at Dartmouth College. Ms. Friedman is the author/editor of the book Making Choices: Ethics Issues for Health Care Professionals.

Does a high-quality corporate culture require organizational ethics? Indeed, *can* a high-quality corporate culture require organizational ethics? We would all like to think so, but we nurse secret fears of going too far. We worry that ethics is somehow incompatible with efficiency and success. Or we fear that ethics constitutes a barrier to effective action: "Just when we thought we had this thing iced, some bozo came in and started talking about doing the right thing, and the whole plan fell apart."

These are not persuasive arguments. To say that ethics and success cannot co-exist is to condemn every organization that has succeeded as unethical. This is not the case, as we know from a burgeoning literature on organizational quality. And to say that ethics prevents effectiveness is really another way of saying that effectiveness is the same as expediency. It has been said that the right thing and the expedient thing are seldom the same thing; true enough, but that does not mean that the right thing and the effective thing are seldom the same thing.

To argue that ethics is inexpedient is, in fact, to argue in favor of including ethics in the corporate agenda. For as philosopher John Ruskin pointed out, in a statement that was posted under the portrait of J. C. Penney that once hung in every Penney's store: "There is hardly anything in this world that a man cannot make a little worse and sell a little cheaper, and those who consider price alone are this man's lawful prey."

There is much more sense in the words of ethical philosopher Michael Josephson, who has said, "The notion that nice guys finish last is not only poisonous but wrong. In fact, the contrary is true. Unethical conduct is always self-destructive and generates more unethical conduct until you hit the pits. . . . The challenge is to be ethical and get what you want. You can do that almost every time."

Furthermore, an ethical corporate culture is critical to the healthcare organization because healthcare executives are similar to the clergy: They are held to a higher standard. Much more is expected of them. From a pornographer, the public does not expect much; from people who hold other people's lives in their hands, the public expects a whole lot. So it is with healthcare organizations; only by fulfilling the public's expectations of proper ethical behavior can such organizations retain the unique privileges society has given them. Thus ethical management is good management, and ethical corporate culture is a good corporate culture—and both are critical to the provider's survival.

What constitutes an ethical corporate culture? It has two components: organizational and individual. An ethical organization has the following characteristics:

1. Honorable leadership that is at least as committed to the community and the organization as it is to its own professional and personal concerns. The leadership must also be known to have those commitments. As Henry VIII tells Sir Thomas More in the play *A Man for All Seasons,* he needs More's support more than that of others because "not only are you honest; you are *known* to be honest."

2. Protection of and responsiveness to those within the organization who bring up ethics problems and questions. Organizations are often reluctant to act, even when someone blows a whistle. The arguments are: a) We don't do that to our own; b) The person will sue; and/or c) He or she is a power in the organization, so he or she is above the law. However, if those who expose ethical problems and wrongs are ignored, hushed up, or worse yet, punished, the obvious lesson will spread rapidly through the organization: We claim to have ethics, but we do not use them.

3. Encouragement of ethical achievement, not just avoidance of ethical failure. Too much organizational self-assessment is based on one politician's Rule of Guilt: "I was not indicted, so therefore I am innocent." However, just sneaking by is not sufficient for ethical success. It is true that too often it is not committing the crime but getting caught that is seen as the real sin. But as sociologist Robert Coles has observed, "character consists of how you behave when no one else is around."

4. Avoidance of hypocrisy. It is foolhardy to include material in the mission statement that is not true or to ignore what is in the mission statement. It is hypocritical to describe the organization, market services, or tout accomplishments in dishonest or misleading ways. And it is not healthy to have two standards: one for how patients are treated and another for how employees are treated.

But the organizational elements are only half the story; an ethical corporate culture is equally dependent on the commitment of individuals. What is required of the individual executive in order to achieve such a culture?

1. Other people's ethical beliefs and standards cannot be controlled, regulated, legislated, or managed. As an old grandmother once observed, "many people don't even like to be rubbed the right way." A manager cannot announce to employees: "We have a new guest relations program. Therefore, you will be nice to the employees—or you're fired!" When such demands are made, and in such a manner, employees either resent being ordered to do what they are already doing, or they resent an unkind manager demanding kindness of them. Employees are more likely to be nice to patients if they see leaders being nice to patients—and to employees. As Sandra Fenwick, vice-president of the Beth Israel Hospital in Boston, says, "Nurtured employees provide nurturing care."

Good managers teach ethics by example; ethics can't be taught by fiat. Unethical behavior must be prevented, of course, even by fiat, if gentler means fail. But to produce positive ethical behavior, one can only create an atmosphere that is conducive to and rewards such behavior.

2. Ethical behavior is the product of a process; it is not a pat solution. Ethics will not tell one what to do in every situation. Ethics simply establishes a moral framework for decision making by providing guidance, clarification, and insight. Ethics also aids the development and strengthening of individual and organizational values. That creates more refined judgment. Indeed, David Kinzer of Harvard University says that Ray Brown, the father of health administration education, defined judgment as "facts passed through values."

A corporate culture that is sensitive to ethics allows executives to tap the expertise and advice of others in a morally acceptable way. It does not obviate conflicts with peers. It does not obviate conflicts involving different value systems. It does not obviate barriers posed by logistics, finances, or current realities. But it helps the leader try to do the right thing, and that is all that can be expected. Embracing ethics and operating in an ethical manner should help the good guys win, but it does not guarantee they will.

3. Pick your fights. Executives can try to fight every ethical battle that comes along, but sooner or later they will get saddle sores from the high horses they are riding around. We all fail our own moral standards; none of us lives a morally integrated life. I suspect that somewhere, at some time, even Albert Schweitzer, Mother Teresa, and Bambi told a little lie.

So you have to pick your fights. It is not worthwhile to start World War III over whether someone copied a recipe on the office photocopier. But by the same token, you should be willing to stand your ground when the issue is of major concern to you. Yet we often find it easier to take on photocopying of recipes than we do a breach of confidentiality involving the president of the medical staff. Meaningless fights are easier, because the risk is low. Thus organized medicine has spent far more time debating the ethics of physician advertising than the ethics of allowing impaired physicians to perform.

To take the easy way, the path of least resistance, is tempting; but it spreads a toxin of ethical laziness throughout the organization. Then, when the tough battles come, no one may feel like fighting them.

4. No manager is an island. It is easy to focus one's good deeds on the relatively few employees, issues, and patients that command attention. But what we don't see and don't do can be as ethically problematic as more obvious challenges.

For example, the U.S. infant mortality rate of 10.2 per 1,000 live births is among the highest in the developed world. Yet the publicity around this ongoing tragedy is not a thousandth of the coverage given the mad young woman who in 1988 walked into a school in a wealthy Chicago suburb and started shooting. She killed one child and wounded several others. On that same day, 10 or 11 American infants also died, probably half of preventable causes. We heard nothing of that. Was it because the child who was shot lived in an affluent suburb, and most of the dead babies likely did not? Was it because the one child died as the result of an act, whereas most of the infants died as a result of inaction? Yet there is no ethical difference between crimes of omission and crimes of commission. What we do not notice can be just as ethically questionable as what we do notice and act on.

Thus one characteristic of an ethical organizational culture is encouraging leaders to stretch the borders of responsibility. For some of the toughest problems in healthcare ethics are the people who are not treated, the prenatal care that is not available, the mental health services that are not provided, and the immunizations and primary care that are not delivered. In the end, as songwriter Si Kahn has observed, "It's not the fights you dream of/But those you really fought."

5. If the patient died, the operation was probably not a complete success. Physician and ethicist Edmund Pellegrino, M.D., has said that healthcare should be "technically correct and morally good." In fact, the two are one and the same. Healthcare quality and healthcare ethics have been treated as though they belong on two different planets; yet they are intimately tied to one another.

The technical quality, appropriateness, and outcomes of care have all ethical overtones—and ethical problems. For example, study after study has shown that many treatments, ranging from cesarean section to radiation therapy, are provided far more to patients with lavish private insurance than to patients with Medicaid coverage. Other studies show that in some instances, black Americans—even if they have private insurance—do not receive as much care as white Americans. We have always claimed that once patients enter the healthcare system, they are treated equally, regardless of insurance status or race. Yet we seem to base some clinical decisions on extraneous, nonclinical factors.

Other studies have raised profound questions about the need for all the cesarean sections, hysterectomies, radiation therapy, cardiovascular surgery, prostatectomy, and many other treatments that are being provided at escalating rates. Are they always indicated? Are they provided too often in marginal cases? Are they offered for nonclinical reasons?

Hippocrates' first admonition was to do no harm to the patient. Many procedures, such as surgery and use of radioisotopes, represent potential harm; yet we often overuse them, or use them inappropriately, just as we deny care inappropriately to those without adequate sponsorship. This is a bedrock ethics issue and deserves discussion in terms of its moral importance, not simply its

financial implications. Many executives prefer to see healthcare as a business, pure and simple; it is not a view shared by the American public. What is relevant is that when the quality, appropriateness, and results of healthcare are taken lightly by providers, it is patients who pay the price.

6. Resource management must be based on some concept of social justice and priorities. Because, by somebody's standards, there is never enough healthcare, providers must always ration care. The ethical test is in how it is done and why. Those who cut up the pie should do it rationally, remembering that *rationing* and *rationality* come from the same root word, which means "reason." Rationing must be based on some sense of priorities, but, equally important, it must be rooted in some sense of fairness. There are many ways to ration care, but the worst way is to do it by default, so as to avoid accountability.

7. We are responsible for both identified and statistical lives. There is a profound difference between an individual who is known to us and the nameless and faceless masses whose plight is unimportant to us. An excellent recent example was in 1988, when, after the monumental effort to save two gray whales trapped in Alaskan ice, the government of Japan announced that its ships would not kill those two particular whales. Japan would continue to kill whales; it would just spare those two. We scoff at that hypocrisy; but the fact is that the identified life usually wins out over the statistical life in our country as well. This becomes more true as news media herald the celebrity of the moment, whether trapped whale or sick child.

Would we not be better off to rethink our neglect of the unnamed? Had the world been more sensitive to the plight of whales earlier on, those two whales would not have become so symbolic that everyone felt a moral compulsion to save them, because there were so few whales left. Similarly, if healthcare providers spent more time seeking coverage and support for early intervention and appropriate treatment for all, they would not have to agonize over which woman with preventable end-stage kidney disease would receive a transplant, once it is too late for less radical care. Statistical lives are no less valuable because we have not put names to them; after all, each of us is only a statistic to most of the world.

In addition, within the organization, the ethical executive must be a voice for the voiceless and unseen. That includes the lower-echelon employee, who may not be heard above the din of more articulate and powerful professions. Everyone in a healthcare organization—not just clinical caregivers, but also security guards, parking attendants, the folks in finance, dietary and housekeeping staff—is also a provider. How they are treated is reflected in how they behave with patients. And most patients see much more of the housekeeper than the CEO.

8. Embracing ethics may require taking risks. We glorify risk-taking in this country, and as a result, we sometimes gloss over the obvious: risk-taking behavior means going against the odds. Despite what we read in the literature of entrepreneurship, for every person who mortgaged his home to produce a better peanut butter and became a millionaire, there are a dozen people who mortgaged their homes to produce a better peanut butter and became homeless. Integrating ethics into a corporate culture is not always easy. To develop values through which pass the facts that become your judgments, and to stick to those values in the face of opposition, can be risky. Sometimes the risk lies in easy temptation, especially when it appears harmless, although it is still wrong. One must tread a narrow line between upright behavior and self-righteous behavior.

Sometimes the risk is in accepting the consequences of one's actions. The ability to understand and accept such consequences is the basis of the legal definition of competence; yet we all try to get away with things. And when we do get caught, it is difficult to accept our due with any kind of grace. Sometimes the risk is not in getting caught, but in *not* getting caught. Then we must live with ourselves, confessing our sins around the office or home,

irritating people who would really rather not hear about it. We often seek an informal confessional, when it would be a lot easier all around if we just turned ourselves in.

There are other risks—humiliation, moral discomfort, losing one's job. Perhaps the most useful knowledge one can have is that there are also risks associated with *not* doing the right thing. They are less obvious, and appear less frightful, but they can pack a wallop. Perhaps the greatest of these risks is the poisoning of the culture in which one works, of which we want to be proud. An ethical corporate culture cannot rest on cowardice.

A man named Utivich once said that education is the process of moving from cocksure ignorance to thoughtful uncertainty. That process is one of three elements necessary for a corporate culture that successfully integrates ethics. The other two are courage and creativity. Without courage, the effort is doomed, for ethics cannot permeate a culture in which leaders only act when it is safe to do so. Without creativity, we do not move ethics or corporate culture forward; we remain engrossed with reinventing the fire engine while Rome burns. In an era in which the ethics of providers, individual and organizational, face ever more questions and greater scrutiny, we no longer have the luxury of such inaction.

Chapter 18

Marginal Missions and Missionary Margins

Emily Friedman

Reprinted, with permission, from *Healthcare Forum Journal*, January/February, 1990, pp. 8–12. Published by The Healthcare Forum.

Emily Friedman is a healthcare writer, lecturer, and policy analyst based in Chicago. She is a regular columnist for the Healthcare Forum Journal.

It became one of the stock hospital phrases of the 1980s, having first been used (so legend has it) by the sisters who govern Catholic hospitals: "no margin, no mission." If the hospital cannot cover its costs and get a little bit ahead in order to have reserves, it cannot remain open, and its ability to fulfill its mission will, of necessity, be destroyed.

But the phrase moved beyond concerned religious orders to become a commonly used, and soon overused, capsule defense of hospital economic behavior. Today it is a glib—indeed, smug—rebuke to anyone who suggests that hospitals might not be doing all they can to husband the resources society has granted them.

It seems to me that a closer examination of the mission-margin relationship is in order, for three reasons. First, when the inspector general of the Department of Health and Human Services, assorted congressmen and senators, consumer advocates, and, increasingly, the press continue to suggest that hospitals are profiteering on Medicare and other programs, it behooves hospitals to respond with something more persuasive than dubious margin statistics and [a] perfunctory "no margin, no mission."

Second, the fact that some sort of margin is necessary, which few people would dispute, does not mean that any margin, no matter how inflated or how cruelly achieved, is automatically necessary and morally justified. Doing well is not necessarily the same as doing good. There is quite a spectrum between the need for a hospital to balance its books and the Machiavellian pursuit of the highest possible margin. Margin and mission are related, but to claim that the margin is the mission is to pervert the notion of mission.

Third, providers can no longer claim the high moral ground simply by virtue of being providers. This is a dearly held self-deception throughout healthcare; I am a doctor (or nurse, or hospital administrator, or HMO executive, or clinic director), and therefore anything I do is morally good because I am doing it. This delusion has allowed physicians to commit butchery, hospitals to engage in sociopathic behavior, and nurses to violate the rights of patients, without guilt. Similarly, hospitals like to think that anything they do in pursuit of their missions is automatically good, because their missions (which are defined in eloquent and high-minded language on a plaque in the lobby) are good. Whether its mission is relevant or appropriate to the community the hospital serves, and whether the mission is honored in a more than casual manner (if at all) is not important. It is the form, not the substance, that counts.

With American hospitals at a crossroads in terms of their future (including, in the eyes of some pessimists, the issue of whether they *have* a future), it is not sufficient to say, "I gotta have a margin because I must fulfill my wonderful mission, so give me more money and leave me alone." They will neither give you more money nor leave you alone. And it is entirely possible that they should not do either, because you may not deserve it.

Trappings of Charity

This change in public attitudes has been difficult for hospitals, because they have long worn the trappings of charity—the mission to serve the sick and the poor, the white cloak of voluntarism, the high principles of social service, the ivoried morality of science. And, to be fair, it is not entirely hospitals' fault that they still see themselves in this light. This was the light in which society saw them for a long time.

In her brilliant portrait of the American hospital in the 20th century (*In Sickness and in Wealth,* Basic Books, 1989), Professor Rosemary Stevens points out that hospitals today are still often seen as what they were at the beginning of the century: "institutions through which the moral values of American society are expressed." Americans still have great hope for the moral purity of their hospitals—on the social level, because these are great social institutions with a proud heritage, and on the individual level, because we are all potential patients, and we want to feel safe within their walls.

But if hell hath no fury like a woman scorned, a society scorned is a close runner-up. And society is beginning to think that the moral purity of hospitals ain't what it used to be (it probably never was what society thought it was, but that's another story). To a degree, this is a bum rap; as Professor Stevens also notes, it is unfair to encourage hospitals to behave like businesses, imbued with market mania and primed for cutthroat competition, and then to condemn them when they succeed in doing so. Nevertheless, hospitals were eager to undertake the role of hard-edged business enterprise, and very easily slid into the use of industrial terminology, marketing campaigns, and disdain for and avoidance of the poor, insured and uninsured alike.

The Tax Man

No sane observer could have truly believed that this embracing of mercenary attitudes would go unchallenged, and it has not. The tax man has responded with a simple and logical equation: Act like a business, pay taxes like a business. It is really quite sad that it has taken the Internal Revenue Service, certainly one of the most hated institutions in the country, to remind what were once some of the most beloved institutions in the country of what they are supposed to be about.

Government has played another key role in the confusion over margin and mission. In undertaking the subsidy of hospital care of virtually all the elderly and between one-third and one-half of those living in poverty, government seemed to obviate the need for broad charitable behavior on the part of hospitals.

In sparking this "death of charity," as Professor Stevens dubs it, government greatly lessened what had been seen as the primary charitable mission of hospitals: care of the poor and vulnerable. Then what were they supposed to do? It reminds me of the question asked by Henry James after Karl Marx alleged that God was dead: "What is the role of faith if there is no God to have faith in?"

Confused about which god to follow, hospitals fell in with bad company and embraced Mammon. Too often, mission became marginal, a set of knee-jerk phrases that could not be fulfilled—a discrepancy that went unnoticed because no one was trying to fulfill them. Likewise, in the absence of a mission to guide its use, the margin began to be spent in inappropriate ways. Far from being used in a missionary manner, margins were frittered away on risky new ventures, servicing of unnecessary debt, and bloated administrative overhead.

All this was a warning; but we do not always heed warnings. The development of the atomic bomb was code-named "Trinity." Years later, asked when talks on nuclear arms control should have begun, J. Robert Oppenheimer, the physicist who ran the project, said, "The day after Trinity." Similarly, discussion of the relationship of margin and mission should have begun 25 years ago, as Medicare appeared on the horizon and promised to change hospital financing forever.

Start The Discussion

Well, better late than never; let's start the discussion now, in every organization, *beginning on the board level.* Ownership is not an issue; public, volunteer, and proprietary organizations alike need to engage in this kind of introspection. Whether an organization pays taxes or not is an issue of tax status, not a measure of its commitment to mission or its right to a margin. I suggest the following thoughts to help frame the discussion.

Does the organization know what its losses and margin really are? I recently completed a study of hospital uncompensated care for the *Journal of the American Medical Association,* and my greatest frustration was the constant use of inflated figures for uncompensated care, based on billed charges (which virtually no one pays) and listed as "deductions from revenue." Hospitals also report two margins, one for patient care revenue and one for non-patient care revenue. This statistical sleight of hand is self-serving and vaguely dishonest; it is also unpersuasive evidence in the court of public opinion. Every organization should know how much it is making and losing, and should share that information openly and in an understandable way.

Margins involve both revenue and expense. One of the manifest ironies of the 1980s is that healthcare expenditures have increased more than 100 percent in this decade, and no one can really explain why. Even someone as notoriously pro-hospital as I cannot defend that rate of increase, especially when I see the massive architectural projects, the boutique services, the vice-presidential limousines, the lavish expense accounts, the advertising budgets, the estimated $25 billion going into the passive hands of stockholders, and the duplication, everywhere the duplication of services and technology. If an organization needs to increase its margin, it should ask itself whether the first sacrifices should be care of uninsured pregnant women — or the retreat and golf outing at the Ritz-Carlton.

Doing as little as possible is not mission fulfillment. Somewhere along the line, hospitals convinced themselves that if they fulfilled their Hill-Burton obligations, they were fully honoring their mission of serving the poor and downtrodden. However, charity and mission fulfillment are not simply what you can get away with. Minimum requirements are just that: minimal. They are floors, and should not become ceilings.

A social service mission extends beyond the self-interest of the organization. I once knew a cynic who explained the conservatism of foundations by saying, "The purpose of any foundation is to protect the assets of the foundation." Similarly, most hospitals believe the single most important issue in the mission-versus-margin debate is the survival of the organization: "We can't help anybody if we're closed." This assumes that every institution's survival represents an ethical good.

I would be the first to claim, with passion, that some needed hospitals have closed; I *know* that some needed hospitals have closed. But I would also be the first to claim that quite a few unnecessary hospitals are still around.

Despite institutional pride, tradition, the hospital-as-employer argument, and, often, community support, some hospitals could probably best fulfill their missions by closing and freeing up resources for other health and social services. To state unequivocally that the first loyalty of a healthcare organization must always be to itself is to state a highly questionable mission. I reminds me of the famous Vietnam War comment: "It was necessary to destroy the village in order to liberate it." If a healthcare organization purchases its survival at the price of its own honor or the community's health, then one must ask whom it thinks it is serving.

Any organization's mission is inextricably tied to the missions of its brethren. I find it amazing that at this point in the development of hospital consortia, alliances, and systems, the members of these organizations turn pale and gasp at the idea that the stronger ones should perhaps share resources with the weaker ones. I find it amazing that wealthy hospitals in affluent areas resist the notion that they owe something to the poor and the hospitals that serve them. Having fat reserves and big margins in upscale suburbs is not necessarily evidence of superb management; it may be evidence of market area. It should be apparent by now that either hospitals are going to voluntarily support each other (and yes, that includes the public hospitals), or government will force cross-subsidization.

Does the organization see itself as a vendor or as a charity? Professor Stevens argues that most hospitals play both roles. However, to claim to be a charity and to act only as a vendor is unacceptable. The organization has to know what it is, what it wants to be, and what its community wants it to be. Even if it cannot immediately fulfill all of its own and the community's expectations, the organization can at least give itself a star to shoot for.

Is the organization being honest about what it is and what it wants to do? I know of institutions with the usual pretty mission prose hanging on the wall whose CEOs say their real mission is to provide good care to the middle and upper classes. Period. I know of hospitals with little interest in serving the medically indigent; however, they pretend to care because they don't want it known that they do not care.

If you want to be strictly a business, without charitable pretension or intent, say so — and take the consequences. If you're afraid to do that, perhaps you should re-examine what you have chosen as goals. If you can't be proud of them, maybe you shouldn't be pursuing them. Mission cannot be a hidden agenda.

Are the uses to which the margin is put appropriate? The crux of the matter, of course, is the assumption that the margin that is obtained through effort, sacrifice, and brilliant management is carefully husbanded and used with innovation, conscience, and care. Is it? Too often, much of it is misspent. Or the margin is socked away, along with millions of dollars from previous years' margins, saved for a rainy day that somehow never comes, even as the infant mortality rate rises, the low-income elderly suffer, and epidemics eat their way through the poor. There never seems to be a need worthy of risking the accumulated funds.

It is precisely that attitude that got us into this mess. Too many hospitals made an inordinate amount of money, especially on Medicare, and then used it in questionable ways while access to care declined. Payers, unimpressed with how providers used their largesse, cut back to the point that many hospitals now are truly suffering. But as we blame the payers for their penury, let us remember that we squandered much of what we had, and now seem hypocritical in complaining that we are broke.

Delicate Equilibrium

The equilibrium between mission and margin will always be delicate. Some hospitals that have husbanded resources splendidly and served their communities generously and wisely will close. Some organizations that have been completely irrelevant since the day they started will prosper. Nevertheless, the best chance hospitals have to retain and/or reclaim the margins they need will be through meaningful, realistic missions that guide operations and budgeting. As Donald Berwick, MD has said: "no mission, no margin."

The poet Louis MacNeice once wrote a magnificent love poem, "Flowers in the Interval." I would like to borrow that thought. For all those hospitals that have been missionary in the use of their margins and resistant to the marginal mission: flowers to you all, until justice comes to healthcare. For those who think that margin is more important than mission, or that margin *is* mission: May you understand that you are not only failing yourselves; your failure may drag all that is good in healthcare down with you.

Chapter 19

Leprosy: A Disease of the Heart

Ralph Crawshaw, M.D.

Reprinted, with permission, from *JAMA* 248(5):573–76, Aug. 6, 1982. Copyright ©1982, American Medical Association.

Ralph Crawshaw, M.D., is in private practice, Portland, Oregon.

While in India last summer, I was invited by Dr Shubhada Pandya to join her at the Acworth Leprosy Hospital, Bombay, and then to accompany Dr R. Ganapati, a public health officer, on his rounds in Bombay's Dharavi slum.

The taxicab ride to Acworth Leprosy Hospital passes through some prosperous sections of Bombay, yet the ride, as in every city of the Far East, is a battering encounter with masses of people. In addition, the ride had the eerie quality of a submarine dream, for the drenching monsoon with its oppressive humidity had me soaked in my own sweat as I peered through the steamy, rain-streaked windows. The sidewalks were crowded with makeshift cardboard and plastic hovels that seemed like barnacles growing along the base of the buildings. The underwater effect was reinforced by the swirl of bicycles passing like schools of fish and clusters of umbrellas hopping up and down over curbs like scallops over a rough seabed.

The hospital itself did nothing to relieve the illusion of being underwater. It sat behind its dilapidated walls like some inundated ruin, complete with a wavering file of patients, some clutching children, some on crutches, some with torn pieces of plastic held over their bent cramped bodies, like a line of fiddler crabs limping and scurrying through the hospital's gate for shelter.

Inside the scarred two-story building, Dr Pandya greeted me. She is a youngish woman, slim in her white coat, who obviously does not spend afternoons over tea and pastry. Her penetrating gaze conveys a gentleness continually challenged by the violence of a world of intransigent disease. From her glowing dark eyes to her sandaled feet she is the picture of the focused intensity that uniquely marks the Indian intellectual. The formalities of greeting took but a moment, and we quickly moved through a series of rooms, meeting pharmacists, technicians, nurses, and fellow physicians, while she explained in the clipped accent of Indian English, "You must understand from the beginning that this disease is a socioeconomic one. Leprosy is on the increase in this country and should anyone tell you that it will be eliminated by the year 2000, poppycock! Our hospital treats 5,000 cases a year, and each day 250 new patients are seen, even though they may have been diagnosed elsewhere. All patients get treatment; in fact, the sulfones can be supplied for a patient in adequate doses at a cost of only 50 cents a year. However, it must be taken for a lifetime, and patient compliance here, as the world over, is a sometimes thing."

We made our way out a back door onto a sheltering veranda where a small group of men and boys were busy hammering and sawing, making chairs and desks. Dr Pandya explained that although they were not economically competitive, since it was a sheltered workshop, the state had agreed to buy the furniture made by patients with leprosy. However, as in all things connected with leprosy, arrangements are never easy. She had been unable to find anyone in the city of Bombay to supervise these young men, who in turn were reluctant to learn, since patients could make more in the established trades that support 80% of Bombay's patients with leprosy:

prostitution and bootlegging. Only a few dedicated patients stay long enough to become carpenters.

The rain had let up, so we stepped from beneath the dripping veranda for Dr Pandya to demonstrate the symptomatology of the young men in better light. "This lad has a rash over his lower arm and hand which could easily pass as impetigo, and yet he is in the infectious state. He has responded well to medication and if he sticks with it, the rash will subside and he will probably suffer no serious complications. Probably, that is, but only if he sticks with the medication and cares for himself. Remember, this is a socioeconomic disease. Once he is diagnosed as a leper he is fired from his job. The government punishes him for something he has not done. He is continually tempted to conceal his disease, both from his employer and himself, simply to make enough to eat." She directed my attention to an older man. "Here, look at the nodules around the ears. These are like the tubercles of tuberculosis, each loaded with Hansen's bacteria. With adequate treatment this will subside. We seldom see what was once the characteristic leonine face; disfigurements are not as prevalent as they used to be, though the disease is on the increase. Here is a claw hand," and she pointed out a man holding a chisel between two stumps of hands. "The ulnar nerve has been attacked. Notice how difficult it is for him to work, yet he works. The most important part of our work—and it seems like we never can accomplish it—is to have the patient learn to protect himself. He must not pick up anything hot; he must wear special shoes, but telling a patient to get special shoes is like telling him to buy a Rolls Royce. The disease causes the loss of pain fibers, so stepping on a nail, cutting a foot, or burning a finger goes unnoticed until a secondary infection produces the ulcers you smell when you enter the hospital." She called over an older man with leonine features. "Zemil has worked here for three years and is helping us teach carpentry. You see his nose has collapsed. The cartilage is gone. Incidentally, most of the transmission of leprosy is through the nose."

I asked her if she was not afraid of leprosy for herself. There was no question in my mind but that I was afraid of leprosy for me, as I hesitated to touch a patient or shake any hands even when proffered out of clean, white coats. She answered, "No, I know I've had leprosy. It's like tuberculosis. Most of us have had tuberculosis as a primary tuberculosis focus; the same is true of leprosy, a primary eruption. It is a matter of immunology, and so much of that is nutrition and as I say, this is a socioeconomic disease. It happens to the rich as well as the poor, but it happens mostly to the poor, and it will disfigure and destroy the poor who cannot protect themselves properly. Shoes, clothing, cleanliness, and food. Oh yes, I'm quite sure I've had leprosy."

We moved back to a room where female patients were being trained as seamstresses. Dr Pandya continued, "You see, if we can get our women to make any sum of money, just the least, they will immediately be taken back by their families. However, when they have no money to contribute to their families, they are forever outcasts. It really makes little difference whether they are lepers or not; it's whether they are adding to the family's food. Incidentally these sewing machines were given to us by a group of ladies who come regularly with a check, but you can be sure that once they give us the check, they never shake hands with anybody in the hospital and touch no one as they quickly leave. There are ancient feelings about leprosy which are unchanged today. Come, we'll go upstairs to the treatment clinic."

We made our way up a back stairway, through a crowded corridor—dark except for a lone neon tube flickering against the ceiling—and attempted to turn into a long room. In the doorway a knot of people had formed about a young doctor who was lecturing a dark-skinned, apathetic, youngish man. It was more an argument than consultation and after perfunctory introduction, the doctor turned back to the patient, explaining to me over his shoulder that the man had just been diagnosed as having Hansen's disease. "Look," he pointed to the butterflylike configuration of inflamed skin shaded ever so lightly redder than the rest of the man's face, but distinct once pointed out, "He is telling me that he doesn't want to come back to be treated, and he is in the infectious stage. He says that if he takes the treatment his employer will find out and he will no longer be able to support himself and his family. He has to protect his job, but his disease is sure to spread, not only to him but to his children. What is there to do? How loud should I shout at him to tell him that he has to come back?" He knew there was no answer and desperately, more to reassure himself than to inform me, abruptly changed the subject, "Look over here; we have some work at hand." Anxiously, he pointed out a vial of a newly developed vaccine. A nurse was injecting it into a row of patients. "We're doing everything we can to stimulate the immunologic response. It seems strange that some people are protected and others are not. We do not understand. It is not a simple thing by any means, because leprosy produces so many different reactions." When we turned back, his patient had slipped away and disappeared into the mass of flowing patients, crowding in and out of the doors.

As though in relief to the pervasive despair, Dr Pandya drew in a father and daughter for me to see. The short gray-haired father, in a Western three-piece suit and tie, had obviously come on important business, and his daughter, probably 16 years old, in a shimmering blue sari, stood sullenly beside him. He was elated, as Dr Pandya explained, "He thought his daughter had leprosy. See, look, this discoloration around the mouth, a loss of pigment, we see that at times, and I know it's not leprosy, and I told him so but he is having trouble believing.

Understand that in this country marriages are arranged, and if the woman is damaged — and there is no doubt that leprosy is a damage — it will be very difficult for her father to marry her off. You can see, he has trouble believing that such good fortune could happen to him, that his daughter does not have leprosy." The man's face was alternately lighting with smiles and darkening with frowns as he looked first to one and then another doctor, hoping that each and all would concur with him in beating down the fear that his beautiful daughter was damaged property.

"Come and see our dressing station," suggested Dr Pandya, and we elbowed our way into the center of the long room where a wall of half-open jalousies did nothing to relieve the stench of putrid flesh. Rows of disfigured patients seated on the long benches proclaimed the final stages of leprosy: arms missing, faces askew, hands clawed, stumps dripping pus from what was once an ankle. The floor was a litter of blood-soaked gauze and mud. "They are not infectious, probably; none of them are infectious at all, but they have lost most sensation in their bodies and secondary infection is killing them all," she remarked. As if in response to her attention a creature without name or shape detached itself from the line against the back wall and like some misbegotten error of evolution snaked toward me on its belly. It had neither ears nor a nose, and what had been a face was the color and consistency of burned meat surrounding a slobbering slit lined with broken teeth. It approached close enough to grab at me, with its claw alternately outstretched and pointing to the remnants of a leg, but Dr Pandya, staring the horror down, explained, "He is only trying to use you," which confirmed that it was a man, and that he was begging for a shoe to cover the stump of his left leg. "Money, money," he screamed, at least I presumed he said money, since his Hindi was unintelligible to me. But the pleading claw eloquently expressed his whole tale of filth, disease, and ignorance. He was begging for a share of my strength and knowledge. My blunt "No," turned him away cursing. No one took heed, for the other patients busily continued dressing their own wounds, searching among the piles on the floor for cleaner rags than the ones they had torn off. Behind me, he cursed again and again, but his cries eventually were lost in the turmoil.

Leading me downstairs and back to the entrance, Dr Pandya explained, "Now, I'll turn you over to Dr Ganapati who will take you into the field." As she spoke, an attendant rushed up with a note that caused her face to light up. "See, we are having some effect. Here is a referral from a doctor. For so long doctors have not even referred patients to us for treatment for leprosy," and then with a sobering second thought, "but perhaps it is that some doctors are willing to recognize leprosy now simply to rid their practice of lepers."

Dr Pandya pointed out the microbus. Thanking her, I climbed in, and met Dr Ganapati, who proved to be an unprepossessing middle-aged man, with a short-sleeved white shirt open at the neck, neat slacks, thick horn-rimmed glasses, receding hairline, and gray about the temples — the type of man who might have been class treasurer throughout medical school, collecting dues, yet never expecting and always surprised by any recognition of a lifetime devoted to hard work. As we lurched along, he shouted over the unmuffled roar of our microbus that we were headed for the Dharavi slums, where the Bombay Leprosy Project had one of its stations in case detection, treatment, and public education. The leprosy project, which is supported by funds from the German Leprosy Relief Society, is staffed by two doctors, 15 paraprofessionals, and a few support personnel. It focuses on the million people living in Bombay's wards "H" and "G." Today, we were delivering drugs and other supplies to the Dharavi middle school, where the principal had generously allowed the project to undertake a health survey.

Before we reached the turn-off, he explained that this slum was reputed to be one of the worst; the inhabitants lived in degradation, eating, sleeping, defecating, urinating, and copulating in the open. The dangers for children are fierce; many drown in open septic tanks, while the most common source of child abuse and murder are frantic mothers who break into uncontrollable fury at the unrelieved cries of their starving children and beat them, sometimes to death.

Unexpectedly, we veered off the viaduct onto a side road that became a byway straggling down to a lane, which contracted to a passageway barely wide enough to allow our microvan to squeeze through as it rubbed against improvised shops and splashed the bystanders with the filthy mud of the Dharavi. Up close, poverty is a gigantic, socially propelled slime mold, without form, yet an inexorable force that defiles everything it touches with malignant degeneration. Poverty's essence is trash, and with the exception of a very few faces lighted with dignity despite a life of suffering, everything else in the slum was broken, torn, marred, grimy, and filthy. There are not even rocks as such, for a rock would have had wet moss or at least some surface of clean rain-washed sheen. Everything was besmirched, mismatched, or worn: pieces of glass, rusted cans, piles of offal, garbage, shattered barrels, crushed plastic bottles, sickly chickens, thin pigs looking to eat the chickens, small, weak children, shreds of human beings, yet beating the pigs with sticks. Everywhere a trash of expressions: scowls, threatening stares, disgust, and surprised hostility at the presence of an invading "European." As though expressing the ultimate example of trash, a garbage pile was pointed out in which a live, discarded baby had been uncovered the week before.

Slowly we made our way to the school, which could be heard before it was seen, since this one massive building in the Dharavi was filled to bursting with screaming students (school attendance is discouraged, since there are more children than seats and a high dropout rate—which might better be called a forceout rate—is necessary). It was filled to overflowing with a trash of discordant noise.

Dr Ganapati led me up to the roof and then to the final crest of the water tank, from which the rusty tin roofs and infinite squalor of the Dharavi could be seen in every direction. Directly below a woman was squatting, defecating, at the edge of the school way. Further off, the people were less distinct, and Dr Ganapati pointed our [out] narrow chimneys belching steam and smoke, explaining that these illicit distilleries were the main support of the people.

Convinced that I had had the broad view, Dr Ganapati led me back down the ladder of the water tower, through the door, down the stairway, to an airless room on the third floor—Bombay Leprosy Project's station. The windows were closed to lessen the piercing racket of the classes. The doctor gave me a "close" view of the project, complete with slides—again, photographs of leprosy and, inadvertently, a picture of a physician who is fighting leprosy. When one slide announced "leprosy can be cured," I did not confront the doctor with my doubts. Perhaps it may be arrested, but it cannot be cured, particularly as it is a socioeconomic disease. The doctor accentuated repeatedly the paradox of Hansen's disease, the undamaged infectious nose disseminates, while the disfigured but noninfectious face repels; the carrier easily passes in society as simply having scabies or an innocuous red rash, while the burned-out noninfectious patient causes the people to shrink. Slide after slide, some showing how symptoms can be contained, some showing how prevention can work; statistics showing how the sheer mass of people makes contagion inevitable. It is madness to think the disease can be eliminated by the year 2000. If I needed convincing, which I did not, the slide showing the yearly incidence of new cases—55 a year—among children in the school we sat in was the clincher.

When the lecture ended, we made our way out of the school, and our talk turned to the role of the medical profession in fighting leprosy. Dr Ganapati's voice, although not penetrating, had a clarity of understated conviction that carried through rather than over the turmoil. "I do not hold it against medical students who seek to become surgeons. They are taken up with the glamour of the specialty and realistically want to enter a field where they can make money. Like it or not, medical schools teach what is important to a successful career. A bright student does not take long to see where the profession gives recognition and know that with the recognition goes freedom from the insecurity of living on state budgets which are always endangered by political whim. No, I can understand why medical students are not attracted to working with a disease that lacks glamor and continually threatens your own health."

His explanation continued as our bus moved out of the Dharavi and into the wider streets of Bombay, but my eyes were open to a different matter, for when the bus stopped at an intersection, or a traffic light, and I saw those countless hands shoved in through the half-open window—the begging hands of children and adults, all imploring money—I was now alert to the leper's claw, the subtle rash of Hansen's disease, and the meaning of stumps for fingers. Despite this distraction, I listened closely to the doctor, trying hard to understand his forgiveness of medical students, hoping it included traveling physicians such as myself.

The microbus eventually wended its way back to my five-star hotel. I gratefully thanked my guide and the driver, who cheerfully waved me up the marble steps as the doorman, a formidable uniformed Sikh, threw open the door to my immaculate, air-conditioned palace. I turned to wave back only to see them submerging into the flow of traffic milling about the "Gateway of India." Few would question why I immediately made for the hotel pharmacy to purchase a bottle of methyl alcohol. The bored clerk informed me that medicinal alcohol was illegal in India; however, when I explained I had just returned from a leprosy hospital and wanted to disinfect my camera and myself, he instantaneously called the manager and after considerable rummaging the two of them produced a bottle of Listerine. I said, "No thanks," and went to my room, where I removed my shoes before entering. Balancing my camera carefully on the edge of the bathroom sink, I stripped naked, rolled all my clothes into a tight bundle, placed them in a plastic laundry bag, and plunged beneath a hot, soapy shower, where I remained for 30 minutes.

Once my body was cleansed as only a scrubbing with soap and hot water can do, I slipped into a fresh robe, retired to the sitting room of my suite, and in the silence of the dark room, I slumped into a large chair, chin on chest, arms splayed, staring straight ahead into the cool shaded dimness, the picture of a defeated Roman general sorting through a lost campaign. All I had were thoughts, thoughts to be arranged and rearranged and rearranged yet again, until at last the diagnosis of leprosy, that grim socioeconomic disease, would make sense to me.

What did I think? I thought my eye sharp enough to see the lesions, the loss of pigment, the fine macular quality of the infected skin, the nodules around the ears that would never again go unrecognized by me, but those were niggardly clinician's thoughts. What did I think? I thought it curious that there is no physical pain connected with this disease. There is no squeezing chill or overbearing fever as in malaria, just the faintest touch—so easily denied—of dread death. What a strange psychology for an illness. Diabolically, leprosy preserves the illusion of health by destroying the pain fibers that lead to the brain. Only those fibers that run to the heart remain intact. The pain of leprosy originates in the eye of the beholder and becomes pain for the patient as he is shunned and ostracized, as he loses the humanness he once possessed. The pain of leprosy is not inflicted by the bacillus but by his fellow man. And I knew not what to make of this.

A terrible equation appeared before my eyes. If I am a human being and patients with leprosy are human beings, we are of the same flesh, therefore some part of me is a leper. Gradually, I realized I had become one with the perverse disease. I had it in my heart. Had I not, as a priest of science, spent the day cutting the hearts out of a thousand people, cutting them out just as surely and deftly as an Aztec priest standing on the heights of his holy pyramid? Had I not been holding a thousand hearts as far as I could from my own, using all my clinical skill to see them as parts of human beings, as less than human beings, as fascinating specimens? Had I not committed the most despicable sin of a physician, silently reserving myself to myself and denying what compassion I might have, holding back from the profferred hand of a patient in need? Had I not told myself, the whole day through, that when night fell I would leave the leper's hell, as when a medical student, I had left the body on the anatomy table, left the slide of syphilitic tissue beneath the microscope, had left the caged rats in the physiology labora-tory, left them to enjoy myself in the living world. Had I not contracted leprosy in the very act of fending it off? My heart felt weak.

What to do? How can I act as a physician now that I saw leprosy for what it is? I had asked Dr Pandya if there was anything I could do. She had hesitated a moment, as though a bit embarrassed and said, "I know you are from the States and you said your wife is meeting you by way of Hawaii. Should she go to Molokai, I would appreciate a picture of Father Damien's grave. I know they dug up that leper's body and shipped it back to Europe, but I believe his heart is still there. If you could get me a snapshot of his grave—it doesn't have to be in color—it would help."

And there it was—I could do something, but I could do nothing. I could do nothing directly to relieve the lepers of Bombay, but I could recognize that there are some who do help. There are some, very few, who touch the spirit of mankind as deeply as leprosy repels it. Perhaps there is a cure for leprosy, but it will only come from those few who have the heart to be greater than the disease. As though released by that flash of belief, a great sob welled from within me, and almost as though I would wash my spirit as I had washed my body, I found myself crying, and I cried, and cried, and cried, and cried. Leprosy is truly a disease of the heart.

Part V

The Practice of Bioethics

Until recently, bioethics was such a new field that there were few, if any, parameters or standards for its practice; most of the rules were made up as ethics committees and ethics counselors went along. Slowly, a body of experience was compiled that has produced, if not standards, then at least models—good and bad—that others could emulate or avoid. Now, also slowly, bioethics is beginning to examine its own practices.

In this section, Renée C. Fox, Ph.D., and Judith P. Swazey, Ph.D., challenge the individualistic focus of much of bioethics, arguing that favoring the individual has trivialized or even ignored equally important questions of social ethics and communitarian values. In a series of articles and letters, George Annas, J.D., Barbara Mishkin, J.D., and George Washington University Hospital provide a case study of a deeply troubling patient care incident, the litigation it spawned, the ultimate legal resolution, and the revised patient care procedures that resulted. William Nelson, Ph.D., and Andrew Pomerantz, M.D., examine the practice of bioethics in rural settings, including common problems and their possible remedies. And Donald F. Phillips chronicles the community health decisions movement, its origins, its accomplishments to date, and why it has been so successful.

Chapter 20

Medical Morality Is Not Bioethics—
Medical Ethics in China and the United States

Renée C. Fox, Ph.D., and Judith P. Swazey, Ph.D.

An earlier version of this paper was presented by Renée C. Fox as the Fae Golden Kass Lecture at Harvard Medical School and Radcliffe College, February 22, 1983. The authors are indebted to Judith Berling and David Smith, Indiana University; James Gustafson, University of Chicago; and Willy De Craemer, Setha Low, and Nathan Sivin, University of Pennsylvania, for their critical reading of the manuscript.

Renée C. Fox, Ph.D., is Annenberg Professor of the Social Sciences, University of Pennsylvania, Philadelphia. Judith P. Swazey, Ph.D., is president of the College of the Atlantic, Bar Harbor, Maine.

Confiants dans les "lumières de la raison naturelle" . . . ils n'ont pas vu qu'ils étaient en présence d'une conception du monde et de modes de pensée fondamentalement différents des leurs et que ces modes de pensée étaient en rapport avec la morale, les attitudes religieuses, l'ordre social et politique des Chinois.[a,1]

Drawing in part on a medical sociological journey that we made to the People's Republic of China in 1981, this paper examines what the Chinese call "medical morality": the form currently taken by medical ethical interest

and activity in their society. But our reason for having explored and written about medical morality is not confined to things Chinese. Another primary goal has been to obtain some cultural perspective on what we in the United States term "bioethics." Bioethics is the neologism coined in this country in the 1960s to refer to the rise of professional and public interest in moral, social, and religious issues connected with the "new biology" and medicine and to the emergence of an interdisciplinary field of inquiry and action concerned with these issues. Medical morality not only exemplifies the at-once ancient and contemporaneous "Chinese-ness" of Chinese medical ethics. Seen in a comparative framework, it also helps to illuminate what is characteristically Western about "our" bioethics and highlights some of the ways that it is specifically American.

Our title—"Medical Morality Is Not Bioethics"—is a rather mischievous one. It was provoked by an article, "Bioethics in the People's Republic of China," that we read before we went to China in 1981 and reread upon our return.[2] It is a "traveller's report" written by a professor of the philosophy of medicine, on behalf of a group of prominent bioethicists (mainly associated with the Kennedy Institute of Ethics, Georgetown University) who made a 2-week-long trip to China in 1979. In his report, H. Tristram Engelhardt attributes solely to Maoism-Leninism-Marxism what he loosely terms the "moral viewpoint" of the Chinese scientists, professionals, and intellectuals with whom he and his companions discussed questions of medical ethics. No allusion is made to possible Confucian, Taoist, or Buddhist origins of what the Chinese define as ethical matters or of how they think

Renée C. Fox, Ph.D., and Judith P. Swazey, Ph.D.

about them. Instead, Engelhardt expresses puzzlement over what he experienced as the "resistance" of his Chinese interlocutors to "intellectually justifying" their moral outlook within the framework that he considers properly and logically philosophical.

In this regard, Engelhardt's reaction resembles that of the first Christian missionaries who lived and worked in China in the late sixteenth and early seventeenth centuries, and who assumed that the Chinese "do not have logic." Even the most culturally learned and responsive of the Jesuit missionaries, Father Matteo Ricci, did not fully recognize that his Scholastic notion of Reason was not universal or that the Chinese also reasoned systematically within their own internally consistent modes of thought [Gernet, p. 327 et passim[1]].

Engelhardt's failure to discern the pattern and logic of today's Chinese thought is related to the inadvertent ethnocentricity of the implicit premises on which his article rests. Bioethics, particularly its philosophical aspects, is viewed as largely *a*cultural and *trans*cultural in nature. The author does not seem to appreciate the extent to which the way that he and his fellow voyagers reason about ethics is imprinted with Western and American cultural influences. Furthermore, he, his colleagues, and the editors of the *Hastings Center Report* who allowed him to retain the title of his article took it for granted that bioethics is a sufficiently neutral and universalistic term for it to be applied to medical morality in China or, for that matter, to medical ethical concern in whatever society or form it may now occur.

This kind of cultural myopia disturbs us. Such myopia is not confined to those occasions when American bioethicists venture forth to other lands. Rather, it is a more widespread characteristic of the field of bioethics, one that generally manifests itself in the form of systematic inattention to the social and cultural sources and implications of its own thought.

We consider this cultural nearsightedness, with its implied distortion of vision, to be serious because, from a sociological viewpoint, bioethics is not just bioethics. What we mean by this is that, using biology and medicine as a metaphorical language and a symbolic medium, bioethics deals in public spheres and in more private domains with nothing less than beliefs, values, and norms that are basic to our society, its cultural tradition, and its collective conscience. If this is indeed the case, we have reason to be concerned when bioethicists ignore or misperceive the social and cultural matrices of their ideas.

Introduction to Chinese Medical Morality

In the summer of 1981, we spent 6 weeks doing medical sociology fieldwork in the People's Republic of China, primarily in the city of Tianjin. Our trip was arranged by the program of scientific exchanges created by the American Association for the Advancement of Science in Washington, D.C., and the China Association of Science and Technology (CAST) in Beijing. The focal point of our work was a miniethnographic study of a profoundly Chinese urban hospital that is energetically committed to modern scientific and technological medicine. (With characteristically ironic but affectionate wit, the nurses and physicians of Tianjin First Central Hospital, where we did our research, continually referred to us as "the 'Team of Two,' rather than the 'Gang of Four.' ")

The hospital that our Chinese colleagues chose as the base for our research and teaching proved to be the center of medical modernization that we had asked to study—and more. It contained the only freestanding Critical Care Unit in China,[3] conducted hemodialysis for acute renal failure, included a bioengineering-oriented absorbent artificial kidney group, and had made some forays into the transplantation of human organs. It was also highly active in matters pertaining to our work in medical ethics—an interest which we had not thought of pursuing in a Chinese setting.

In retrospect, it seems far from accidental that the hospital we were sent to turned out to be as notable for its leadership in what the Chinese term medical morality as in the "fourth modernization" of (medical) science and technology. We soon learned that the First Central Hospital's intensive involvement in medical ethics was partly due to the influence of its vice-director, Madame She Yun-zhu, a remarkable 75-year-old woman who is one of the pioneers of modern nursing in China. "Grandmother-Nurse," as she is respectfully and fondly called, personifies the indissoluble bond that she believes exists between the observance of certain ethical principles, virtues, and rules, and the achievement of greater technical excellence, humanity, and commitment to service, in nursing and in medicine.

But even without the dynamic presence of Madame She, we probably would have been introduced to medical morality as representatives of what our Chinese colleagues conceived to be medical sociology and expected from it—albeit in a somewhat more tentatively conceptualized and less vigorously uplifting way. For, in a number of medical and nursing schools that we visited or about which we were told, first steps were being taken to develop courses that were alternately called "Medical Sociology," "Medical Psychology," and/or "Medicine, Morals, and Society." As the last course title suggests, in China, medical sociology and medical ethics are not only interrelated— they are virtually synonymous. Social relationships and a conception of what one of our hosts termed "the individual as a social community" are at the heart of what the Chinese have always defined as ethics. And ethics is the center of the Chinese world view—its very core and essence in Chinese society today as it has been for thousands of years. What is more, participant observation—which the Chinese recognized as a guiding principle as well as a major technique of our research—is also inherent to their own inductive, humanistic approach to ethics. For them, thinking in an entirely abstract or speculative way about moral or social questions runs the risk of what Chinese scholars historically have called "playing with emptiness." What seems to them more "practical" and "right," as well as comfortably familiar, is to work from everyday, empirically observable human reality, focusing particularly on the relationship between specific, identifiable persons, and on their "lived-in," reciprocal existence.

It was both surprising and satisfying to learn in a first-hand way that, despite the thousands of geographical miles and historical years that separate Chinese society and our own, and their very different cosmic outlooks, these aspects of Chinese thought are compatible with the conceptual and methodological framework in which we observe, analyze, interpret, and evaluate as sociologists. It was also unsettling to feel that (although cross-cultural resemblances can be very deceiving), in these particular respects, we might have more in common with Chinese than with many American colleagues in medical ethics. For, as we will subsequently show, it is the individual, seen as an autonomous, self-determining entity rather than in relationship to significant others, that is the starting point and the foundation stone of American bioethics. Herein lie some of the deepest intellectual and philosophical difficulties that we have experienced as two of the relatively few social scientists who have been professionally associated with bioethics since its inception.

The Components of Medical Morality

Medical morality is "the kind of morality that doctors and nurses should have." It is concerned with three sets of interconnected goals and with the obligation of "medical workers," individually and collectively, to do everything possible—"sparing no effort"—to attain these goals. Repairing the moral and intellectual as well as the economic and political damage of the Cultural Revolution (1966–1976) is one of the primary objectives of medical morality. Supreme importance is given to restoring the basic "order" that was "smashed" by the Cultural Revolution (and its personification in the Gang of Four): the "task of straightening things out in every field of [medical] work" that must be accomplished, especially the reteaching of "what is right and wrong." A second basic aim of medical morality is to "scale the heights" of modern medicine and thereby achieve the "golden-dream" benefits that come from applying advanced science and technology to problems of health, illness, and the care of patients. This is the medical facet of the national policy of "Four Modernizations" (agriculture, industry, defense, science and

technology) that currently prevails in China. In turn, "order" and "modernization" are part of the third general goal of medical morality: the dynamic and creative continuation of the "Great Liberation," the revolution that established the People's Republic of China in 1949.

As this implies, medical morality fits into a larger societal frame. "Work ethics" and "civic virtues" and their relationship to the integrity and development of the whole society are constantly stressed, ideologically and politically, in every sphere of Chinese life. Nationwide campaigns like the civic virtues month and the *Wujiang Simei* ("Five Efforts" and "Four Beauties") movement have been organized around these themes. Workers of all kinds are continually reminded that they are expected to pay attention to morality. Medical workers are among those who have special ethical responsibilities because their job is to care for patients, "relieve them from pain," help them to recover from their illnesses, and "save them from death." Leading nurses and doctors, in particular, are exhorted to demonstrate "the highest level of ethics" in their own behavior—to be "the first to observe the principles and disciplines" entailed—and thereby to set an example that is "a silent order" to those who work with them.

Medical morality is rooted in a conception of the individual in relation to statuses and roles, enmeshed in the network of human relationships that this involves. In this conception, the individual steadfastly strives to meet his responsibilities and carry out his duties ever more totally and perfectly, guided by certain principles, inspired by particular maxims and exemplars, and in conformity with concrete rules. At the vital center of this morality is the continuous effort that each person is expected to make to perfect his at-once individual and social self through relationships to significant others and the fulfillment of obligations to these persons. The relationships encompassed by medical morality include those of physicians, nurses, other medical workers, and hospital administrators with each other and with patients and their families. It also concerns the relations between the unit or *danwei*[4] to which medical workers belong and the local bureaucrats and Communist party officials associated with their professional activities. The bedrock and point of departure of medical morality lie in the quality of these human relationships: in how correct, respectful, harmonious, complementary, and reciprocal they are. Here, for example, is the way that Madame She Yun-zhu expresses some of these "relationship" aspects of medical morality in the set of "Requirements for Training Quality Nursing" that she drafted: "Do a good job in building close relationships among physicians, nurses, and patients. Be good at uniting your colleagues to work together. Unite not only those who share your point of view, but particularly those who have different opinions from you. . . . Appoint people on their merits. Treat colleagues equally." In this series of ordered and interconnected relationships that medicine entails (as Madame She goes on to articulate), it is the relations to the patient that have the highest moral status and importance: "Serve the patient whole-heartedly. . . . Put the interests of the patient first all the time. . . . Try to build deep proletarian affection with the patient. Think what the patient thinks, be as eager as the patient is, and be as worried as the patient feels. . . . We should treat our patients as our sisters and brothers. . . . Treat the patient even better than your relatives."

The development and enactment of good moral character, attitudes, and thoughts, and of exemplary professional conduct, are embedded in this skein of relationships and contingent on the way they are handled by medical workers. Scientific knowledge and technical skill are considered to be important ethical as well as intellectual components of excellent medicine. They are morally mandatory. But medical morality and its attainment require more. In the words of Dr. Wang Chin-ta (director of the Critical Care Unit of Tianjin First Central Hospital): "No matter how good doctors and nurses are technically, if they do not have noble thinking, they cannot serve the patient, the people, and the country."

"Noble thinking" is an epigrammatic way of referring to the moral virtues that good medical professionals are ideally expected to demonstrate in their work and work relations. Foremost among these medically relevant virtues are the following:[b]

> Humanity, compassion, kindness, helpfulness to others;
> Trust in others;
> A spirit of self-sacrifice;
> A high sense of responsibility;
> A good sense of discipline, good order;
> Hard, conscientious work that is also systematic, careful, precise, punctual, and prudent;
> Devotion, dynamic commitment;
> Courage to think, act, innovate, blaze new trails, overcome difficulties;
> Alertness, high spirits, optimism, a positive attitude;
> Patience;
> Modesty;
> Self-control, a sense of balance and equilibrium;
> Politeness, good manners, proper behavior;
> Cleanliness, tidiness, good hygiene, keeping healthy;
> Lucidity, clarity, intelligence, wisdom;
> Honesty, integrity;
> Self-knowledge, self-examination, self-criticism, self-cultivation, self-improvement;
> Frankness about difficulties, limitations, shortcomings, and mistakes—admitting them, and working to overcome them.

Seen as a whole, these virtues have a number of patterned characteristics. They are relatively concrete ethical qualities, close to the empirical reality of medical practice and patient care. They are formulated as responsibilities and duties, generally stated as positive "musts" and "can do's," rather than as admonitory "must nots" and "do nots." They are punctuated by aphorisms and proverb-like political slogans. A "we shall overcome" moralistic optimism pervades the outlook that they represent. But seen in closer detail, the dynamic nature of these moral virtues is a product of the balancing and blending of the active and passive, traditional and innovative, intellectual and emotional, personal and interpersonal, individual and collective qualities that their fulfillment requires. They are as neo-Confucian as they are Maoist, and more of both than they are Marxist or Leninist.

Particular individuals are singled out because they personify the virtues of medical morality. They are considered to be models whose "example will inspire and encourage others to follow them." At Tianjin First Central Hospital and in the Chinese nursing profession at large, Madame She—"Grandmother-Nurse"—is considered to be such a model. She is esteemed for her pioneering contribution to the establishment and development of modern nursing in China and its rehabilitation after the Cultural Revolution; for her role as "Teacher" (with the ethical as well as intellectual connotations that the term carries in Chinese); and for her unwavering, lifelong commitment to nursing and to improving its quality (even when, at age 62, during the Cultural Revolution, she was sent to the countryside for 9 years of "reeducation"). Other valued qualities are her hard, "independent and loyal work"; the "strict demands" she makes on herself and her staff and her "strict sense of responsibility"; and her "concern for the pain and suffering of patients." Madame She is also recognized for her "obedience to rules and regulations" while "breaking the traditional frame of mind" sufficiently to generate "new ideas"; for her energy and optimism, courage and resiliency; and for her capacity for self-criticism and self-improvement.

One of Madame She's closest younger colleagues, Meng Bao-zhen, the hospital's vice-director of nursing, is another such morally emblematic figure. She is often called *Doctor* Meng by the nurses and physicians with whom she works, because during the Cultural Revolution she became a physician and practiced medicine in Inner Mongolia for 9 years. Meng was chosen as "Model Worker" of her province in 1974, for which she was awarded a medal and a special diploma by the Committee of Inner Mongolia. In 1979, she was called back to Tianjin and First Central Hospital to help "reconstruct" its nursing. She willingly rebecame a nurse to do so, and it is for this, as much as for her self-sacrificing ardor and "revolutionary humanism" in Inner Mongolia, that she is seen as outstandingly virtuous.

But in keeping with the virtues of modesty, candid self-criticism, and generosity toward others, both Grandmother-Nurse She and Nurse-Doctor Meng insist that they "have not done so much in the First Central Hospital . . . only what our duty required us to do." They cite still another colleague, Guan Xiao-ying, the director of nursing, as a person whose heroic medical morality surpasses their own (letter from Madame She to the authors, March 27, 1982):

. . . It has been only more than three years since we came back from the countryside. We couldn't do much work in such a short period of time. Most work was done by Guan Xiao-ying, the director of the nursing department, and nine middle-aged supervisors who have both ability and political integrity, and thirty-four head nurses. They led over three hundred nurses fulfilling the task of straightening things out in every field of work.

I want to say something about Guan Xiao-ying. She is 53 years old and suffers from coronary disease. She is rich in clinical experience in [a] career of 30 years. She loves her work and usually works 12 hours a day. Really, she takes the hospital as her own home, even pays more attention to her work than to her family. During the period when her husband suffered from cancer, we could still find her working in her post. Compared with her, we still fall far behind.

In the particular settings where nurses, physicians, and their coworkers carry out their medical duties, the principles and virtues of medical morality are translated into specific sets of rules. The ethical importance of these rules is aesthetically expressed through the high quality of their calligraphy, the care with which they are framed, and the prominence with which they are displayed. Here, for example, are the rules of the Critical Care Unit of Tianjin First Central Hospital. Composed by the members of the unit out of their shared experiences, they are written in elegant black script under the title, "Regulations of the Critical Care Unit," which is written in contrasting red ink. Enclosed in an ornate green frame, they hang alone on a wall adjacent to the unit's doorway. The nine sets of regulations are explicit and detailed statements of the unit's work norms, and also of the problematic attitudes and behaviors—the persistent "shortcomings" at work—that have been identified as needing improvement:

1. Patients in this room need critical care. When they are better, they should be transferred to the recovery ward.
2. Care should be given to these patients day and night.

3. The work should be done strictly by the medical workers. They should cooperate. In these ways, they will be able to serve the people wholeheartedly.
4. Medical workers must check the equipment, drugs, and machines on every shift, e.g., ventilator, EKG, tracheal tubes, IV, catheters, abdominal dialyzer, suction, extension cord. Everything must be kept in its place. Do not lend things out.
5. Adhere strictly to regulations. Visiting doctors should make rounds twice a day, in the morning and in the afternoon. Doctors on duty should carefully observe the patients. They should make careful observations at the bedside in order to discover any developments, and be prepared to give emergency treatment if necessary.
6. The staff on one shift should tell the staff on the next shift about any changes that have taken place with the patients. Explain things clearly for continuing with the next shift.
7. For emergency treatment, use Western and Chinese medicine together. There are four principles to follow in administering Chinese medicine—four things that must be done in time:
   a. Prescription;
   b. Fetching of drugs;
   c. Cooking of prescription;
   d. Administering of prescription.
8. Check regulations, and carry them out strictly, in time. Carry out the doctor's orders, to do well and avoid complications.
9. Perform a case history in time.

The First Central Hospital's various sets of rules, regulations, and requirements are now being organized into a centralized system of total quality control (called TQC) under the direction of the hospital's medical administration office and the Party dialectician who is attached to it. The TQC is an elaborate moral accountancy system, designed principally to apply to nurses and doctors and to raise the overall level of medical care. One of its major features is a "shortcomings control" classification scheme which identifies and categorizes various kinds of "technical" and "responsibility" errors and mistakes that physicians and nurses can make in giving care. It then attaches quantitative weights to them according to how major or minor they are considered to be. "Responsibility shortcomings" are viewed largely as moral errors. They are therefore defined as more grave than are shortcomings judged to be primarily technical in nature and are correspondingly subject to more severe penalties and punishments. Eventually, First Central Hospital hopes to translate the variables of its TQC system into a computer program for calculating individual and group "medical quality scores" in a sophisticated, modern way. The hospital regards the computer not only as an important technological tool in this effort but also as a powerful empirical and symbolic expression of the medical modernization toward which it strives.

Medical morality, with its goals, principles, virtues, rules, and human exemplars, plays an important role in the continuous process of "walking on two legs," a process that dynamically shapes and reshapes the orientation of the whole society [Fox, pp. 700–701[3]]:

> A chain of dualities is involved: an intricate balancing of modern Western and traditional Chinese medicine, community public health and individual patient care, central control and institutional autonomy, preventive and curative medicine, primary and tertiary care, acute and chronic illness, rural and urban needs, mental and manual labor, being "Red" and being "expert," proletarianism and elitism, the old and the new, and the balancing of ideas and resources imported from abroad and "made in China." A series of dilemmas . . . are contained in these dualities. Societal precepts constantly shift concerning how the dilemmas ideally should be resolved and what combination of binary elements and states of equilibrium between them this implies. Proper "two-leggedness" in the medical as in all spheres of Chinese society is not only defined and monitored but repeatedly altered by the flow of minor and major national policy directives that emanate from the political leadership in Beijing. In part, these fluctuations in policy are transforming consequences of the interaction between still another set of basic dualities: the canons of Communist Party doctrine and the dictates of Chinese pragmatism.

The "Chinese-ness" of Medical Morality

Nothing could more fundamentally epitomize the profound Chinese-ness of medical morality than the kind of two-legged dualism that underlies it. What it entails is an essentially yin-yang relationship between opposed but complementary opposites. They are the constituent elements and the dynamic force in a moving equilibrium that is continually established and reestablished through their interaction.

The same Chinese principle of dynamic complementarity is also basic to the view of the relationship between self and others, and the individual and society, in which medical morality is grounded. In this view, what it is to be a person and what it is to be in relationship to other persons complete each other and form part of a larger, vital whole.

The central status that medical morality attaches to the primary ethical importance of fulfilling one's duties to specified others in commonplace settings and in everyday acts, and to the continual improvement and perfecting of self in and through these relations and duties, is also anciently and quintessentially Chinese. These are core ideas in the traditional morality: of how striving to perfect one's individual and social being expresses the principle of immanent order in the cosmos and contributes to a society that embodies it.

The "noble" ethical virtues emphasized by medical morality are also closely related to the Confucian virtues that structured the ongoing ethical effort required by traditional Chinese morality (*ren* [humanity], *li* [sense of rites], *yi* [sense of duties], *zhi* [wisdom]). Rules were one of the principal forms in which these ethical obligations were made explicit, as is the case with medical morality. In China's past, they were often developed out of the group experience of a guild or a clan and were posted in temples, clan halls, and schools in a manner comparable to the way that medical morality rules are currently displayed in First Central Hospital.

The stylistic features and ambience of medical morality—with its emphasis on orthodoxy, righteousness, and propriety, its concern about "moral sympathy," its stress on the power of didacticism, its ritualization and bureaucratization, and its preeminently public nature—all have their counterparts and origins in Chinese tradition.

Tianjin First Central Hospital's TQC system has significant antecedents in Chinese history and tradition. It could be said that ancestral versions of TQC existed in the "morality books" (*shanshu*) and the "ledgers of merit and demerit" (*gongguoge*) that were kept by individuals and families in the sixteenth- and early seventeenth-century years of China's Ming dynasty [Gernet, pp. 193–196,197[5]]. These were moral account books, based on the self-examination of conscience, the written confession of wrongdoing, and the recording of both good and bad thoughts and acts. Not only were thoughts and deeds morally classified in this positive and negative way, but they were sometimes weighted by a point system. In some ledgers, good points were recorded in red ink, bad ones in black ink. (Since at least the time of the Han dynasty, red had been the color of positive numbers and black of negative ones.) At periodic intervals, the person keeping this moral audit added up the points, thereby arriving at a quantitative score of his current state of ethicality and his cumulated "moral capital." Sinologists identify Taoist and Buddhist influences in these morality books, including concepts of judgments meted out by a "cosmic bureaucracy" that involved one's present life, life span, and rebirth.[6]

This is not to imply that medical morality is a pure emanation of Confucianism, Taoism, and Chinese Buddhism, or that Marxism-Leninism-Maoism has played a negligible role in shaping its form and content. Certain precepts of medical morality constitute radical departures from the concepts on which the traditional system of Chinese ethics was built. Most notable are the ways in which the egalitarian and universalistic principles of Marxism have strongly influenced the tenets of medical morality. Doctors and nurses are urged to unite, to work closely together professionally and "transprofessionally," and to treat colleagues equally. This egalitarian view runs counter to the traditional Chinese thesis that morality and public order consist of, and depend on, a series of hierarchically structured relationships and the fulfillment of the duties associated with them. The archetype and the ethical keystone of these superordinate-subordinate relationships was that between father and son; filial piety (*xiao*) was regarded as the model and the source of all other virtues.

Seen from this traditional perspective, perhaps the most revolutionary and un-Chinese aspects of medical morality are those centered on the relationship of nurses and physicians to patients. Medical workers are not only asked to treat their patients as coequals and to identify with them feelingly, "in deep proletarian affection." They are also exhorted to accord such supreme moral importance to their relations with patients that they surpass what have always been the first and ultimate relationships in Chinese society—family relationships, beginning with those between father and son.

The fact that nurses and women, like She, Meng, and Guan, rather than physicians and men, are the leading architects and representatives of medical morality is still another indicator of the impact of Marxist ideas on a society that has been patriarchally as well as hierarchically oriented for thousands of years.

This does not mean that equality between women and men, and the nurses and doctors who work in medicine, is now a de facto achievement in China, or that the ancient and strong cosmic, moral, and social sense of hierarchy has been eliminated from the medical sphere. Chinese nurses complain much the same way that American nurses do about how inequitably they are treated by many physicians—"like servants," they say. An elaborate formal and informal status-rank hierarchy still characterizes work units like First Central Hospital, accompanied and supported by a considerable amount of everyday ritual. Furthermore, hospitals are ranked vis-à-vis each other on a local and a national scale of excellence and prestige. Even medical morality itself is premised on certain hierarchical assumptions, such as the notion that it is "the leadership" of the nursing and medical professions that should set an example for other (nonleaders) to follow. Nevertheless, Marxist ideas of egalitarianism and universalism have made more than a doctrinal difference in medical morality and its implementation.

In the end, it is the essential Chinese-ness of the way that Marxist, along with Taoist, Confucian, and Buddhist, ideas have been blended into medical morality that is the most striking. A distinctively Chinese outlook has been as powerful a determinant of the phenomena and questions that are *not* included under medical morality as of those that are. In contradistinction to American bioethics, as already indicated, Chinese medical morality is not preoccupied with social and ethical problems associated with the advancement of medical science and technology. At the present time, medical modernization—enriched by its incorporation of traditional Chinese medicine—is viewed as morally good, socially desirable, economically necessary, and politically obligatory. Substantive issues that *do* fall under the aegis of medical morality include the population's response to the new, one-child-per-family policy; the wisdom of telling or not telling seriously ill patients (particularly those with cancer) about the gravity of their illness;[c] the role that the family ought and ought not to play in the care of ill relatives who are hospitalized;[d] the causes, prevention, and treatment of suicide attempts;[e] and the problem of obtaining blood donations. All are issues that are encountered by nurses and doctors in the various medical milieus where they currently work. Prominent bioethical concerns, such as human experimentation, the "gift of life" and "quality of life," the termination of treatment, and questions about the allocation of scarce resources associated with therapeutic innovations like organ transplantation and hemodialysis in our own society, are not yet considered to be problems in China. Chinese nurses, physicians, and relevant officials are aware that, as the process of medical modernization goes forward, they may face comparable difficulties. But, in accord with Chinese pragmatism, they are disinclined to engage in abstract speculation about hypothetical problems that may (or may not) develop, and about how they should be handled if they do. It is not until the Chinese face such issues in a firsthand way, and can meet and analyze them as "lived-in experiences," that these matters will become part of their medical morality.

* * *

From all the foregoing, it is amply clear that medical morality is not bioethics. It is as Chinese as bioethics is American. We now turn to bioethics, an arena in which we have worked and observed since the mid-1960s.[f] In the final analysis, as we shall see, American bioethics and Chinese medical morality are so culturally dissimilar that they are not sufficiently related to form a yin-yang (opposing, but complementary) pair.

American Bioethics

In contrast to medical morality, the phenomena with which bioethics is primarily concerned are related to some of the ways in which modern, Western, American medicine has already *succeeded* in what the Chinese call "scaling the high peaks" of science and technology. Bioethics is focused on what we consider serious *problems* associated with these advances, rather than on the achievements they represent or the "golden dream" promises that they hold forth:[7]

> Actual and anticipated developments in genetic engineering and counseling, life support systems, birth technology, population control, the implantation of human, animal, and artificial organs, as well as in the modification and control of human thought are principal [areas] of concern. Within this framework, special attention is concentrated on the implications of amniocentesis, abortion, *in vitro* fertilization, the prospect of cloning, organ transplantation, the use of the artificial kidney machine, the development of an artificial heart, the modalities of the intensive care unit, the practice of psychosurgery, and the introduction of psychotropic drugs. Cross-cutting the consideration . . . given to these general and concrete [spheres] of biomedical development, there is marked preoccupation with the ethicality of human experimentation under various conditions. . . .

Bioethics has also been concerned with the proper definition of life and death and personhood and with the humane treatment of "emerging life and life that is passing away"[8] — especially with the justifiability of forgoing life-sustaining forms of medical therapy. One of the most significant general characteristics of this ensemble of bioethical concerns is the degree to which they cluster around problems of natality and mortality, at the beginning and at the end of the human life cycle.

The chief intellectual and professional participants in American bioethics are philosophers (above all, those who are called "ethicists" in the United States, and "moral philosophers" in Europe), theologians (predominantly Catholic and Protestant), jurists, physicians, and biologists. Lately, the thought and presence of economists have been strongly felt in the field; but relatively few other social scientists are actively involved or notably influential in bioethical discussion, research, writing, and action. The limited participation of anthropologists, sociologists, and political scientists in bioethics is a complex phenomenon, caused as much by the prevailing intellectual orientations and the weltanschauung of present-day American social science as by the framework of bioethics.[9]

The disciplinary backgrounds of bioethicists contrast sharply with those of the key participants in medical morality because of historic differences in the American and Chinese cultures as well as current differences in our respective political and economic systems. For example,

although one could argue that there are functional parallels between the role of a Chinese dialectician and that of an American theologian, one would hardly expect a theologian trained in the Judeo-Christian tradition to define value and belief issues and make decisions in the same way as someone whose world view is shaped by Confucian, Taoist, and Buddhist thought. Nor does the pivotal place of lawyers and judges in bioethics have its counterpart in medical morality. The status and role of jurists in bioethics are integrally connected with the singular importance that Americans attach to the principle as well as to the fact of being "a society under law, rather than under men."

On the other hand, the control in degree and kind over medical morality exercised by the central government in Beijing is not only an emanation of the Chinese Communist party, its present-day leadership, and its current doctrine. It is thoroughly compatible with the at once profane and sacred power over the order and organization of the entire society accorded to the emperor and his imperial bureaucracy throughout all the dynasties of Chinese history. In the United States, quite to the contrary, the fact that bioethical questions, with their moral and religious connotations, have been appearing more frequently and prominently in national and local political arenas — in our legislatures, courts, and in specially created commissions — constitutes a societal dilemma. Although ours is a "society under law," it is also a nation founded on the separation of church and state as one of its sacredly secular principles. What ought we to do, then, about the fact that bioethics (like Mr. Smith) has gone to Washington? In the light of the religious and even metaphysical, as well as moral, nature of bioethical issues, is it legitimate or wise for our government to deal with them? If so, at what level, through what branch, using what mechanisms? If not, are there other means through which we can try to resolve such matters of our collective conscience, on behalf of the whole society? These are distinctly American questions that are decidedly not Chinese.

The pluralism of American society and its voluntarism have contributed to the development of the numerous centers, institutes, and associations of varying orientations that have been organized around bioethical activities in the United States over the course of the past 20 years, both inside and outside university settings. Most of the persons who are professionally active in the field of bioethics belong to one or several of such groups and participate in their interconnected and to some extent overlapping activities (discussions, research, teaching, consultations, meetings, publications, etc.). In this sense, they form a sort of "invisible college," although not a unified school of thought.[8]

Such a plethora of voluntary associations, organized around common interests, but with somewhat different origins, auspices, memberships, and outlook, is a very American configuration. It embodies a set of culture patterns and social traits, not confined to bioethics, that always have been strikingly characteristic of American society and its conception of democracy. As early as the 1830s, Alexis de Tocqueville, the astute French observer-analyst of our new nation-state, identified our tendency to form and join voluntary associations as one of our most notable societal attributes. Again, for reasons broader, deeper, and older than the particular contemporaneous circumstances that have given rise to bioethics and medical morality, this is not a pattern that exists in China or that one would expect to find there.

But above all, it is in the values and beliefs emphasized and deemphasized by bioethics, and in its cognitive framework and style, that its Western and American orientation is both most evident and most fully articulated.

* * *

To begin with, as already indicated, individualism is the primary value-complex on which the intellectual and moral edifice of bioethics rests. Individualism, in this connection, starts with a belief in the importance, uniqueness, dignity, and sovereignty of the individual, and in the sanctity of each individual life. From this flows the assumption that every person, singularly and respectfully defined, is entitled to certain individual rights. Autonomy of self, self-determination, and privacy are regarded as fundamental among these rights. They are also considered to be necessary preconditions for another value-precept of individualism: the opportunity for persons to "find," develop, and realize themselves and their self-interests to the fullest—to achieve and enjoy individual well-being. In this view, "individuals are entitled to be and do as they see fit, so long as they do not violate the comparable rights of others."[10] "Paternalism" is defined as interfering with and limiting a person's freedom and liberty of action for the sake of his or her own good or welfare. It is regarded as ethically dubious because, however beneficent its intentions or outcome, it restricts autonomy, involves coercion, implies that someone else knows better what is best for a given individual, and may insidiously impair that individual's ability to decide and act independently.

The notion of contract plays a major role in the way relations between autonomous individuals are conceived in bioethics. Self-conscious, rational, specific agreements by persons involved in interaction with one another, that explicitly delineate the scope, content, and conditions of their joint activities, are presented as ethical models. They are considered to be exemplary expressions of the way that moral relationships, protective of individual rights, can be structured. The archetype of such contractual relations is the kind of informed, voluntary consent agreement between subjects and investigators in medical research which the field of bioethics helped to formulate and that is now required by all federal and most private agencies funding this research. The informed consent contract, though mutual, is asymmetric. It is principally concerned with the rights and welfare of one of the two partners—the human subject, often a patient—because he is the most vulnerable, disadvantaged, and least powerful of the pair. The special contractual obligation to watch over and safeguard the rights of the person(s) most susceptible to exploitation or harm in this type of exposed and unequal situation is a part of the bioethics conception of individualism and of moral relations between individuals. But little mention is made by bioethicists of what sociologist Émile Durkheim termed the "noncontractual aspects of contract": that is, the more implicit and informal commitment, fidelity, and trust aspects of social relationships that reciprocally bind persons to live up to their promises and their responsibilities to one another.

Veracity and truth-telling, the "faithfulness" dimension of relationships on which bioethics fixes its attention, is more specific and circumscribed than the Durkheimian concept. In keeping with the overall orientation of bioethics, what is stressed is the right of patients or research subjects to "know the truth" about the discomforts, hazards, uncertainties, and "bad news" that may be associated with medical diagnosis, prognosis, treatment, and experimentation. The physician's obligation to communicate the truth to the patient or subject is derived from and based on the latter's presumed right to know. Discerning what is the truth and what is a lie is seen as relatively unproblematic. And there is a decided tendency to look on the use of denial by the patient as an undesirable defense, because it complicates truth telling and blocks truth receiving. Here, the affirmation that patients have the right to know the truth veers toward insistence that they ideally ought to face the truth consciously and deal with it rationally (in keeping with the particular definitions of "truth" and of "rationality" inherent to bioethics).

Another major value preoccupation of bioethics—and one that it has increasingly emphasized since the mid-1970s—concerns the allocation of scarce, expensive resources for advanced medical care, research, and development. What proportion of our national and local resources should be designated for these purposes, in what ways, and according to what principles and criteria? The resources with which bioethics is chiefly concerned are material ones, mainly economic and technological in nature. The allocation of nonmaterial resources such as personnel, talent, skill, time, energy, caring, and compassion is rarely mentioned. Bioethics situates its allocation questions within a rather abstract, individual rights-oriented notion of the general or common good, assigning greater importance to equity than to equality.

The ideally moral distribution of goods is defined as one that all rational, self-interested persons are willing to accept as just and fair, even if goods are allotted unequally. "Cost containment" is also an essential value-component of this view of rightful distribution. In the bioethical calculus, it is not just a practical or necessary response to an empirical situation of economic scarcity. It has become a more categorical moral imperative.

Finally, what is usually referred to as "the principle of beneficence" or "benevolence" is also a key value of bioethics. This enjoinder to "do good" and to "avoid harm" is structured and limited by the supremacy of individualism. The benefiting of others advocated in bioethical thought is circumscribed and constrained by the obligation to respect individual rights, interests, and autonomy. Furthermore, rather than being seen as an independent virtue, doing good is generally conceived to be part of a "benefit-harm ratio" in which, ideally, benefits should outweigh costs. "Minimization of harm" rather than "maximization of good" is more strongly emphasized in this bioethical equation.

These values are predominant in American bioethics and are considered to be the most fundamental. They are accorded the highest intellectual and moral significance and are set forth with the greatest certainty and the least qualification. Other values and virtues and principles and beliefs that are part of the ethos of bioethics occupy a more secondary and less secure status. They are less frequently invoked and when introduced into ethical discussion and analysis are likely to elicit debate or require special justification.

The concept and language of "rights" prevail over those of "responsibility" and "obligation" in bioethical discourse, and the term "duty" does not appear often in the bioethical vocabulary. As already indicated, the strongest appeals to responsibility are concentrated on requirements for the protection and promotion of individual rights.

The emphasis that bioethics places on individualism and on contractual relations freely entered into by voluntarily consenting adults tends to minimize and obscure the interconnectedness of persons and the social and moral importance of their interrelatedness. Particularly when compared with Chinese medical morality, it is striking how little attention bioethics pays to the web of human relationships of which the individual is a part and to the mutual obligations and interdependence that these relations involve. Concepts like reciprocity, solidarity, and community, which are rooted in a social perspective on our moral life and our humanity, are not often employed. Characteristically, bioethics deals with the "more-than-individual" in terms of the "general good," the "common good," or the "public interest." In the bioethical use of these concepts, the "collective good" tends to be seen atomistically and arithmetically as the sum total of the rights and interests, desires and demands of an aggregate of self-contained individuals. The fair and just distribution of limited collective resources is the major dimension of commonality that is stressed, often to the exclusion of other aspects, and usually with a propensity to define resources as material (primarily economic), and quantitative. In this view, private and public morality are sharply distinguished from one another in keeping with the underlying essential dichotomy between individual and social. Social and cultural factors are largely seen as external constraints that limit individuals. They are rarely presented as enabling and empowering forces, *inside* as well as outside of individuals, that are constituent, dynamic elements in making them human persons.

The restricted definition of "persons as individuals" and of "persons in relations" that pervades bioethics makes it difficult to introduce and find an appropriate place for values like decency, kindness, empathy, caring, devotion, service, generosity, altruism, sacrifice, and love. All of these involve recognizing and responding to intimate and non-intimate others in a self-transcending way. Although these principles and qualities are esteemed in bioethics as exemplary and meritorious, they do not fit neatly and logically into its moral framework. There is a real sense in which they fall outside the tight range of variables that are defined as generically "ethical" by this field. For values like these, that center on the bonds between self and others and on community, and that include both "strangers" and "brothers," and future as well as present generations in their orbit, are categorized in bioethics as sociological, theological, or religious rather than as ethical or moral.

These assumptions about what is and is not purely moral are integrally related to the major cognitive characteristics of bioethical thought: to how participants in bioethics actually *do* think, and especially, to what they define as ideal standards of ethical thinking. A high value is placed on logical reasoning—preferably based on a general moral theory and concepts derived from it—that is systematically developed according to codified methodological rules and techniques around select, analytically designated variables and problems. Rigor, precision, clarity, consistency, parsimony, and objectivity are regarded as earmarks of the intellectually and ethically "best" kind of moral thought. Flawed logical and conceptual analysis is considered to be not only a concomitant of moral error but also, to a significant degree, responsible for producing it. This way of thought also tends toward dichotomous distinctions and bipolar choices. Self versus others, body versus mind, individual versus group, public versus private, objective versus subjective, rational versus nonrational, lie versus truth, benefit versus harm, rights versus responsibilities, independence versus dependence, autonomy versus paternalism, liberty versus justice are among the primary ones. Even the field's own self-defining conception of what is and is not a moral problem is formulated in a bipolar, either/or fashion.

Bioethics is an applied field that brings its theory, methods, and knowledge to bear on phenomena and situations deemed ethically problematic. It seeks to identify and illuminate points of moral consideration and provide a way of thinking about them that can contribute to their practical moral resolution through concrete choices and specific acts. Bioethics attempts this by proceeding in a largely deductive manner to impose its mode of reasoning on the phenomenological reality addressed. The amount of detailed investigation of the actual situations in which the ethical problems occur varies. But what philosophers call "thought experiments" are more often conducted in bioethics than is empirical, in situ research. This ordered, cerebral, armchair inquiry is given precedence, partly because the formalistic "data" it generates more closely fit the norms of bioethical logic and rationality than information gathered through firsthand research. Thought experiments are one of an array of cognitive techniques used in bioethics to distance and abstract itself from the human settings in which ethical questions are embedded and experienced, reduce their complexity and ambiguity, limit the number and kinds of morally relevant factors to be dealt with, dispel dilemmas, and siphon off the emotion, suffering, bewilderment, and tragedy that many medical moral predicaments entail for patients, families, and medical professionals.

Within its rigorously stripped-down analytic and methodological framework, bioethics is prone to reify its own logic and to formulate absolutist, self-confirming principles and insights. These tendencies are associated with the disinclination of bioethics to critically examine its own moral epistemology: to searchingly identify and evaluate the presuppositions and assumptions on which it rests. In a scholastic sense, the field of bioethics is knowledgeably aware of the traditions of Western thought on which it draws (e.g., act and rule utilitarianism and various theories of justice). But there is a more latent level on which it nevertheless considers its principles, its style of reasoning, and its perceptions to be objective, unbiased, and reasonable to a degree that not only makes them socially and culturally neutral but also endows them with a kind of universality. Paradoxically, these very suppositions of bioethical thought contribute to its inadvertent propensity to reflect and systematically support conventional, relatively conservative American concepts, values, and beliefs.[h]

These value, belief, and thought patterns of bioethics have developed within an interdisciplinary matrix. But particularly since the mid-1970s, when philosophers began "arriving by the score" in bioethics (and "in applied ethics more broadly"),[11] moral philosophy has had the greatest molding influence on the field. It is principally American analytic philosophy — with its emphasis on theory, methodology, and technique, and its utilitarian, Kantian, and "contractarian" outlooks — in which most of the philosophers who have entered bioethics were trained. Defined as "ethicists" who are specialized experts in moral problems associated with biomedicine, they have established themselves, and their approach to matters of right and wrong, as the "dominant force"[13] in the field.

This is not to say that all analytic philosophers who actively participate in bioethics think and write in a uniform way, or that every philosopher-bioethicist is grounded in this analytic tradition. Major contributors to bioethics, for example, also include a number of highly esteemed philosopher-scholars whose work incorporates more phenomenological, social, and religious dimensions rooted in the traditions of moral theology and American social ethics. The respect that such individuals are accorded notwithstanding, the perspective that they represent has had far less influence on the predominant ethos of bioethics than has analytic philosophy.

The conviction of analytic philosophers that value questions and ethical problems can and should be handled objectively, rationally, and rigorously, with specialized targeted competence, is shared and supported by many jurists, professionally involved with bioethical issues, whose intellectual and moral authority in the field is second only to that of the philosophers. The intricate and controversial, but nonetheless significant, connection that has always existed between law and morality in American society, and the increasing extent to which bioethical issues have been coming before our courts and into our legislatures since the mid-1960s, have contributed to the important status of the law and of lawyers in bioethics. In turn, the rationalism of American law, its emphasis on individual rights, and the ways in which it has been shaped by Western traditions of natural law, positivism, and utilitarianism, overlap with and reinforce key attributes of the philosophical thought in bioethics.

The principles and rules of "being scientific" that physicians and biologists have been educated and socialized to apply to their own professional work, and that they have brought to bioethics, are highly compatible with the positivism of philosophers and jurists. Within the framework of bioethics and its scientistic assumptions, this parallelism confers a semblance of "scientific-ness" on the philosophical and legal aspects of its thought and in so doing enhances the validity that it is believed to have.

These same tendencies in the currents of thought that underlie bioethics have played a major role in framing its operational conception of "the moral," in which religious, cultural, and social variables are not only sharply distinguished from ethical ones, but their relevance is minimized. In these respects, despite the significant contributions of theologians to bioethics, its overall orientation is decidedly secular as well as unsociological. When questions of a religious nature do arise in bioethics, there is a marked tendency either to screen them out or to logically "reduce" them, so they can be fitted into the field's circumscribed definition of ethics and ethical. Through a comparable process of intellectual laundering and reductionism, the social is taken out of its larger cultural, historical, and societal context by bioethics, as well as out of what the field defines as ethical.

The applied pragmatism of bioethics strengthens the common tendency among its participants to cleave to a conceptual framework that focuses on individuals, plays down their interrelationships, rationalizes and simplifies the emotional and social milieus of which they are a part, and limits the range of facts and values considered germane to ethics. Bioethics is oriented to problem solving, decision making, and policy formulation. Bioethicists are continually called upon to serve as expert consultants in numerous biomedical, legal, political, educational, and industrial arenas. In these arenas, physicians, nurses, and other medical professionals, hospital administrators, patients, families, biologists, lawyers, judges, legislators, politicians, business executives, and their associates must make up their minds about what to do or not to do in real-life settings and then act on the basis of their determinations. This advisory role to decision makers has reinforced the cognitive predisposition of bioethics to distill the complexity and uncertainty, the dilemmas and the tragedy out of the situations they analyze. The fact that bioethicists are being asked to help professional practitioners and policymakers arrive at reasonably specific and clear ways of resolving the concrete medical-moral problems they face has given a new, expedient justification for the forms of intellectual and moral reductionism in which it engages.

Bioethics Is Not Just Bioethics

In our sociological view, the paradigm of values and beliefs, and of reflections on them, that has developed and been institutionalized in American bioethics is an impoverished and skewed expression of our society's cultural tradition. In a highly intellectualized but essentially fundamentalistic way, it thins out the fullness of that tradition and bends it away from some of the deepest sources of its meaning and vitality.

In the prevailing ethos of bioethics, the value of individualism is defined in such a way, and emphasized to such a degree, that it is virtually severed from social and religious values concerning relationships between individuals; their responsibilities, commitments, and emotional bonds to one another; the significance of the groups and of the societal community to which they belong; and the deep inward as well as outward influence that these have on the individual and his or her sense

of the moral. Social dimensions of ethicality are largely compressed into and meted out through a "do good" and "avoid harm" idea of beneficence. To this narrowly gauged conception of individualism, bioethics attaches an inflated and inflationary value. Claims to individual rights phrased in terms of moral entitlements tend to expand and to beget additional claims to still other individual rights. In these respects, the individualism of bioethics constitutes an evolution away from older, less secularized and communal forms of American individualism.

The outlook of bioethics is also based on a principle of rational calculation set forth as a standard of moral as well as intellectual excellence. Qualities and considerations that do not easily fit into a logico-rational and cost-conserving framework of ethicality are either excluded from bioethics or relegated to a secondary or peripheral status within it. "Qualities of the heart" like compassion and caring that elicit generosity have a lesser place in bioethics than the reason-guided "qualities of the mind" that support frugality. The moral economy of bioethics, like its cognitive system, is governed by a notion of parsimony that borders on penury.

The positivism and the materialism of bioethics integrate it around a narrow range of variables and values. These tight and exclusionary properties of bioethical thought heighten the tension traditional in Western culture and American society between certain pairs of principles. Bioethics splits them further apart and drives them into conflictful dichotomies. Individual and social, self and other, rights and responsibilities, thoughts and feelings, the rational and the nonrational, the material and the nonmaterial, what is ethical and what is religious—all become irreconcilable opposites, among which absolute choices have to be made. We already know the choices bioethics epitomizes. But, "How does one balance a total focus on the needs of the individual with one's responsibility to the whole community? How does one hold together in a kind of creative tension the assurance of faith with the flexibility of tolerance? It is as if one were continually putting up two different poles and letting the sparks fly between. The truth is that we must preserve a readiness to ask new questions add seek new truths in all spheres. . . ."[14]

The reluctance of bioethics to let "the sparks fly between . . . two different poles," to ask such questions, and to "seek new truths in all spheres," is connected with its secularism: ". . . What I am referring to is a process of reductionism that 'thins down' and 'flattens out' the meaning of the individual and person, family and kinship . . . self-giving and sharing, kindness and sympathy, caring and mercy, equality and justice, mutuality and solidarity, communion and community, responsibility and commitment, birth and life, joy and suffering, mortality and death, so that they are progressively stripped of both their primal and transcendent significance, and of their relationship to the common good, the human condition, and the vaster-than-human. . . ."[15]

Bioethics has "sprung loose from that broader [religious] framework"[15] in which the values of our cultural tradition are historically embedded. In turn, the particular forms that the secularism, the rationality, and the individualism of bioethics take, and the ways in which they interact with each other, contribute to another of the field's constricting features: its provincialism. Bioethics is sealed into itself in such a way that it tends to take its own characteristics and assumptions for granted. It is relatively uncritical of its premises and unaware of its cultural specificity. It is this sort of parochialism, with its mix of naiveté and arrogance, that makes it difficult for bioethicists not only to recognize medical morality and its Chinese-ness when they encounter it but also to perceive the "American-ness" of their particular value-concerns and of how they approach them.

It is unclear whether bioethics truly reflects the state of American medical ethics today and whether it can—or ought to—serve as the common framework for American medical morality.

Beyond this, if, as we suggested at the outset, "bioethics is not just bioethics" and is more than medical—if it is an indicator of the general state of American ideas, values, and beliefs, of our collective self-knowledge, and our understanding of other societies and cultures—then there is every reason to be worried about who we are, what we have become, what we know, and where we are going in a greatly changed and changing society and world.

References

1. Gernet, J. *Chine et Christianisme.* Paris: Gallimard, 1982.
2. Engelhardt, H. T., Jr. Bioethics in the People's Republic of China. *Hastings Cent. Rep.* 10 (April 1980): 7–10.
3. Fox, R. C., and Swazey, J. P. Critical care at Tianjin's First Central Hospital and the fourth modernization. *Science* 217:700–705, 1982.
4. Henderson, G. E. Danwei: the Chinese work unit: a participant observation study of a hospital. Dissertation submitted in partial fulfillment of the requirements of the Ph.D. (Sociology) at the University of Michigan, Ann Arbor, 1982.
5. Berling, J. Religion and popular culture: the management of moral capital in *The Romance of the Three Teachings.* In untitled work edited by A. Nathan, D. Johnson, and E. Rawski. Berkeley and Los Angeles: Univ. California Press.
6. Sivin, N. Ailment and cure in traditional China (unpublished manuscript).
7. Fox, R. C. Ethical and existential developments in contemporaneous American medicine: their implications for culture and society. In *Essays in Medical Sociology.* New York: Wiley, 1979.
8. Bok, S. In discussion at the Conference on the Problem of Personhood, organized by Medicine in the Public Interest, (MIPI). New York City, April 1–2, 1982.
9. Fox, R. C. Advanced medical technology—social and ethical implications. In *Essays in Medical Sociology.* New York: Wiley, 1979.
10. Gorovitz, S. *Doctors' Dilemmas: Moral Conflicts and Medical Care.* New York: Macmillan, 1982.
11. Callahan, D. At the center: from "wisdom" to "smarts." *Hastings Cent. Rep.* 12:4, 1982.
12. Noble, C. N. Ethics and experts. *Hastings Cent. Rep.* 12: 7–9, 15, 1982.
13. Callahan, D. Minimalistic ethics. *Hastings Cent. Rep.* 11: 19–25, 1981.
14. Saunders, C.; Summers, D. H.; and Teller, N. (eds.). *Hospice: The Living Idea.* Colchester and London: Arnold, 1981.
15. de Craemer, W. See[8].

Notes

a. Description of the problems that the first Jesuit and Franciscan missionaries to China, in the late fifteenth and early sixteenth centuries, had in understanding and analyzing the Chinese way of thought—and their own thought in relation to it. See [Gernet, p. 274[1]].

b. This list of virtues was compiled from the firsthand data we collected through our participant observation, interviewing, and analysis of relevant documents in China, particularly in Tianjin and at the First Central Hospital. The language used is as close to the original as possible—to the Chinese or the English used by our informants and respondents.

c. We had the decided impression that the predominant tendency was *not* to tell patients about serious illness. The expert knowledge that the patients at the Cancer Hospital in Beijing possessed about their conditions, and the pride with which they displayed it to visitors, was a dramatic exception to this general inclination. Nevertheless, there was considerable discussion among doctors and nurses about this "to tell or not to tell" issue. Nurses seemed to us to be more concerned about this problem than doctors, more prone to believe that patients ought to be told, and more disposed to believe that many patients know without being told, particularly when they have cancer.

d. At First Central Hospital, family members were sometimes allowed and even asked to help take care of a relative who was an inpatient, particularly during the night when nursing personnel was more sparse. However, in this hospital and in a number of others that we visited in Tianjin, the days of the week and the hours when patients' families were permitted to visit them were very restricted. From what we could discern, this policy partly stems from the shared sentiment of nurses and doctors that families contributed to the disorder that existed in hospitals during the Cultural Revolution by challenging their medical professional expertise and authority. In addition, many nurses and physicians seemed to feel that the presence and participation of relatives in hospital care introduce "superstitious" and folkloric medical notions into what ideally should be scientific, predominantly modern, medical care in this era of the Four Modernizations.

e. We do not know how great the incidence of suicide attempts and of successful suicides is in China. However, partly because First Central Hospital has a Critical Care Unit, a number of dialysis machines, and absorbent artificial kidney treatment capabilities, it is not uncommon for such cases to be sent to the hospital for emergency care. They are of great concern to the medical staff. One particularly interesting thing that we learned in this connection is that nurses and physicians divided suicides and suicide attempts into two different moral categories: those that were attributed to mental illness and therefore were not considered to be "the fault" of the individual involved; and those that were considered blameworthy, even criminal. These latter included suicide attempts motivated by "lost love," problems with schoolwork and/or in relations to teachers, and difficulties in family relations. Patients who had engaged in blameworthy suicide attempts received severe moral lectures from nurses and doctors, as well as medical care. They and their families were also expected to pay for the medical care given to them.

f. The discussion of the cognitive, value, and belief components and characteristics of American bioethics that follows is based on our extensive and intensive work in a variety of bioethical contexts and roles, on a close and continuous knowledge of the bioethical literature, and on a content analysis of the recurrent themes in that literature. As part of this content analysis, we have also been interested in identifying themes that are notable for the infrequency with which they occur in bioethical discussion and publications, or for their consistent absence from bioethics.

g. Among the best-known and influential bioethics organizations are: The Hastings Center (Institute of Society, Ethics, and the Life Sciences), which publishes the *Hastings Center Report,* one of the most important bioethical journals in the United States; the Center for Bioethics, Kennedy Institute of Ethics, Georgetown University; the Society for Health and Human Values; and the Institute for the Medical Humanities, University of Texas Medical Center, Galveston. Among these associations, the Hastings Center is probably the most interdisciplinary and eclectic in perspective, the Kennedy Institute the most theological and Catholic, and the Society for Health and Human Values the most humanistic, Protestant, and focused on medical education. The Hastings Center and the Kennedy Institute are also strongly influenced by analytic philosophy and analytically trained philosophers; the Society for Health and Human Values is less so.

h. Several major critiques of the emergence of the new philosophical subdiscipline of applied ethics on the American scene have been published in the *Hastings Center Report* during the past 2 years, which coincide in numerous respects with our characterization of bioethics, particularly its "seeming indifference to history, social context, and cultural analysis."[11-13]

Chapter 21

She's Going to Die: The Case of Angela C

George J. Annas, J.D., M.P.H.

George J. Annas is Utley Professor of Health Law and Chief, Health Law Section, Boston University Schools of Medicine and Public Health.

Angela C was a twenty-eight-year old married woman who was approximately twenty-six weeks pregnant. She had suffered from cancer since she was thirteen years old, but had been in remission for approximately two years before she became pregnant. The pregnancy was planned, and she very much looked forward to the birth. Her health seemed reasonably good until about the twenty-fifth week of pregnancy, when she was admitted to George Washington University Hospital, and a tumor was found in her lung.

Within a few days the physicians determined that her condition was terminal and she would die within weeks. At approximately 4:00 p.m. on June 15, 1987, she was told that she might die much sooner. Because her fetus would have a much better chance to be born healthy at twenty-eight weeks or more gestation, she agreed to treatment that might help her survive longer, but insisted that her own care and comfort be primary.

Ms. C's husband, her mother, and her physicians agreed that keeping her comfortable while she died was what she wanted and that her wishes should be honored. The next morning this information was communicated to hospital administration. Legal counsel was consulted, who decided to consult the university's outside counsel. Outside counsel asked a judge to come to the hospital to decide what to do.

The Hearing

Judge Emmett Sullivan of the District of Columbia Superior Court summoned volunteer lawyers, and with a police escort rushed to the hospital where he set up "court." Legal counsel was, of course, present for the hospital. In addition, lawyers were appointed to represent Ms. C, and her fetus, and the judge invited the District of Columbia Corporation Counsel to participate as well. The lawyer for the hospital opened the proceeding:

> [T]he apparent desire of the patient and her family is that if the patient is to die, that no intervention be done on behalf of the fetus. . . . The hospital is seeking declaratory relief from the court to direct the hospital as to what it should do in terms of the fetus, whether to intervene and save its life.

The lawyer for the fetus expressed the view that the fetus was "a probably viable fetus, presumptively viable fetus, age twenty-six weeks," and that the court's task was to "balance" the interests of the fetus "with whatever life is left for the fetus's mother. . . ." Ms. C's lawyer argued simply that she opposed surgical intervention to remove the fetus.

Her attending physician, Louis Hamner, testified that Ms. C had agreed to have the child at twenty-eight weeks, but that because the odds of a major handicap were much higher at twenty-six weeks gestation, she did not want the fetus delivered earlier. He said Ms. C was heavily sedated, and would likely die within twenty-four hours.

A neonatologist testified hypothetically, having "had no direct involvement with the mother or the family." She strongly supported intervention on the basis that for any individual fetus, survival and morbidity are "very difficult to predict." When pressed she put the likelihood of fetal viability at 50 to 60 percent and the risk of serious handicap at less than 20 percent.

The patient's mother testified that the previous day, after her daughter had been informed that her condition was terminal, she said, "I only want to die, just give me something to get me out of this pain."

Hospital counsel then asked the court to decide "what medical care, if any, should be performed for the benefit of the fetus of [Ms. C]." The lawyers' arguments focused not on what Ms. C wanted or even on her best interests, but on the best interests of the fetus and on Ms. C's terminal condition. The lawyer for the fetus, for example, urged that a cesarean be performed because, "sadly, the life of the mother is lost to us no matter what decision is made at this point." Ms. C's lawyer, on the other hand, argued the case on the basis of Ms. C's wishes, noting (correctly) that "we can't order abortions even to protect the post-viability and potentiality of life if a woman objects." The lawyer for the District of Columbia argued that Ms. C's interests need not concern the court because of the "sad fact" that "the mother will die regardless of what we do. . . ." A subsequent exchange between Ms. C's lawyer and Judge Sullivan captures the essence of the hearing:

Mr. Sylvester: As I see this, as I understand the medical testimony, if we were to do a C-section on this woman in a very weakened medical state, we would in effect be terminating her life, and I can't—
The Court: She's going to die, Mr. Sylvester.

The lawyer for the fetus concluded: "All we are arguing is the state's obligation to rescue a potential life from a dying mother." The judge took a short recess and then issued his opinion orally. The decisive consideration was Ms. C's terminal condition: "The uncontroverted medical testimony is that Angela will probably die within the next twenty-four to forty-eight hours." He did "not clearly know what Angela's present views are" respecting the cesarean section, but found that the fetus had a 50 to 60 percent chance to survive and a less than 20 percent chance for a serious handicap. The judge concluded: "It's not an easy decision to make, but given the choices, the court is of the view the fetus should be given an opportunity to live." He cited only one case, an unreported 1986 opinion from the District of Columbia Court of Appeals (the only case anyone present had a copy of). That case was based in large part on dicta from a New Jersey case that had previously been largely overruled and was, in any event, easily distinguishable.

After the Hearing

Shortly after the court recessed at 4:15 p.m., Hamner informed Ms. C of the decision. Ms. C was on a ventilator,

but was able to mouth agreement. The court reconvened upon learning that Ms. C was awake and communicating.

The chief of obstetrics, Alan Weingold, reported a more recent discussion with the patient in which she "clearly communicated" and after being informed that Hamner would only do the cesarean section if she consented to it, "very clearly mouthed the words several times, I don't want it done. I don't want it done." Hamner confirmed this exchange. Weingold concluded:

I think she's in contact with reality, clearly understood who Dr. Hamner was. Because of her attachment to him wanted him to perform the surgery. Understood he would not unless she consented and did not consent. This is, in my mind, very clear evidence that she is responding, understanding, and is capable of making such decisions.

The judge indicated that he was still not sure what her intent was. Counsel for the District of Columbia then suggested that her current refusal did not change anything because the entire proceeding had been premised on the belief that she was refusing to consent. In his words, "I don't think we would be here if she had said she wants it." The judge concurred, and reaffirmed his original order.

The Appeal

Less than an hour later three judges heard by telephone a request for stay of at least fifteen minutes so that arguments could be heard. Ms. C's lawyer told the judges that the cesarean section had been scheduled for 6:30 p.m., which gave them approximately sixteen minutes to hear arguments and make a decision. He argued that the cesarean section would likely end Ms. C's life, and that it was unconstitutional to favor the life of the fetus over that of the mother without the mother's consent. The lawyer for the fetus argued that Ms. C had no important interests in this decision because she was dying: "unintended consequences on the mother" are "insignificant in respect to the mother's very short life expectancy." The state's interest, she said, "overrides any interest in the mother's continued very short life, which is under heavy medication and very short duration."

A discussion ensued about the possibility of the fetus surviving, which the chief judge cut short by asking: "Let me ask you this, if it's relevant at all. Obviously the fetus has a better chance than the mother?" The lawyer for the fetus responded, "Obviously. Right." A few minutes later, the court denied the request for a stay, reserving the right to file an opinion at a later date. The proceeding was concluded at 6:40 p.m.

What Went Wrong?

The cesarean section was performed and the nonviable fetus died approximately two hours later. Ms. C, now confronted with both recovery from major surgery and the knowledge of her child's death, died approximately two days later. Five months later the Court of Appeals issued its written opinion (*In re A.C.,* D.C. Ct. Appeals, No. 87-609, Nov. 10, 1987). The opinion reads more like a Hallmark sympathy card. Its first paragraph, for example, concludes: "Condolences are extended to those who lost the mother and child." The court acknowledged that its opinion might "reasonably" be seen as "self-justifying" and then went on to rationalize the denial of the stay.

The opinion rests on a number of false assumptions. The most serious error is the statement that "as a matter of law, the right of a woman to an abortion is different and distinct from her obligations to the fetus once she has decided not to timely terminate her pregnancy." This is incorrect as both a factual and legal matter. Ms. C never "decided not to timely terminate her pregnancy," and because of her fetus's effect on her health, under *Roe v. Wade* she could have authorized her pregnancy to be terminated (to protect her health) at any time prior to her death. In essence, the court forced Ms. C to have an abortion prior to her death, doing so on the false premise that a terminal diagnosis strips a pregnant woman of her constitutional rights.

The second basis for the opinion is that a parent cannot refuse treatment necessary to save the life of a child (true) and therefore a pregnant woman cannot refuse treatment necessary to save the life of her fetus (false). The child must be treated because parents have obligations to act in the "best interests" of their children (as defined by child neglect laws), and treatment in no way compromises the bodily integrity of the parents. Fetuses, however, are not independent persons, and cannot be treated without invading the mother's body. There are no "fetal neglect" statutes, and it is unlikely that any could withstand constitutional scrutiny. Treating the fetus against the will of the mother degrades and dehumanizes the mother and treats her as an inert container. This *is* acceptable once the mother is dead, but is never acceptable when the mother is alive. The court seems to understand this, at least at the instinctive level, and thus ultimately justified its opinion on the basis that Ms. C was as good as dead and had no "good health" to be "sacrificed." "The cesarean section would not significantly affect A.C.'s condition because she had, at best, two days of sedated life. . . ." But this reasoning will not do. It would, for example, permit the involuntary removal of vital organs prior to death when they were needed to "save a life." But if the child had already been born, no court (not even this one) would require its mother to undergo major surgery for its sake (for example, a kidney "dona-

tion") no matter how dire the potential consequences of refusal to the child. And certainly no court would ever require the father of a child to undergo surgery, even to save the child's life. The ultimate rationale for the decision may be purely sexist: this situation could never apply to males like these judges; they are unable to identify with the pregnant woman and thus need not concern themselves about the future application of their decision to themselves.

This is a cavalierly lawless and unprincipled opinion that merits condemnation and reversal. The proper question the opinion poses is not whether the patient was competent, but whether the lawyers and judges were competent. What went wrong with the judicial process? At least three things: (1) the emergency nature of the hearing and the question asked of the judge; (2) the refusal to recognize the patient as a person with rights; and (3) the self-justifying nature of the appeals court's opinion.

This case illustrates the general rule that judges should never go to the hospital to make emergency treatment decisions. First, judges know nothing about treatment decisions. Judges can render an opinion about the lawfulness of a proposed course of treatment or nontreatment (although even this is seldom needed). But to ask judges to make the treatment decision to protect the hospital from some speculative potential liability simply invites them to play doctor; something they might enjoy, but something about which judges possess no more competence than the average person on the street. Rushed to an unfamiliar environment, asked to make a decision under great stress, and having no time either for reflection or to study existing law and precedents, a judge cannot act judiciously. Facts cannot be properly developed and the law cannot be accurately determined or fairly applied to the facts. The "emergency hearing" scenario invited arbitrariness.

The only reason a judge should ever go to a hospital is to determine the competence of a patient. This *is* a proper judicial task. Thus it is astonishing that the judge never even bothered to go the short distance to her hospital room to talk directly with Ms. C. The reason, of course, is that he viewed her simply as an inanimate container and so didn't care what the container's wishes were; this is what makes the decision so offensive. Angela C was legally presumed competent, did not consent to the surgical intervention, and surgery was ultimately performed over her express objection. She was totally dehumanized, her wishes and best interests ignored.

Finally, the appeals court did not act like an appeals court. It initially heard brief arguments over the phone and made a snap decision. It did not wait for the "trial" judge to write a more formal opinion before issuing its own; did not hear or invite arguments from the parties; and ultimately wrote a "self-justifying" opinion instead of a neutral and fair rendering of the law.

George J. Annas, J.D., M.P.H.

When asked how he would make decisions on the U.S. Supreme Court in his confirmation hearings, Judge Anthony Kennedy replied that he would carefully consider all of the facts, listen to the legal arguments, review all of the legal precedents, and then reflect long and hard about the case and how to apply the law to the facts properly to arrive at a fair and just opinion. Many commentators were disappointed in this response, noting that it was just a summary of what judges do. In fact, it is a summary of what judges *should do,* but unfortunately does not in any way reflect what the judges involved in Ms. C's case did. They treated a live woman as though she were already dead, forced her to undergo an abortion, and then justified their brutal and unprincipled opinion on the basis that she was almost dead and her fetus's interests in life outweighed any interest she might have in her own life or health. This is what happens when judges (and hospital lawyers that call them) forget what judging is all about and combine rescue fantasy with dehumanization of the dying.

This was *not* a hard case. The patient's wishes should have been honored. If there really were facts in dispute, a case conference involving the patient, family, and all attending health care personnel could have been held to assess them. Direct communication with the patient is almost always the most useful and constructive response to "problems" like those presented by this case. Calling a judge was a counterproductive panic reaction.

Letters

But She's Not an "Inanimate Container . . ."

Reading George Annas's article, "She's Going to Die: The Case of Angela C" ("At Law," *Hastings Center Report,* February/March 1988, 23–28) was like glimpsing myself in a house of mirrors. As one who was summoned by the court to assist in the case by representing the fetus, I would like to correct some of the misimpressions created by this article.

First, Annas's assertion that the judge (let alone any of the participants) viewed Angela as "an inanimate container," devoid of legal interests or human value could not be further from the truth. The major focus of the hearing was an attempt to determine Angela's intentions with respect to her baby. The case record reveals that Angela wanted a baby very much and embarked upon pregnancy knowing that it presented a serious risk to her health should her cancer recur. On Friday, June 12, 1987, she "unequivocally" stated in discussions with several physicians that she wanted to have the baby, and agreed to a cesarean at twenty-eight weeks, understanding that she herself would not survive. Regrettably, the question of performing the operation prior to twenty-eight weeks was never discussed with her.

The day before the hearing, prior to being taken to the intensive care unit, she again discussed her treatment with her family and physicians. Her obstetrician acknowledged that in that discussion she agreed to radiation and chemotherapy for the purpose of reaching twenty-eight weeks, at which point she understood that the likely outcome would be the baby's survival (following cesarean delivery) but not her own.

The oncologist who participated in that discussion testified to the same effect. Asked how he thought Angela herself would decide, whether she would refuse permission for the cesarean section at 26½ instead of at twenty-eight weeks to save the baby, he also testified that he had "not heard anything that would support that position."

The Legal Concept of Viability

The Supreme Court observed in *Colautti v. Franklin* (439 U.S. 379, 396 [1979]) that, "different physicians equate viability with different probabilities of survival," noting that expert witnesses had defined viability variously as: 2 to 3 percent, 5 percent, 10 percent, and "10 percent or better" chance of survival. At our hearing, an expert neonatologist testified that Angela's fetus was viable (in the legal sense of having a reasonable likelihood of sustained survival outside the womb) based upon the hospital's record of 80 percent survival of infants delivered at twenty-six weeks. Taking Angela's medical condition into account, she estimated a 50 to 60 percent chance of this fetus surviving, while acknowledging that it is difficult to predict survivability for an individual baby.

The Real Source of Conflict

I argued—and still believe—that the court did not have to balance maternal and fetal rights in this case, because maternal and fetal interests were not in conflict. Rather, the family's interests seemed to be at odds with those of the patient.

Annas wrote that I argued for performing the operation "because sadly the mother's life is lost to us," suggesting that I believe terminal illness vitiates rights. I was making a quite different point: that this was not a forced choice, that is, sacrificing one life to save the other. What I said was: "We are not confronted with the problem of choosing between the life of the mother and the life of the fetus. Sadly, the life of the mother is lost to us no matter what decision is made [with respect to the fetus]" (TR 64). Joining halves of different arguments oddly distorts the transcript.

Angela's attorney never had an opportunity to speak with his client. His impression of what Angela would want was derived from conversations with her family, but the family's position was problematic. Her husband could not bring himself to express either his own wishes or those of his wife. He did not testify. The only family member to testify was Angela's mother, and her statements seemed at odds with the reports about Angela's desires from the attending physicians. My attempts to understand her reasoning produced the following exchange:

Q. This is terribly difficult for you, I know, and I'm sorry to have to ask you some questions, but I think it's important at least to get some sense of how you, as a family, would be able to cope if there were a live baby to come out of this. Do you have, for example, is there medical insurance?

A. Nobody. Nobody would insure the baby. Nobody would insure my daughter. Nobody.

Q. So there is no family insurance that would cover the baby's care?

A. No, that doesn't even enter into it. I don't care about the money. It's just that I know there will be something wrong with this baby. I can't handle it. I've handled [Angela] and myself. . . .

Q. Would you—would you even have the resources to handle a healthy baby?

A. No.

Q. If the baby was not compromised?

A. Not really . . . they have only been married eight months. I mean, he hasn't even had her long enough. It's me and I'm in a wheelchair. I can't put that burden on us anymore. Angela is the only one that wanted that baby to love. She said she wanted something of her very own.

Q. Would you consider placing the baby for adoption?

A. Never. Never.

Q. What would you do if the baby survived?

A. Who wants it?

Q. I guess I'm asking you a terribly difficult question, but I'm trying to determine. . . .

A. I would take care of the baby. I would never put it up for adoption. I would do the best I could but we

don't want it. Angela wanted that baby. It was her baby. Let that baby die with her (TR 60).

The uncontroverted testimony was that Angela could not possibly communicate her present wishes; thus, the proper standard for decisionmaking was substituted judgment. The problem was that the surrogate decisionmaker (Angela's mother) appeared to be making the choice based not upon the patient's known values or previously expressed goals, but rather upon the burden of care that she herself was unprepared to assume.

As understandable as this choice may have been given the circumstances, it was not an acceptable basis for substituted judgment. As a matter of legal precedent and public policy, the implications of permitting the burden of care to influence life and death decisions made on behalf of others, the severely handicapped and the frail elderly, for example, are grave indeed.

The Question of Competence

Why did the court not go to see Angela? Both her attending obstetrician and the chief of obstetrics had testified that she was too heavily medicated to respond, and that there was no possibility of reducing her medication so that we could consult with her. Indeed, we were warned that to try might shorten her survival. After the court had ruled, the doctors went to prepare Angela for surgery and discovered (contrary to their earlier assertions) that her medication had worn off and she was rousable. The attending obstetrician described what happened:

I explained to her essentially what was going on. I said do—I said it's been deemed we should intervene on behalf of the baby by cesarean section and it would give it the only possible chance of its living. Would you agree to this procedure? *She did say yes.* I said, do you realize that you may not survive the surgical procedure? *She said yes. And I repeated the two questions to her again and asked her did she understand. She said yes* (TR 87-89). (Emphasis added.)

Twenty minutes later, when Angela's attorney went with her mother and her husband to verify what she had said, she mouthed several times, "I don't want it done." She gave no explanation for either the "yes" or the "no." Annas quoted testimony of a senior physician that Angela seemed clearly to understand what she was saying, but he quoted only part of the physician's statement, omitting the last two sentences:

I would state the obvious and that is that this is an environment in which, from my perspective as a physician, this would not be an informed consent one way or the other. She's under tremendous stress with the family on both sides [of her], but

I am satisfied that I heard clear[ly] what she said (TR 92-93).

The physician later elaborated that informed consent "has to take place in an environment other than the intensive care unit with a weeping husband and mother and all the paraphernalia." To which the hospital's medical director added, "plus the sedatives" (TR 94-95).

According to case law in the District of Columbia, when a patient vacillates as Angela did "it cannot be said with certainty that a deliberate and intelligent choice has been made" (*In re Boyd,* 403 A.2d 744, 749 [D.C. 1979]; *In re Osborne,* 294 A.2d 372, 374-75 [D.C. 1972]). It was on this basis, together with the physicians' testimony that the context and the medications precluded informed consent, that the trial judge concluded he still was unsure of Angela's present intent.

In summary, this was not a case of overriding a competent refusal of treatment. It was a case in which we had to determine what a dying and heavily medicated young woman would want, in circumstances that no one had foreseen in time to discuss with her. It was a case about whether a family member, primarily concerned about the burden of care, is a proper substitute decisionmaker. It was a sad case and a difficult decision, largely *because we did care about Angela.*

Aftermath

Although Angela's parents have since expressed their belief that the operation hastened her death, her obstetrician has acknowledged that it probably improved Angela's condition by removing the stress of pregnancy (D. Remnick, "Whose Life Is It, Anyway?" *The Washington Post Magazine,* February 21, 1988, 21). When I called the hospital the day after the hearing, I was told Angela was much stronger than she had been prior to the surgery.

More telling, Angela's husband was recently quoted as saying:

> If she knew she was going to die, she probably would have said yes to the cesarean. She knew how much I wanted the baby (D. Remnick, "Whose Life Is It, Anyway?" *The Washington Post Magazine,* February 21, 1988, 41).

The questions raised by this case are important, and should be considered carefully by a court fully briefed by all parties. Questions about the enforced treatment of competent pregnant women are equally important and worthy of discussion, but they were not raised by this case.

One final note: Annas wrote that approximately two hours following the cesarean, "the nonviable fetus" died.

As a matter of fact, a premature infant was born and lived briefly. On her birth and death certificates, the name is Lindsay Marie. She was buried with her mother.

Barbara Mishkin
Hogan & Hartson
Washington, D.C.

George J. Annas replies:

At the hearing, Barbara Mishkin was called upon to represent the fetus. She performed that role vigorously and effectively by persuading both the trial judge and the appeals panel that the fetus's right to life overcame the mother's interests in refusing to have her body surgically invaded. She now asserts that all she was really trying to do was find out what Angela wanted. Her letter demonstrates how an advocate's viewpoint can color one's perspective. Judges must decide cases on the facts and arguments actually presented to them.

At the hearing itself, she summarized her position to the judge as follows:

> The only possible optimism that we have . . . is for that baby. There is no longer any optimism for the mother and therefore the only good thing that can come out of this is the human life, potential human life which I think the state is bound to protect (TR 75).

Perhaps Mishkin really believes that this is a substituted judgment argument, but upon reading the transcript she should be able to understand why the judge, the appeals court, and others present did not see it this way.

Viability

Viability was relevant only to the extent that Angela considered it important in making *her* decision. The judge, nonetheless, concluded that if the fetus was viable, it had a right to live. This was an incorrect conclusion, but flowed from the arguments presented at the hearing. Mishkin quotes *Colautti v. Franklin* for the proposition that different physicians view viability differently. This is, of course, true. The relevant legal question, however, is which physician's view on viability controls. The U.S. Supreme Court answered this question in the paragraph following the one Mishkin quotes: "We affirm . . . that *'the determination of whether a particular fetus is viable is, and must be, a matter for the judgment of the responsible attending physician'*" (at 396, emphasis added). If viability were really an issue in this case, only the "responsible attending physician" had legal standing to make that determination. The testimony of the neonatologist who had never even examined Angela or her fetus was irrelevant and should not have been allowed into evidence. Moreover, the District of Columbia has *no* law restricting a woman's right to an abortion, and Angela's legal right to terminate her pregnancy continued after viability in any event.

The Real Source of Conflict
The notion that it was the family against Angela, and not the fetus against Angela, is not reflected in the transcript. What other conclusion can a court be expected to draw from the statement that "the life of the mother is lost to us no matter what decision is made" except that it should ignore the mother's rights or balance them in favor of life for the fetus?

The argument that no one knew what Angela wanted is even more incredible. Her attending physicians testified that they knew, and were so certain of her wishes that they refused to operate on her even if ordered to do so by the judge. Her mother and father also knew. Her mother presented uncontradicted testimony that Angela had said just the previous day: "I only want to die, just give me something to get me out of this pain." The fact that her attorney did not speak directly to her does *not* mean that he could not speak on her behalf (any more than the fact that Mishkin did not speak with the fetus precluded her from speaking on its behalf). In fact, all parties (including Mishkin) acknowledged in the midst of the hearing that they were willing to assume that they were overriding the wishes of a competent adult (only Angela's lawyer arguing that this was improper). After being informed that Angela was conscious and had refused to be operated on, the issue was put to the judge as follows:

Attorney for the District of Columbia: *I don't think we would be here if she had said she wants it.* The reason we are here is because we have to waive her constitutional—assuming she has clearly indicated that she does not want this procedure, I think that presents the dilemma that the Court saw in *weighing that privacy interest against the rights of the fetus* in this case *and the chances of that fetus being viable versus the imminence of the patient's death. That's the balancing that the Court must make* and that's—that only sets up the dilemma. It does not answer it. The fact that she says she does not want [the c-section] creates the dilemma it does not answer it. *I think we are in the same legal posture that we were before.*
Attorney for the fetus: Your Honor, *I think that time at this point really is of the essence.*
The Court: I think it is too.
Attorney for the fetus: *My sense is that that* [the fact that Angela has refused] *is troubling but has not greatly changed the matter.* I would opt for and urge they pursue their right to appeal . . . (TR 96-97). (Emphasis added.)

The record on this point is unequivocal. It was *assumed* that Angela was refusing, so there was no need to make a "substantiated judgment" determination. The argument that Angela's mother might have had improper motives is irrelevant. It was Angela's rights, not her mother's, that were at stake. We do want to protect the severely handicapped. But *there was only one severely handicapped person in this picture whose rights were violated:* Angela C.

Competence
Angela *was* competent and no one ever questioned her competence. There was no request to declare her incompetent, and no guardian appointed for her. Nor does vacillation indicate either incompetence or consent. The two District of Columbia cases cited do not discuss vacillation, but are very explicit on how a judge should respond in a case like Angela's. The middle part of the paragraph quoted tells judges what to do if the patient's choice is uncertain:

Whenever possible it is better for the judge to make a firsthand appraisal of the patient's personal desires and ability for rational choice. In this way the court can always know, to the extent possible, that the judgment is that of the individual concerned and not that of those who believe, however well-intentioned, that they speak for the person whose life is in the balance (*In re Osborne,* 294 A.2d 372, 374 [D.C. App. 1972]). (Emphasis added.)

If there was any question about what Angela wanted, there is no way around the conclusion that the judge should have talked directly to her. The reason he did not is that the entire case was based on the belief that Angela *was refusing,* and the only legal question was whether her rights should be ignored to try to save her fetus. The excuse that talking to Angela might have shortened her life cannot be taken seriously in view of the judge's conclusion that a major surgical procedure, which had a much greater prospect to end her life, should nonetheless be performed. Cutting without talking is how one would treat an "inanimate container."

Mishkin now concludes that the questions Angela's case raises "should be considered carefully by a court fully briefed by all parties." But at the hearing itself she did not argue for careful consideration by the court, but rather insisted that the court should hurry its decision and not bother to even talk with Angela because "time at this point is really of the essence" (TR 97).

The attorney who represented Angela has described the case as follows:

I think gender bias was present in our case, definitely. In a powerful and subliminal way, it's true that many perceive women, especially pregnant women, as second class citizens, as carriers. What is also compelling about this case is the court was not able to think of this competent individual—and sedation should not be confused with competence—as having vested rights and being capable of exercising them. This case ultimately is about a lack of respect for the individual, and her right to make the medical care decision that's best for herself (*American Medical News,* March 11, 1988, 18).

This has it exactly right. And it is worth noting that at the request of forty organizations, including the Ameri-can Medical Association, the American College of Obstetricians and Gynecologists, and the American Civil Liberties Union, who thought this case was wrongly and dangerously decided, the full bench of the D.C. Court of Appeals has "vacated" the appellate decision discussed in my column, and has said it will rehear the entire case at a later date. The District of Columbia, whose lawyer argued for surgical intervention on behalf of the fetus, has since repudiated its own position and joined in the request for a rehearing by the full court. All of this is, of course, too late for Angela; but it is a victory for all pregnant women who insist on making decisions for themselves, the views of would-be fetal rescuers notwithstanding.

Foreclosing the Use of Force: A. C. Reversed

George J. Annas, J.D., M.P.H.

William Carlos Williams relates how he once used force to pry open the mouth of a recalcitrant child who, he suspected, had diphtheria that could only be diagnosed by viewing her throat.[1] The little girl resists his coaxing, and when, with the father's help, he finally manages to jam the wooden tongue depressor between her teeth, the child opens her mouth just enough to crunch down on the blade to "reduce it to splinters." The doctor becomes furious with the child, whose mouth is now bleeding and who is "screaming in wild hysterical shrieks." But he knows he must see her throat for her own good, and it actually becomes "a pleasure to attack her. . . . The damned little brat must be protected against her own idiocy. . . ." Using a metal spoon and all his strength, he overpowers the child "in a final unreasoning assault. . . ." He learns her secret: she has diphtheria.

We can agree that Williams lost control and brutalized his child patient, yet still sympathize with him. Diphtheria was a life-threatening disease, and the child could not make a competent decision to refuse to have the doctor look at her throat. Moreover, her parents were present, and consented to the entire proceeding. It was the means not the rationale that was wrong.

The Right Track

The use of force has little, if any, role in the practice of medicine, although it may sometimes seem necessary in treating children and mentally incompetent patients. The 1980s, a decade not known for its compassion, saw some physicians and judges moving beyond children and the mentally incompetent to encompass pregnant women in the group of patients for whom forcing compliance was sometimes seen as justifiable. The rationale was not that pregnant women were incompetent to make their own decisions, but rather that some of the decisions they made might take inadequate account of the possible consequences of those decisions on the soon-to-be-born child.

Although there have been dozens of lower court opinions involving attempts to force treatment, usually cesarean sections, on pregnant women, only two have reached appeals courts. The first, *Jefferson v. Griffin Spalding Hospital Authority,*[2] was at the beginning of the 1980s. The second opens the 1990s on an entirely different note and is the most important case to be decided in this area to date: the case of Angela Carder, known simply as *In re: A.C.*[3] This new en banc decision, issued by the District of Columbia Court of Appeals almost three years after the original hearing (and two years after the original three-judge appeals decision was vacated), firmly reverses the original decisions (7 to 1) and sets forth the legal principles that should govern all doctor-patient relationships with pregnant patients: "We hold that in *virtually all cases* the question of what is to be done is to be decided by the patient—the pregnant woman—on behalf of herself and the fetus. If the patient is incompetent . . . her decision must be ascertained through . . . substituted judgment" (emphasis added).

Angela Carder was twenty-six-and-a-half weeks pregnant and near death from cancer when the hospital's lawyer decided to ask a judge to come to the hospital to tell the hospital what to do. The request was made because

Angela's attending physicians had informed the hospital administrator that they intended to honor the patient's wishes to keep her comfortable while she died, and not perform an immediate cesarean section. The patient, all members of her family (her husband and her mother), and all her attending physicians agreed on this course of action. The issue at the hearing was not what Ms. Carder wanted, but centered instead on whether the state had a compelling interest sufficient to force immediate surgery for the sake of the fetus. Accordingly, the testimony focused on the likelihood of fetal survival if surgery were performed immediately, rather than waiting until after Ms. Carder died (she was expected to die within forty-eight hours in any event) to deliver the fetus. The trial court found that her fetus had a 50 to 60 percent chance to survive an immediate cesarean, and that delay would greatly increase the risk to the fetus.

The D.C. appeals court has now ruled that it was improper for the lower court judge to weigh the mother's interests versus the state's interest in the fetus to decide what to do. Instead, the appeals court concluded that the proper procedure would have been for the judge first to determine if Ms. Carder were competent (a step that would at least have required the judge to see Ms. Carder), and if she were competent, to permit her to make the decision herself. The appeals court reached this conclusion because it could find no persuasive rationale to justify depriving women of their constitutional and common law rights as citizens because they become pregnant, carry a fetus to viability, or continue pregnancy with a terminal illness.

If the pregnant patient is incompetent, the trial judge is to determine what she would decide if she could decide, i.e., to apply the substituted judgment doctrine. To make this determination the judge should examine previous statements by the patient, the patient's value system, and what family members, loved ones, and even treating physicians think the patient would want.

Appeals courts cannot find facts, and this court accordingly did not determine what Ms. Carder wanted. On the other hand, the court did make it clear that judges are to do what patients in situations like this want done, and it could think of no "extremely rare and truly exceptional" case in which the state might have an interest sufficiently compelling to override the patient's wishes. The court also concluded unequivocally that the state had no interest sufficiently compelling to force surgery in the *A.C.* case itself.

All of this is solid and reasonable, and essentially concurs with the August 1987 opinion of the American College of Obstetrics and Gynecology's Ethics Committee. ACOG's committee concluded that when disagreements occur the physician should "convey the reasons for the current recommendation to the pregnant woman, encouraging responsible behavior through education and counseling," and that "resort to the court is *almost never* justified" (emphasis added). Law and medicine are on the same track here, and in honoring the pregnant patient's decision as outcome-determinative, both are on the right track.

The case was remanded, but *not* for further fact finding, an exercise that appeals court labeled "inappropriate and futile." To litigate competence and substituted judgment without Ms. Carder would be little more than a vulturous act of vengeance on the part of those who treated her as if she were already dead at the original hearing.

The Footnotes

One potential for misunderstanding and underestimating the importance and strength of this opinion are some of its twenty-three footnotes. Footnotes in legal opinions are an old problem. It is often stated, for example, that "footnotes are for losers." This implies that the judge writing the majority opinion will put material in footnotes at the request of other judges who will join the opinion only if he does. Some of the footnotes in *A.C.,* read separately from the opinion, could easily be taken out of context to present a misleading view of the opinion itself.

The opinion holds that in "virtually all" cases the decision should be made by the pregnant woman herself or through substituted judgment. Footnote 2, however, seems to suggest that a separate "tribunal" of some sort be formed to make the final decision on unspecified grounds: "Because the judgment in such a case involves complex medical and ethical issues as well as the application of legal principles, we would urge the establishment — through legislation or otherwise — of another tribunal to make these decisions, with limited opportunity for judicial review." Of course, there are no "complex medical and ethical issues" to resolve if the only relevant issue is what the woman wants done.

This suggestion should not be taken any more seriously than legislatures and others have taken suggestions from a string of courts since the Karen Ann Quinlan case to establish quasi-administrative agencies to resolve conflicts that should have been resolved in the doctor-patient relationship. The central idea in *A.C.* is not that an alternate decision-making "tribunal" or committee should be established; rather it is that judges should not be called to hospitals to make emergency decisions. As this case so well illustrates, rushed to an unfamiliar environment, asked to make a decision under great stress, and having no time either for reflection or for study of existing law and precedents, a judge cannot act judiciously. Neither the facts nor the law can be accurately determined. The judge in the hospital in an emergency situation will ultimately act arbitrarily, and the exercise will become one simply of using raw force. The court has made the law

George J. Annas, J.D., M.P.H.

crystal clear; it is now the obligation of physicians, hospitals, and hospital lawyers to follow it.

Prior Decisions

Footnotes 7 and 23 try to distinguish this case from *Jefferson,* the only other appeals court decision in this area, and from a previously decided lower court opinion in the District of Columbia, *In re Mayden.*[4] In both of these cases the pregnant woman was "unquestionably competent," and both women refused to submit to cesarean sections based on religious objections. Even though the court refuses either directly to challenge *Jefferson* or directly to overrule *Mayden,* it should be emphasized that neither decision can any longer be considered good law in the District of Columbia. The appeals court spent little time on *Jefferson* because it found the facts distinguishable. In *Jefferson* the court relied completely on the testimony of one physician that because of placenta previa, without a cesarean section there was a 99 percent chance that the soon-to-be-child would die, and a 50 percent chance that the mother would die. Legally, the *Jefferson* court wrongly equated an almost child *before* birth with an actual child after birth. Reliance on medical "evidence" also proved misplaced. The child was ultimately delivered vaginally, without any surgical intervention, and both mother and child did fine.[5]

The *Mayden* case is more important because it is a District of Columbia case, and the trial judge in *A.C.* relied on it. In footnote 23 the appeals court says it is neither "approving or disapproving" *Mayden;* nonetheless, its opinion overrules it. In *Mayden,* the chief resident at the public hospital wanted to perform a cesarean section on a woman whose labor was not progressing. The woman, a Muslim who was specifically determined to be competent, refused and her husband agreed with her. She instead wanted to stand up or walk to assist delivery naturally. The stated basis of the physician's wish to perform a cesarean was that an infection could begin at any time and could kill the baby or cause brain damage. The likelihood of an infection increased every hour. On this basis alone the court ordered the cesarean. A healthy child was born, with no evidence of infection. The *Mayden* decision also contains two revealing statements: "All that stood between the Mayden fetus and its independent existence, separate from its mother was, put simply, a doctor's scalpel"; and "Neither parent . . . is a trained physician." In short, *Mayden* seemed to hold that if a doctor believes a surgical procedure is necessary, and has the means to perform it, he should be able to perform it even if the woman competently refuses, a result precisely opposite to that in *A.C.*

Moreover, in *A.C.* the pregnant woman was dying, and the judge believed that the *only* chance for the fetus to live was an immediate cesarean. In *Mayden* there was *no evidence* of medical problems to either the mother or the soon-to-be-child. It appears that the majority of the appeals court decided to discuss *Mayden* at all only because the lone dissenting judge opted to append the text of this previously unreported decision to his dissent. Rather than ignore it altogether, the majority apparently decided to add a final footnote to their already finished written opinion.

Three other footnotes are also relevant. The first is note 17, in which we learn for the first time in the court proceedings to date the views of Ms. Carder's personal physician, who had been treating her cancer for years. The court tells us that he was not notified by the hospital about the hearing, but if he had been "he would have come to the hospital immediately and would have testified that a cesarean section was medically inadvisable *both for A.C. and for the fetus*" (original emphasis). The court says this shows that the record was deficient, but it shows much more. It shows that emergency hearings in hospitals are inherently unfair and arbitrary because it is impossible to prepare for them adequately and even to assemble, much less consider, the relevant facts and individuals.

The Use of Force

In footnote 3 the court notes that even though Angela Carder's attending physicians refused to perform the cesarean, and another doctor who was willing had to be found, "no physician was ordered to perform surgery or to provide any treatment against his or her will." Likewise, the trial judge in this case indicated that he didn't believe he had the authority to order a physician to operate against his will. Everyone at the original hearing seemed to concur. Nonetheless, none of the judges to date has commented on the radical asymmetry: forcing invasive surgery on a competent adult had, until this opinion, seemed perfectly acceptable; forcing a physician to perform such surgery was always unthinkable. Both should be unthinkable. Even the lone dissenting appeals judge, who defines "the viable unborn child" as "literally captive within its mother's body" (transforming the mother-fetus relationship into a warden-prisoner relationship), would draw the line at the use of physical force to perform surgery on an unwilling pregnant woman.

The dissenting judge, just as the trial judge in *A.C.,* apparently thinks that because a major surgical procedure such as a cesarean section must be done by a trained physician, it does not constitute the use of force, whereas holding someone's hands down does. This is probably because judges are very familiar with restraining one's physical liberty, but have little familiarity with medical procedures. It may also, of course, be simply that because judges are predominantly male and cesarean sections will never be performed on them, it is a surgical intervention they cannot see as offensive.

The use-of-force argument, if taken seriously, would lead to the repulsive conclusion that it is acceptable to force unwanted procedures on defenseless competent patients, such as the anesthetized or quadriplegic, but not on those who can physically fight back. This is just one reason why the ultimate justification for surgical intervention must be the consent of the patient, not the patient's ability to fight the doctor. William Carlos Williams's language in "The Use of Force" is again helpful: force fouls the doctor-patient relationship, subverting it into an assailant-victim relationship. He asks his small patient, "Will you open it [her mouth] now by yourself or shall we have to open it for you?," and without her agreement, their relationship rapidly deteriorates to a point where medical "treatment" can only be termed "unreasoning assault." It is thus not surprising that all the judges in *A.C.* find the use of force unacceptable.

The *A.C.* opinion and the ACOG standards come as close to saying that the decision of a pregnant woman, even one in labor, should *never* be overridden by a judge as any court or medical professional association can. It is almost impossible to think of any case where a competent pregnant woman's decision might be appropriately overruled by a judge that would be consistent with the *A.C.* opinion that "force" should never be used to physically restrain a competent woman. Not only surgery, but blood transfusions, injections, and even forcing a pill down a woman's throat, are to be prohibited.

The conclusion thus seems inescapable: the use of the judiciary to force women to undergo medical treatments against their will is not only counterproductive, unprincipled, sexist, and repressive, it is also lawless. Instead of trying to develop better procedures to force "treatment" on a few unwilling pregnant women, we should be trying to improve consensual prenatal and perinatal care for everyone.

Williams opens another of his *Doctor Stories* with the words, "That which is possible is inevitable."[6] Forcing pregnant women and those in labor to undergo surgery and other interventions against their will is certainly possible, as we have seen. If the decision in *A.C.* and the guidelines of ACOG are taken seriously, however, the use of force in the delivery room will no longer be inevitable.

References

1. William Carlos Williams, "The Use of Force," in *The Doctor Stories* (New York: New Directions, 1984), 56–60.
2. 247 Ga. 86, 274 S.E.2d 457 (1981).
3. *In re: A.C.*, D.C. Ct App., April 26, 1990 (en banc, slip op.). The story of the 1987 in-hospital hearing and appellate decision that ordered Ms. Carder to undergo a cesarean section was reported previously in "She's Going to Die: The Case of Angela C," *Hastings Center Report* 18:1 (1988), 23–25.
4. 114 Daily Wash. L. Rptr. 2233 (D.C. Super. Ct. July 26, 1986).
5. George J. Annas, "Forced Cesareans: The Most Unkindest Cut of All," *Hastings Center Report* 12:3 (1982), 16–17, 45.
6. William Carlos Williams, "Danse Pseudomacabre," 88.

Policy on Decision-Making with Pregnant Patients at The George Washington University Hospital

Decision-Making with Adult Patients Generally:

Health care decision-making is a joint enterprise between patient(s) or surrogate(s) on the one hand and caregiver(s) on the other. Ethics, law and sound medical practice emphasize both patient autonomy and professional standards. No party should be the mere instrument of another. In shared decision making, the act of informed consent or informed refusal affirms and protects patient autonomy while acknowledging the physician's commitment to professional standards.[1]

We base our policies regarding decision making on this hospital's (and the medical profession's) strong commitment to respecting the autonomy of all patients with capacity. Respect for autonomy does not end because an adult patient with capacity refuses a course of action strongly recommended by an attending physician. Nor do professional standards require that patients comply with every physician recommendation or that physicians agree to comply with every patient's request. From this respect for both patient autonomy and for professional standards flows our strong preference for maintaining decision making within the physician-patient relationship rather than having outsiders (e.g. courts) impose health care decisions on unwilling patients.

Some patients are not capable of consenting to or refusing treatment in an informed fashion, either because they have lost capacity (such as an adult who becomes comatose) or because they never had capacity (such as infants and children, or adults who have been mentally disabled from birth). These patients' preferences as to health care decisions should be determined through the doctrine of "substituted judgment". Under this doctrine, the surrogate decision-maker attempts to determine what the patient would have decided if capable, based upon the surrogate's knowledge of the patient's value system, expressed wishes or other reasonably reliable evidence of the patient's desires.

When no reasonably reliable evidence exists from which a surrogate and the care-giver can determine a patient's desires relevant to a particular treatment decision, the surrogate and the care-giver together must consider what would be in the patient's "best interest".

Decision-Making with Pregnant Patients:

These ethical, legal and medical standards also govern the decision-making process with a pregnant patient. But the uniqueness of the maternal-fetal relationship may occasionally create special considerations in the application of these principles.

The American College of Obstetricians and Gynecologists ("ACOG") and the American Academy of Pediatrics ("AAP") both recognize that a pregnant woman and her fetus comprise "two patients". Both organizations recognize as well that the unique characteristic of this situation is that one patient (the fetus) is accessible only through the other (the woman). ACOG advises that the "obstetrician should be concerned with the health care of both the pregnant woman and the fetus within her, assessing the attendant risks and benefits to each during the course of care."[2] AAP similarly suggests that pediatricians "formulate treatment recommendations that balance the best interests of the fetus and the potential risks to the woman."[3]

Consistent with the ACOG and AAP statements, it is the policy of this hospital that obstetricians must consider the health of the pregnant patient and her fetus in assessing the range of medically reasonable treatment options, and must communicate this information to the pregnant patient to enable her to make informed health care decisions. The difficulty in evaluating a degree of benefit or risk to the fetus requires great care in presenting such information. That evaluation often will be enhanced by input from pediatric and other appropriate specialists.

Our usual expectation is that the welfare of the fetus is of enormous, if not primary, importance to the pregnant women, and that conflicts between a pregnant woman's medical treatment decisions and fetal well-being are unusual. Both the obstetrician and the pregnant woman work together for the well-being of both the woman and fetus. When the decision serves both maternal and fetal interests, there is no need to question the basis for the patient's decision.

When a pregnant patient with capacity is properly counseled by her attending physician about the risks and benefits to her and her fetus of a particular course of care, the decision of the pregnant patient to consent to or refuse that care may be inconsistent with the welfare of the patient or her fetus. When a pregnant patient's decision appears unnecessarily to disserve her own or fetal welfare, great care should be taken to verify that her decision is both informed and authentic. When a patient's choice appears to conflict with her own values or when her decision conflicts with our usual expectation, special attention to the decision and process of decision-making is warranted.

In such a situation, the attending physician should explore the reasoning behind the pregnant patient's decision. Such a decision may result from the patient's inadequate understanding or misconstruing of the relative risks and benefits to herself and to her fetus of available treatment alternatives.[4] It may result from pressures by family members, who in turn may have an inadequate understanding of these risks and benefits.

Additional counseling (by the obstetrician and by pediatric and other appropriate specialists) may correct inadequacy of information or misunderstanding. The attending physician may suspect, however, that the pregnant patient's decision stems from emotional or psychological difficulties. In such circumstances, a psychiatric consultation should be requested since treating impaired

mental functioning may restore the patient's decision-making capacity. Discussions with family members also may be appropriate. The attending physician is encouraged to bring such matters to the attention of the hospital ethics committee, which is available to consult with the attending physician, the pregnant patient, family members and other interested parties.[5]

When a fully informed and competent pregnant patient persists in a decision which may disserve her own or fetal welfare, this hospital's policy is to accede to the pregnant patient's preference whenever possible (see paragraphs on Withdrawal from Participation by an Individual Caregiver and by an Institution). As noted earlier, our respect for autonomous adult patients' decisions is not altered simply on the basis of disagreement between the patient and her caregivers regarding the appropriate course of treatment.

Assessing Decision-Making by a Pregnant Patient's Surrogate:

When a pregnant patient is not capable of consenting to or refusing treatment in an informed fashion, her preferences should be determined through the doctrine of "substituted judgment". When a properly-selected or legally-recognized surrogate insists that the pregnant patient, if capable, would have decided to act in a fashion which appears unnecessarily to disserve the welfare of the mother or her fetus, the care-giver must scrutinize each element of the surrogate's participation, to evaluate, for example, (a) the possibility of conflict of interest, (b) the reliability of the evidence of the patient's desires upon which the surrogate purportedly is relying, (c) the surrogate's knowledge of the patient's value system and (d) the surrogate's responsible commitment to the decision-making process.

The caregiver should enlist the assistance of appropriate consultants, including the hospital Ethics Committee, in undertaking this evaluation. This policy contemplates that a surrogate's decision to act in a fashion which appears unnecessarily to disserve the welfare of the pregnant patient's fetus will be honored only if the care-giver and the hospital are convinced that the surrogate's decision is well-founded under the criteria articulated above. The hospital will accede to a well founded surrogate's decision whenever possible (see paragraphs on Withdrawal From Participation by an Individual Caregiver and by an Institution).

Withdrawal from Participation of an Individual Care-Giver:

This policy also recognizes that professional standards do not require individual care-givers to comply with every patient decision. When an individual care-giver believes that compliance with a pregnant patient's refusal of or request for treatment would cause that care-giver to violate his/her professional standards, it may be appropriate for the care-giver to withdraw from the relationship with the pregnant patient. As in any other treatment situation, withdrawal from the care of a pregnant patient is appropriate only where that patient is given adequate notice and assistance in obtaining competent substitute care.

Withdrawal from Participation by the Institution:

Whenever a conflict in such cases arises which cannot be resolved within the caregiver/patient relationship, all other intra-institutional resources, including the Ethics Committee, must be utilized. The remote case may still ensue that a pregnant patient's decision continues to appear to disserve fetal welfare and is so ethically unsettling that it may justify an institutional decision to withdraw from the case. Such justification normally would exist when there was unanimity or overwhelming consensus among the attending physician and assisting members of the health care team that:

- There is near certainty of substantial and imminent harm to the fetal patient absent the proposed treatment; and
- The proposed procedure has a very high possibility of reversing or preventing the anticipated harm to the fetus; and
- Risk to the mother is minimal; and
- Withdrawal from the case is not likely to cause harm to the pregnant patient or cause her to abandon medical care for herself and her fetus.

Seeking Judicial Intervention:

Courts are an inappropriate forum for resolving ethical issues. Resort to court for the purpose of resolving such issues should rarely occur. We recognize there may be legal motivations to seeking judicial intervention in certain situations.

When Time Is Short:

The activities encouraged by this policy presume the availability of time: for a care-giver to explain his/her professional standards to the pregnant patient; for a care-giver to engage in a substantive and meaningful dialogue with the pregnant patient calculated to enable that patient to consent to or refuse treatment in an informed fashion; for the pregnant patient to contemplate the reasonable medical options and to consult with the care-giver and family members; for the care-giver to enlist the assistance of appropriate consultants, when necessary.

Every effort should be made to address treatment decisions as early as possible. We recognize, however, that there will be times when decisions need to be made under emergent circumstances. In those cases, as in other emergency situations, the principle of therapeutic privilege[6] ought to apply. Therapeutic privilege should only be invoked when it is virtually impossible to apply the process outlined earlier in this document.

Conclusion:

1. Health care decision making is a joint enterprise between patients (or their surrogates) and their caregivers, with patient autonomy and professional standards respected as complementary values.

2. Respect for patient autonomy compels us to accede to the treatment decisions of a pregnant patient whenever possible. When a pregnant patient makes a decision which unnecessarily disserves maternal or fetal welfare, caregivers must undertake to ensure that the decision is not the result of inadequate information or a correctable misunderstanding before acceding to the decision, withdrawing from the case if the care giver feels compelled by professional standards or seeking resolution of the problem outside the patient/ physician relationship.

3. Respect for patient autonomy and professional standards engenders a strong commitment to keeping health care decision-making within the patient-physician relationship. When a caregiver's questions about a patient's treatment decision require input from outside the immediate relationship, that input should be solicited from other elements of the hospital community, including individual consultants in appropriate specialties and the Ethics Committee. It may occasionally, for ethical reasons, be appropriate for the hospital to withdraw from a case. It will rarely be appropriate to seek judicial intervention to resolve ethical issues.

16autonomy.2
11-13-90
Approved by the Executive Committee 11/16/90

References

1. President's Commission for the Study of Ethical Problems in Medicine and Biomedical and Behavioral Research, *Making*

Health Care Decisions, US Government Printing Office, Washington, 1983.

2. ACOG Committee Opinion Number 55 October 1987 "Patient Choice: Maternal-Fetal Conflict".

3. AAP Committee on Bioethics "Fetal Therapy: Ethical Considerations".

4. Brock, D. W.; Wartman, S. A.. 1990. Sounding Board: When Competent Patients Make Irrational Choices, *New England Journal of Medicine.* 322:1595–1599. Eraker, S. A.; Politser,

P. 1982. "How Decisions are Reached: Physician and Patient. *Annals of Internal Medicine.* 97:262–8.

5. The George Washington University Hospital Ethics Committee, *Ethics Committee Structure.*

6. Therapeutic privilege is defined as the right of a physician to act in what he or she judges to be in the best interest of the patient(s) involved in the absence of the opportunity to obtain informed consent.

Chapter 22

Ethics Issues in Rural Health and Hospitals

William A. Nelson, Ph.D., and Andrew S. Pomerantz, M.D.

William A. Nelson, Ph.D., is codirector of the National Ethics Center, Veterans Administration Hospital, White River Junction, Vermont. Andrew S. Pomerantz, M.D., is an assistant professor of clinical psychiatry at Dartmouth Medical School, Hanover, New Hampshire.

Much of the focus of medical ethics is on the sophisticated, technology-related problems that arise in the academic medical center. Newspapers feature stories almost daily on health care dilemmas in the urban setting. However, ethical issues in the delivery of health care have become commonplace whether one practices medicine in urban or rural settings, in academic or solo practices. More rural physicians than academic physicians have general medical practices, but, nonetheless, medical care has changed dramatically for both. Three factors have influenced this change, neither of which is unique to the physician practicing in a large urban medical center.

The first factor is the rapid advance in medical technology and drugs. Along with the new possibilities for diagnosis and treatment of illness have come new ethical dilemmas. Just because we can do something does not necessarily mean we should do it. The care of the chronically and terminally ill is an obvious example of this problem. There are few deaths today that do not involve decision making at the end of life. According to a 1986 study and a brief prepared by the American Hospital Association, 70 percent of the deaths in this country involve some negotiated agreement not to use life-prolonging technology.[1] This situation emphasizes the ethical questions of who lives, who dies, and—of growing concern—who pays.

The second major factor is that patients today expect more from physicians in resolving medical problems and seek more involvement in decision making. Through the media, the general public is exposed to news of the latest medical advances, which they believe will be readily available to them and will resolve their health care problems.

The third factor is an outgrowth of the patients' rights movement, patients want to make their own decisions. A recent article from the *New York Times* series "Doctors in Distress" attributed the deterioration of the physician–patient relationship to a lack of trust, malpractice suits, and policies and regulations dictating care. Many patients have the feeling that medicine is just a business. They, therefore, want to take greater control over decision making, especially treatment decisions that relate to their personal values.[2]

Although rural physicians may not often face "exotic," highly sophisticated ethical issues related to such high-tech procedures as organ transplantation and in vitro fertilization, they struggle with many of the same ethical dilemmas as urban and academic physicians. However, there are two major differences: The frequency of various ethical dilemmas differs in the two settings, and the dilemmas of rural health care are more strongly influenced by cultural characteristics. For the rural health care provider, issues involving withdrawal of life-support technology are less common than issues of confidentiality.[3] What seems most significant in examining ethical issues in the rural practice setting is understanding the unique sociological factors that affect the nature of the ethical dilemmas. The following case highlights these issues:

Early on a Tuesday afternoon I [Dr. Pomerantz] received a message to call Dr. Gibson, a cardiologist at a nearby community hospital. I didn't know this physician, who had arrived in the area shortly after I had left my general practice. When I returned the call, he told me that a former patient of mine, Carolyn, had apparently suffered a heart attack and most likely a massive stroke. He informed me that she was on life support and that there was essentially no chance she could recover. After thanking him for letting me know, I discovered that he was doing more than just informing me.

Dr. Gibson told me that Michael, a friend, brought her in. "He was pretty upset, partly because she had always told him that if anything ever happened to her, she wanted him to 'call Andy,' but he didn't think you would be able to do much for her." I told Dr. Gibson I agreed that there wasn't much I could have done and that Michael had acted wisely.

"Michael said you knew what she'd have wanted done if she got into this condition. I'm calling to ask you whether we should leave her on life support."

"Shouldn't her family make that decision?" I asked, though I knew full well that her closest relative, a grandniece, had not had any interaction with her for 20 years.

Dr. Gibson continued, "I figured that the decision ought to be made by someone who knows her. I understand you were her doctor for 10 years or more. I'd rather have you decide. From what Michael told me, I think she'd want you to be the one."

Although I knew the law might suggest otherwise, he was right. Carolyn had made no secret of the fact that she trusted me to make the important clinical decisions for her, which I documented in her record. She was from the "old school" of doctor–patient relationships. She fully accepted the model that designated the physician as the one who knew best what was needed. Such patients, when asked by their doctors to make a choice, always answered, "You're the doctor; you tell me what to do." I had begun my general practice in a rural village of 900 inhabitants with an approach to the doctor–patient model that emphasized a shared decision process. I envisioned a partnership with my patients. Carolyn was one of the first to challenge that idea.

When I first arrived in town, there was a bit of hesitancy to see the new physician. My partner, who had been there for 20 years, still saw almost all the patients, while I mostly waited. When Carolyn developed some shortness of breath, she told my wife—whom she met in a ceramics class—that she was going to have me examine her.

One week later she called and asked me to make a house call.

I examined her and found she had signs of heart failure. With some prodding she agreed to come to my office for a chest X ray, an EKG, and some lab work. I eventually started her on digoxin and her condition improved. Soon I had no problem getting new patients.

Following that first visit, several people stopped me on the street or in the store and wanted to know what had happened to Carolyn and how was she doing. I knew it was unethical to share confidential information and generally mumbled something about how they ought to ask her. They looked at me strangely. I asked Carolyn how I should respond to such questions and she asked me why I didn't just tell them how she was doing. She said that anyone in town would know sooner or later and they might as well hear it from the doctor.

Over the years I made house calls to her apartment every month or two. We'd sit in easy chairs, talking about Watergate, the weather, Reaganomics, or whatever was most important at the time. We also talked about her heart and lungs, the swelling in her feet, and her intense fear of someday "being a vegetable." Although she had very little money, she often sent my children a five-dollar bill on their birthdays. We got to know each other very well.

I was Carolyn's doctor for 12 years. During that time news of modern medical advances finally made it to our town. Carolyn was one of the few who understood the limitations of my house calls. She often remarked that she still believed the stethoscope was just as good as the CT scanner, and she understood that the latter would not fit in my little black bag. Many others in the community, although they still wanted me to make house calls, also wanted the same diagnostic precision that they read about in *Reader's Digest.* I found that when I tried to steer people into the office or into the hospital, I was often told I was becoming just like all the other doctors who had given up house calls. I tried to satisfy my own concerns by letting people know that although I was willing to see them at home, they were not going to be getting the same standard of care they were reading about. Although they always said that was fine, if things went sour, my errors kept the town gossip mill grinding for weeks.

Another challenge to practice came from third-party payers. Very often I was unable to limit office calls to the standard 15 minutes. In a small town, many, like Carolyn, still treat the doctor as the all-knowing fountain of wisdom and empathy and share their souls on the way to the examining table.

Others saw me as just another member of the community with whom they would rub elbows at Little League games, church suppers, school concerts, and the like. Some didn't want me to know much about them. These patients were no problem: They came to see me with clear symptoms and received a focused exam, diagnosis, and treatment. Others, however, often needed my shoulder and an hour or so of my time. To provide such care for those who needed it led to two problems: Patients stacked up in the waiting room, and I was reimbursed for only 15 minutes by third-party payers.

A full waiting room was initially a problem for me. I got tired of apologizing to everyone for keeping them waiting. They always said it was okay, but it wasn't until I met Fred that I actually believed them. Fred told me that he didn't mind waiting because he knew that it meant I was spending extra time with someone who needed it and that if he needed extra time he would get it. He viewed the time in the waiting room as an investment of sorts, knowing it would someday come back to him with interest.

The third-party payer part was more difficult. It put me in a bind of knowing I was losing money by providing extra time to people such as Carolyn. There were only three options. I could lie to the insurance company and make up a diagnosis that required an hour's evaluation. I could stop providing the extra time and refer people to psychiatrists. Or I could take the financial loss as a price paid for running a rural medical practice. I chose the last option.

Carolyn's medical care in the last dozen years of her life was probably not much different from what she received in the first dozen. Still, she lived well into her eighties and got the care she wanted. She saw the possibility that I might miss diagnosing an obscure problem as the risk she was willing to take in order to get the kind of medical care she wanted. When Dr. Gibson asked me what to do with her life support, I had no reservations about telling him I knew she would not want to live that way. After treatment was discontinued, she died quickly and quietly.

Rural Care Characteristics

There are many ways of thinking of the term *rural*, ranging from the descriptive (an agricultural community) to population density to distance from population centers. In this chapter rural refers to population size. According to the U. S. Census Bureau, a rural community has fewer than 2,500 people.[4]

Related to the low population density of the rural setting is the low number of physicians. In 1988, rural areas had 97 practicing physicians per 100,000, as compared to 225 per 100,000 in metropolitan areas. In 1988, at least 111 rural counties in the United States had no physician.[5] There is a trend away from family practice, especially in the rural setting, and that trend will likely continue. "The number of medical school graduates entering family practice has remained virtually unchanged for most of this decade," Rakel observes. "At the same time, many other specialties and subspecialties have seen their numbers increase, thereby exacerbating the physician maldistribution problem."[6]

The case of Carolyn highlights many of the characteristics of the rural setting that influence the response to ethical dilemmas, both by the health care provider and the patient. These characteristics include the interplay between the physician's private and professional lives, the physical distance between health professionals, the nonspecialized orientation of the rural practice, and the struggle between conflicting needs.

Interplay between the Physician's Private and Professional Lives

There is a unique interplay between the private and professional lives of rural physicians. There is no buffer between the physician and the patient. In small rural communities, where everyone knows one another, doctor and patient may run into each other frequently in the course of daily life. The physician may be perceived as "community property"— there to be a public servant at all times. He or she may have difficulty getting away from the professional role and is perceived as "the doctor" long after formal office hours, although some patients try to respect set hours. Many physicians leave the rural setting, not because of lack of skills or judgment, but because they insist upon a strict definition of time on and off duty.

Physical Distance between Health Professionals

In rural areas, the physical distance between health professionals can be great. This promotes independence, self-reliance, and, in some cases, alienation. Rural physicians frequently work in solo practices. As a result, consultation with other physicians is often inconvenient or impossible. There is no opportunity to discuss cases informally with colleagues. Consultations usually consist of telephone calls to a specialist in an urban or academic setting.

Another result of the isolated setting is limited opportunity for continuing education. The rural physician cannot easily attend the distant medical center's educational programs, such as medical grand rounds and mortality and morbidity conferences. He or she must depend on medical literature as the main source of education. Although rural physicians can attend conferences lasting several days on a particular topic, the expense of travel and the problem of getting coverage for the time away may present obstacles.

Because of the isolated location, rural patients become dependent on a single provider. Although this is generally satisfactory, some patients may feel that their options are too limited if they lack confidence in or feel uncomfortable with the physician.

Nonspecialized Orientation

Rural medical practice has retained its nonspecialized orientation, in contrast to the rest of the medical community, which emphasizes technology and specialization. Rural care providers practice as primary care physicians, regardless of their training in such areas as family medicine, internal medicine, or general practice. As such, they focus on broad health issues in patient care and get to know the family as well as the patient. Yet some problems require specialized medical skills to provide an acceptable standard of care. There is a clear conflict for the patient, who wants a kindly, "Marcus Welby"-type physician, but also wants the physician to practice at the highest level, using all the newest technology described in the popular press.

Struggle between Conflicting Needs

The physician is frequently caught between conflicting needs, including wanting to make a reasonable income, yet knowing that is not possible if he or she is to remain in rural medicine; needing to be constantly available as a doctor, but wanting and needing personal time; and wanting to serve poor patients, yet needing to fill the economic needs of the clinic or office.

Ethical Issues

Many ethical issues in rural medical practice are influenced by cultural factors. The following are several of the most common issues confronting, in particular, physicians in the private practice setting.

Confidentiality

Confidentiality within the physician–patient relationship is a prevalent issue in medical practice and is particularly complex in the rural setting because the physician is generally the provider for the whole family. Thus the physician must maintain confidentiality while caring for other family members. The fine line between breaching confidence and maintaining truthfulness may become an ethical issue because of family dynamics and the physician's multifaceted role. For example, a parent may not want the physician to inform his daughter about his life-threatening illness. Yet the physician is confronted with questions from the daughter, whom the physician is also treating. Or the physician, who is also a member of the

school board, is treating a science teacher for a severe emotional problem that may be affecting his or her quality of teaching. Does the physician reveal the problem to the board?[7]

In the case of Carolyn, many members of the community were aware of her health problems. The physician behaved appropriately by getting Carolyn's consent before he communicated anything about her situation. Without such confirmation, the physician would be breaching confidentiality.

Quality-of-Care Decisions

A physician's goal is to promote high-quality health care that is in keeping with the patient's desires. Ethical issues surface in rural practice because of limited access to technological medicine and the distance from large hospitals and specialized care. The rural physician routinely makes triage decisions that have an impact on the physician's income, as well as on the patient's perceptions of the quality of care. The patient may have to decide between receiving a low level of care in the rural setting and a specialized level of care in a distant, large, urban medical center. For the patient, the specialized care may lead to significant financial hardships and inconvenience. These issues should be discussed openly with the patient, who must then decide whether he or she prefers to be treated by the primary caregiver or to go to the academic medical center for more specialized care. The physician should present to the patient all options, including the potential benefits and harms of each.

Patient Involvement in the Decision Process

The concept and application of valid consent and refusal are the cornerstones of ethical health care. For a consent or refusal to be valid, the patient must be given adequate information, must not be coerced, and must be competent. If the patient is incompetent, then the person serving as the proxy decision maker should be given the appropriate information and the same process should be applied.[8] However, because of the closeness between patient and physician in rural practice, as in the case of Carolyn, there can be a shared decision process. Physicians should present the patient with treatment options in an unbiased manner, provide the needed information, and foster a discussion of the patient's values regarding the benefits and harms of the treatment. Physicians must be aware of their power in presenting information, which can dominate the decision process. It may be that the bravest thing a physician can say to a patient, if pushed to make the patient's decision, is, "I do not know what is best for you." However, if physicians do accept the decision-making role (which they are not required to do), they should share their thinking with their patients to ensure concurrence.

The physician's role in the consent process is to promote patient self-determination, to help the patient feel some control and participation in his or her own care. Because the primary care provider recognizes that psychological, social, and economic factors influence a patient's thinking, a physician who knows the patient is in an ideal situation to explore these issues as they relate to the medical decision. Developing such a moral role is inherent in primary care medicine, and it leads to a more comprehensive understanding of the physician–patient relationship.[9]

In the case of Carolyn, the physician understood the ethical and legal theory that competent patients can accept or refuse any treatment and that, if the patient is not competent, the patient's advance directive or appointed proxy can serve as the decision maker. When there is no such information or person, a hospital or physician may choose to go to court to have someone appointed the guardian for the patient. That may be the most risk-free process. Carolyn had someone who was aware of her desires and wishes: her former physician. She had indicated previously that she wanted him to make decisions on her behalf, and he had documented the discussion in her medical record. Therefore it was morally appropriate to allow this physician, who knew the patient, to act as a surrogate decision maker.

The surrogate's role is to represent the patient's thinking. Generally the surrogate is a relative or legally appointed agent named in accordance with a durable-power-of-attorney document. In the rural setting, this role is occasionally filled by the physician. It is ethically appropriate to accept such a role, but the physician should document the discussion with and decisions made by the patient and should garner as much specific information as possible regarding the patient's desires, as was done in Carolyn's situation. Physicians should openly seek patients' thoughts long before the occurrence of a crisis, preferably through the use of a living will or a durable power of attorney. Patients generally are willing to share their feelings concerning the extent of care they desire if or when a chronic illness becomes life-threatening.

Referral Issues

Referring patients to a medical center and then receiving them back is an issue that concerns the primary care physician, the patients, and patients' family. The rural physician is often seen by academic medical center physicians as "the outsider." Medical center physicians too frequently have little understanding of rural practice and its cultural features, with the result that referrals frequently are problematic. Furthermore, patients feel rejected when it is suggested they go to the medical center; they are upset when they receive care other than what was explained, and they are confused by a different system. Discharge planning is often ignored or inappropriate; communication with the primary care physician is often inadequate; and in some situations, the patient is not referred back

to the primary physician but instead is sent to multiple specialty clinics within the medical center. In addition, the rural doctor is sometimes openly criticized at the center. Many rural patients do not like being in such a situation and are reluctant to go to a medical center even when their primary care provider believes it is indicated.

What stance, then, should the primary care provider take when discussing the medical center with a rural patient? Past problems with referrals might influence the physician unconsciously, and he or she may not make a referral even when it is indicated. Obviously, the physician should try, in an unbiased manner, to discuss with the patient the need for further care at the medical center. He or she should also try to discuss concerns about the referral process with appropriate medical center physicians and communicate the need for discharge information in order to ensure good follow-up care. In addition, a group of rural physicians with similar referral concerns should meet with medical center officials to develop a reasonable policy to meet the needs of all, especially those of the patient.

Economic Issues

Despite popular mythology, living costs in rural areas are often higher than in urban settings. Food, clothing, fuel, and other necessities must be transported from population and distribution centers in metropolitan areas to these distant sites, thus raising costs. Although the rewards of working so closely with patients are great, the financial needs of both the physician and patient must be met. Commonly the physician is asked to treat patients who have no means to pay or patients who already owe large sums of money. Many patients are too proud to request Medicare or Medicaid coverage, and yet their subsistence funds cover only essentials. Although the village grocer or gas station operator can refuse to provide goods or services to those who are unable to pay, such an option can be used only with great difficulty, if at all, by the rural physician. When a rural resident is faced with multiple bills, the one for medical care is the one most likely to be skipped. Thus the decision to suggest a test may be based on an analysis that includes the cost of the test and an assessment by the physician of how much he or she really needs to know the results.

Third-party reimbursement is a further complication. Rural physicians recognize the preventive health value of extended visits with some patients, and yet third-party payers do not reimburse for time, only for services. In the case of Carolyn, the physician knew the therapeutic value of talking about things beyond her chief complaints and symptoms. He willingly spent an hour doing just that, but he was reimbursed as though he had spent only five minutes taking her blood pressure and listening to her heartbeat in his office.

Hospital-Related Issues

Many primary care providers see hospitalized patients and direct their care at small rural hospitals. These hospitals usually have fewer than 100 beds. The small hospital can provide good care but frequently lacks the variety of specialized services found in the larger medical center. Although ethical issues such as those discussed here are relevant in any hospital setting, the primary physician's ability to provide good care is enhanced by his or her knowledge of the patient's medical history and personal values. Such insights can improve the physician's capacity to serve as a patient advocate and maintain a continuity of care correlated to outpatient treatment. The advocacy role involves both medical and ethical advocacy. The physician advocate seeks to ensure that medical care meets the patient's health care needs in accordance with his or her reasonable desires. Thus, the physician will act on behalf of the patient by protecting what he or she knows to be the patient's best interest.

Occasionally in the hospital setting, there is uncertainty about a mentally incapacitated patient's wishes regarding health care. There may be questions concerning the scope of care for a patient with a limited life expectancy. Such situations raise ethical issues regarding the withholding and withdrawing of life support. We believe that it is ethically permissible to withhold or withdraw life support measures if the patient has clearly directed that this be done, even if doing so hastens the patient's death.[10] Treatment decisions are not mere medical decisions; they reflect the patient's values and perceptions of life and death. Because of their close relationships with their patients, rural physicians are in an ideal position to treat patients according to their desires—a basic goal of medicine.

Coping with Ethical Issues

Physicians and other health care providers have increasingly felt uncertain about how to respond to the growing number of ethical dilemmas they encounter. Fortunately, increasing numbers of physicians have had formal training in ethics because many medical schools now offer such courses. Most of these courses provide a conceptual framework for applying moral theory to ethical dilemmas. Understanding moral theory helps physicians articulate and justify the moral judgments they make when confronted with ethical dilemmas.[11,12]

Self-Education

Rural physicians generally deal with ethical issues with the same self-reliance with which they deal with medical problems: They apply the best knowledge they possess to the problem. Rural health care providers, with and without formal training in ethics, tend to act in accordance with what they believe is morally correct. We believe that physicians who have had a reasonable exposure to medical ethics are able to manage quite adequately the majority of ethical dilemmas encountered in their practices. However, a physician's knowledge of clinical ethics is enhanced by reading case-oriented medical ethics articles found in almost every medical journal. Physicians also should read a basic medical ethics text or an anthology focusing on ethical theory and key conceptual issues. The most important challenge for physicians is to respond to ethical dilemmas only after thoughtful and serious reflection based on moral reasoning, rather than merely on their feelings.

Medical Ethicists

In applied ethics, as in any discipline, some problems are complex enough to justify consulting with people who have specialized knowledge. For rural physicians, this may mean contacting a medical ethicist at a medical center. A growing number of academic medical centers have ethicists on the faculty who teach and offer clinical consultation. The rural physician should be aware of these people and their availability for consultation long before an actual ethics problem arises, just as they should know an available neurologist or oncologist consultant in case of difficult problems in those areas. However, because medical ethicists are not always available, it is important to develop local resources. This could be facilitated through the local hospital's ethics advisory committee (EAC).

Ethics Advisory Committees

Many physicians have sought the advice of a hospital ethics advisory committee for both inpatient and outpatient problems. There is increasing support for and acceptance of such committees from medical associations, rural health care associations, government organizations, and individual clinicians. But probably the most important endorsement is the number of hospitals, large and small, that have formed EACs; currently about 70% of U.S. hospitals have them. In Vermont, where 12 out of 16 hospitals have 100 beds or fewer, a 1988 survey reported that 9 of the 12 hospitals had ethics committees.[13]

The general purpose of an EAC is to provide a forum where health care professionals can discuss ethical issues with other professionals with knowledge in applied ethics. Committee size varies, but 6 to 10 members is enough to allow interdisciplinary discussions. Rural hospitals' ethics committees should comprise physicians, nurses, a chaplain or clergy member, a lawyer, a social worker, and an administrator. Criteria for membership are motivation, knowledge of ethics, and time availability. Because personal commitment is crucial to the functioning of the committee, it is best if members are volunteers. The committee should be formally recognized by the hospital with its own policy indicating the EAC's purpose and functions.

William A. Nelson, Ph.D., and Andrew S. Pomerantz, M.D.

The latter should include the opportunity to bring non–hospital-based dilemmas to the committee for reflection and advice.

The committee should serve only in an advisory role; no one should be required to present an ethical dilemma to the committee, and no one should be forced to follow the committee's advice. The EAC has three specific roles—education, policy review and development, and consultation.

Education

For the committee to achieve its goals, the members must understand basic conceptual issues in ethics as they relate to health care. In a large academic setting, a committee could seek the expertise and knowledge of a medical ethicist to foster its education. But because such a person is unlikely to be available in the rural setting, a local expert in medical ethics must emerge.[14] This expert is usually a respected physician, but he or she could be a member of any health profession. The main criterion is that he or she is willing to take the time for self-education through reading medical ethics literature and attending ethics conferences. This local expert is the key to the success of the committee and should serve as the chairperson. He or she should help other committee members gain a basic knowledge of applied ethics. The committee could also invite an experienced medical ethicist to facilitate a local conference to review the basic medical ethics curriculum.[15] An attorney who is knowledgable about health care issues can familiarize the committee with any relevant state laws.

Once the local expert has enhanced committee members' knowledge of applied ethics, the EAC can promote educational activities within the hospital (case conferences, topic oriented addresses, journal club, and so forth) as well as communitywide educational programs on such topics as living wills and advance directives. The local ethics expert should not be perceived as having "all the answers." His or her most important role in the rural setting should be to dissseminate applied ethics without threatening the independence and self-reliance of rural physicians.

Policy Review and Development

The second role of the EAC is to review and draft ethics-related policy for the hospital. Common ethical problems (such as limitation of therapy, surrogate decision making, confidentiality, and HIV testing) should be covered by established policies. Based on its ethics education, the committee should be able to provide an ethical basis for sound policy that anticipates and encompasses potential problems.

Case Consultation

This role should be undertaken only after the committee feels competent in relating moral theory and basic

conceptual issues—including competency, valid consent and refusal, and justified paternalism—to clinical situations. As Denise Niemira, M.D., suggests, "If the committee has done its homework and is politically astute, the transition from education to policy review and even consultation will be much smoother than anticipated."[16] Any member of the hospital staff and any physician related to the hospital should be able to consult with the committee.

In providing ethics consultations, the following list supplies a useful framework:

1. The committee determines the facts of the case. What is the diagnosis? What are the treatment options? What is the prognosis? What are the patient's or (when patient is incompetent) surrogate's desires? Many ethical problems are really disagreements about the facts of the case. Frequently, clarifying the facts decreases the conflict.
2. The committee determines the moral or ethical dilemma in the case.
3. The committee determines the morally and ethically relevant concepts. Is there relevant health law?
4. The committee decides how the concepts apply to the case.
5. The committee offers its advice, both verbally and, for hospital-based cases, with a chart notation.
6. The committee follows the case and reviews it at scheduled meetings.[17]

Depending on the number and urgency of case consultations, the committee need not always function as a group. The chair and one or two members may serve as consultants on a particular case and then report on it to the entire committee at the next scheduled meeting.

The members of the rural EAC may find it helpful to network with committees from other small hospitals to share common concerns. In many states, chairs of local committees and other interested people gather once or twice a year for education and discussion of shared experiences and problems.

Once EACs have reached a level of competence in applied ethics, they can be invaluable resources for resolving ethical issues in clinical care. Just as rural physicians may want to consult with specialists in cardiology or psychiatry, they may also need consultations on ethical matters. An EAC is not another attempt to reduce the provider's scope of autonomy, but rather is a useful resource to enhance the natural (and ethically appropriate) physician–patient decision-making process. The EAC is important to rural practitioners not only because it helps them think through complex cases, but also because it helps them understand and apply ethics to the basic decision-making process. Thus, the EAC serves as a source of insight and reasoning for the rural physician's practical decision making. This is especially important because "the most frequently occurring ethical issues represent the day-to-day concerns of clinical practice."[18] A local EAC is a valuable resource in creating dialogue about and understanding of ethical issues within basic rural practice.

Conclusion

Despite what many people think, life in the rural setting is not always pastoral and simple. Complex ethical issues in health care are just as prevalent as in urban areas and are dramatically affected by the cultural values of the rural setting.[19] Health care providers must equip themselves with adequate skills to respond to these problems through self-education and should also seek other resources when they face uncertainty.

Acknowledgments

The authors express their appreciation for the helpful comments by Drs. Dale Gephart and Tom Creighton.

References

1. Lipton, H. L. Do-not-resuscitate decisions in a community hospital. *JAMA* 256(9):1164–69, 1986.
2. Kolata, G. Wariness is replacing trust between healer and patient. *New York Times,* Feb. 20, 1990, pp. A1, D15.
3. Dayringer, R., Pavia, R. E., and Davidson G. W. Ethical decision making by family physicians. *Journal of Family Practice* 17(2):267–72, 1983.
4. Purtilo, R., and Sorrell, J. The ethical dilemmas of a rural physician. *Hastings Center Report* 16(4):24–28, Aug. 1986.
5. Study finds medical care wanting in rural U.S. *New York Times,* Mar. 13, 1991.
6. Rakel, R. E. Family practice. *JAMA* 261(9):2845–46, 1989.
7. Purtilo and Sorrell.
8. Rakel.
9. Christie, R. J., and Hoffmaster, C. B. *Ethical Issues in Family Medicine.* New York City: Oxford University Press, 1986.
10. Nelson, W. A., and Bernat, J. L. Decisions to withhold or terminate treatment. *Neurologic Clinics* 7(4):759–74, Nov. 1989.
11. American College of Physicians Ethics Manual. Part I: History; the patient; other physicians. *Annals of Internal Medicine* 111(3):245–52, Aug. 1989.
12. American College of Physicians Ethics Manual Part II: History; the patient; other physicians. *Annals of Internal Medicine* 111(4):327–35, Aug. 1989.
13. Friedman, E., and Niemira, D. A. Grassroots grappling: ethical dilemmas and problem solving in rural practice. Paper presented at National Rural Health Association meeting, Washington, DC, May 1988.
14. Niemira, D. A., Orr, R., and Culver, C. M. Ethics committees in small hospitals. *Journal of Rural Health* 5(1):19–32, Jan. 1989.
15. Culver, C. M., Clouser, K. D., and Gert, B., et al. Basic curricular goals in medical ethics. *New England Journal of Medicine* 312:253–56, Jan. 24, 1985.
16. Niemira, D. A. Grassroots grappling: ethics committees at rural hospitals. *Annals of Internal Medicine* 109(12):981–83, Dec. 15, 1988.
17. Nelson, W. A. Ethics committees provide aid to clinicians. *The Newsletter of the NRHA* 13(3):9, Mar. 1991.
18. Robillard, H. M., High, D. M., Sebastian, J. G., et al. Ethical issues in primary health care: A survey of practitioners' perceptions. *Journal of Community Health* 14(1):9–17, Spring 1989.
19. Dayringer, Pavia, and Davidson.

Chapter 23

Community Health Decisions Programs: The Corporatization of a Grassroots Political Movement

Donald F. Phillips

Donald F. Phillips is the editor of Hospital Ethics, *published by the American Hospital Association, Chicago.*

A grassroots movement in health care emerged in the mid-1980s because of public perceptions that (1) advances in medical care and technology have created complex ethical dilemmas that defy resolution by the old methods of problem solving, (2) decision making by elected government representatives has been stymied by conflicts in values between individual and society, justice and freedom, rights and duties, and benefits and harms, and (3) individual needs and concerns are lost or ignored by a health care system that has become cumbersome and inefficient.

The general public has become dissatisfied with the apparent disregard for ethical issues shown by physicians and health care organizations, elected or appointed government officials, and corporate leaders. The public has also become frustrated with the inability of political bodies to reach agreement on what to do and by its general sense of powerlessness to change the ethical and political climates. These factors have spawned grassroots efforts that encourage people to voice their concerns, values, needs, and wishes and that empower them to influence the political process to accomplish changes in the redistribution of resources and services.

Enter the community health decisions movement, a montage of state and regional programs established to:

- Provide forums for raising public awareness of the link between the ethical, political, and economic choices facing individuals and society and the advances in medical technology and constantly rising health-care costs
- Reflect on the values held by individuals and communities with regard to these choices
- Achieve consensus on specific issues and set priorities for addressing them
- Empower individuals and communities to develop recommendations for policy makers and decision makers

The Community Bioethics Bandwagon

The original grassroots project designed to give citizens a new voice in shaping health policy began in Oregon in 1982 with a series of public meetings to discuss the personal and social choices imposed by technological and economic changes in health care. Word of the Oregon project spread rapidly throughout the country, prompting a number of other grassroots efforts to emerge. The concept gained the attention of the Prudential Foundation, which initiated a first round of community bioethics grants to six projects, identified here by state (California, Hawaii, Idaho, Iowa–Illinois, Maine, Washington). Shortly thereafter, the Robert Wood Johnson Foundation joined in with support for four additional projects (Colorado, New Jersey, Oregon, Vermont).

These 10 initial projects spanned the period from 1985 to 1987. In 1987, Prudential approved continued support with a $400,000 pledge to four projects (California, New Jersey, Oregon, Vermont), by then collectively referred to as the Community Health Decisions program. Several smaller community projects in Indiana and North Carolina, which had been organized with local financial support, also emerged during this period.[1]

Nearly all of these community projects started off with high hopes of becoming ongoing self-sustaining organizations. Of the 10 initial health decisions programs and the two independent projects mentioned above, only four still exist (California, New Jersey, Oregon, Vermont). Jennings attributes program failure to one or more of the following reasons:

1. The project did not establish a secure institutional base.
2. The project remained too dependent on the commitment and energy of one or two key leaders.
3. The project was unable to develop an effective long-term fundraising component.[2]

Since 1988, eight more programs (Arizona, Massachusetts, Kansas–Missouri, North Carolina, New Mexico, Ohio, Tennessee, West Virginia) have come into existence and have initiated activities. Six others (Colorado, Maine, Georgia, Nebraska, New York, Wisconsin) are ready to be launched once funding is secured, and at least five others (Florida, Texas, Delaware, Connecticut) are in the planning stage. Table 1 provides an overview of all projects, their dates of existence, and their sponsoring organizations.

The second generation of community projects reflects a broadened mission and scope of operation and shows greater evidence of adapting to local needs and nuances. Most of the new programs:

- Emphasize the need for coalition building
- Identify themselves as broadly based and nonpartisan
- Develop a separate identity and functional independence from any single sponsoring organization
- Strive for full-time staffs who delegate work, rather than depend on a few individuals

Table 1. Community Health Decisions Projects

Project Name	Duration	Sponsoring Organizations
Arizona Health Decisions	1986–	Independent
California Health Decisions	1985–	Independent
Colorado Speaks Out on Health	1986–88	Center for Health Ethics & Policy, U. of CO, Denver
Georgia Health Decisions	1991–	Independent
Hawaii Health Care, Culture, and Social Values Project	1985–87	Institute for Religion and Social Change
Idaho "No Easy Choices" Project	1985–87	ID Health Systems Agency
IA/IL Health Policy and Bioethics in the Community Project	1985–87	Iowa/Illinois Health Care Alliance
"Just Caring" Project	1985–86	Goshen (IN) General Hospital
Maine Health Care Decisions	1989–	Acadia Institute
Massachusetts Health Decisions	1990–	Massachusetts Health Research Institute
Missouri Heartlands Health Decisions	1989–90	Heartland Health Services & Midwest Bioethics Inst.
Nebraska Health Decisions	1991	Independent
New Jersey Citizens' Committee on Biomedical Ethics	1983	Independent
New Mexico Health Decisions	1989–	Independent
New York Citizens' Committee on Health Care Decisions	1991–	Independent
Bioethics Resource Group of North Carolina	1985–	Charlotte, NC community hospital and county medical society
The Community Dialogue on Values and Health Care, Cleveland, OH	1990–	Case Western Reserve Center for Biomedical Ethics
Oregon Health Decisions	1983–	Independent, quasi-official link to OR Health Services Commission
Tennessee Guild for Ethical Health Decisions	1990–	Vanderbilt University Center for Clinical and Research Ethics
Vermont Ethics Network	1986–	VT Health Policy Council of the VT General Assembly
Washington Health Choices	1985–86	Puget Sound Health Systems Agency
West Virginia Business and Professional Ethics Project	1989–	University of Virginia Center for Health Ethics and Law
Wisconsin Health Decisions	1991–	Lawrence University Program in Bioethics

- Maintain a certain degree of flexibility and adaptability

The Original Model

The seed for the original grassroots project in Oregon was planted in the early 1980s and was nurtured for several years before emerging in 1982 as a private, nonprofit organization known as Oregon Health Decisions (OHD). Ralph Crawshaw, M.D., a Portland psychiatrist, was the project director, and he is often referred to as the movement's godfather. It was his idea that there be public debate on ethical issues.

As chairman of Oregon's Statewide Health Coordinating Council (later renamed the Oregon Health Council) in 1981, Crawshaw was responsible for creating a state health plan. He proposed that there be a study of the state's medically indigent, and in 1982 the Oregon Health Council convened the Governor's Conference on Health Care for the Medically Poor.

The conference heightened participants' concerns about two major questions: (1) What are the relative values society places on curative and preventive services? (2) Given that an implicit rationing of health care already exists, what is the possibility of making such rationing explicit and congruent with community values?

The conference resulted in "a recommendation . . . to form a task force to develop public awareness and consensus on bioethical issues"[3] and in the formation of a Coalition for the Medically Needy. The latter successfully persuaded the state legislature that Oregon should "participate in Medicaid's optional 'medically needy' program—thus adding over $10,000,000 [to the state's coffers] for the care of pregnant women and children."[4]

The council appointed a volunteer steering committee that became the functional head of Oregon Health Decisions, Inc.[5,6] This group held 300 community meetings throughout the state during the latter part of 1983, at which 5,000 people expressed their views about ethical problems in health care. This outpouring was transformed into a number of resolutions that were debated and voted upon at the first Citizens' Health Care Parliament, held in October 1984. The resolutions that passed formed the basis for a report, *Society Must Decide,*[7] and became the formalized goals for future activities of the organization.

Shortly after the release of *Society Must Decide,* Oregon Health Decisions separated from the Oregon Health Council following the council's inaction regarding recommendations made by OHD on the basis of its first public forum. One of these suggestions was that the state legislature establish an ongoing process for defining "adequate" health care that would be the basis for the state's resource allocation decisions. In 1989, the Oregon legislature did so by creating a Health Services Commission (HSC) to "actively solicit public involvement in a community meeting process to build a consensus on the values to be used to guide health resource allocation decisions."[8] OHD became the organization officially responsible for those community meetings.

Ongoing Programs

Many of the new community health decisions organizations adopted the Oregon model, but then branched off into other activities and organizational arrangements.

California Health Decisions

California Health Decisions (CHD) had its beginnings in 1985 as the California Health Decisions–Orange County Project, using a process of citizen involvement patterned on the Oregon model. In 1989, the Orange County Project became the statewide California Health Decisions organization, with financial support coming from more than 3,000 individuals and nearly 50 foundations, health care institutions, insurers, businesses, and professional organizations throughout California.

Policy makers, providers, and the public are invited to serve on the four CHD-sponsored task forces: access to health care, quality and allocation, patients' rights and autonomy, and health promotion and disease prevention. These groups meet from September through May to develop and implement citizen-generated recommendations for action.

The New Jersey Citizens' Committee on Biomedical Ethics

This independent, private, nonprofit organization was established in 1983. It receives approximately three-fourths of its funding from the foundations of 10 large New Jersey corporations and one-fourth from individual contributing members. A nine-member steering committee oversees the management of the committee's office and projects, as well as two regional chapters.

New Active Projects

Following is a description of the nine new projects that are currently active.

Arizona Health Decisions

Arizona Health Decisions (AHD) was established in 1986 by a group of citizens and professionals in the fields of medicine, law, education, nursing, and social work. Located in Prescott, the project serves a population of about 100,000 in Yavapai County in north-central Arizona.

New Mexico Health Decisions

New Mexico Health Decisions (NMHD) was founded as an independent grassroots organization in 1989. Initial foundation funding was sufficient to initiate 34 small group discussions throughout the state on patients' rights and social policy.

Wisconsin Health Decisions

Wisconsin Health Decisions (WHD) was incorporated in 1991 with a major goal of helping "people become better informed about complex health care questions."

The Bioethics Network of Ohio

The Bioethics Network of Ohio (BNO) functions as a health decisions organization for the metropolitan Cleveland area. It was started in late 1989 as an activity of the Center for Biomedical Ethics at Case Western Reserve University under the title of Community Dialogue of Values and Health Care. A group of northeastern Ohio bioethicists filed for incorporation of the group as a nonprofit organization in 1990.

Vermont Health Decisions

Vermont Health Decisions (VHD) is sponsored by the Vermont Ethics Network (VEN), a volunteer group that came into being in February 1986 with the initiation of a special project called Taking Steps: Ethical Decisions for Living and Dying. This special project facilitated 192 community and professional discussions throughout the state on ethical dilemmas and personal decision making in situations involving critical and terminal medical care.

By July 1988, the VEN had become an advisory body to the State Health Policy Council and was responsible for conducting public meetings, performing studies, and writing reports. The VEN's mission is "to promote wider and better public understanding of the ethical issues in modern health care, and to provide public forums [through the VHD process] within which citizens can express the values and principles that they believe should underlie the health care system."

Massachusetts Health Decisions

Massachusetts Health Decisions (MHD) began in 1989 as an official project of the Massachusetts Health Research Institute, a private, free-standing, nonprofit organization dedicated to finding support for research and education programs. A 20-member board of advisors oversees the MHD's activities.

West Virginia Business and Professional Ethics Project

The West Virginia Business and Professional Ethics Project is a nonprofit, nonpartisan consortium of over 20 academic, business, health care, and government groups. It was established in 1990 to promote discussion and public education about applied ethical issues in business, health care, and public service.

Maine Health Care Decisions

Maine Health Care Decisions (MHCD) existed in its first incarnation from 1985 through 1987 as one of the original six demonstration projects funded by the Prudential Foundation for community bioethics projects. It was, and still is, sponsored by the Acadia Institute in Bar Harbor, an independent, nonprofit organization. In addition to its advisory committee, the MHCD draws on the advice and assistance of the institute's board of directors and advisory board and other colleagues in Maine with expertise in long-term care, treatment choices, and institutional ethics committees.

The Tennessee Guild for Ethical Health Decisions

The Tennessee Guild for Ethical Health Decisions (TGEHD) is a newly formed nonprofit organization of about 120 members and has close ties to the Center for Clinical and Research Ethics at the Vanderbilt University Medical Center, Nashville. It operates two study groups— one on the right to die, the other on allocation of scarce resources.

The Bioethics Resource Group

The Bioethics Resource Group (BRG) is a voluntary nonprofit organization formed in 1985 to provide leadership within the community to deal with difficult issues of medicine and ethics. It had its origins in the Mecklenburg County Medical Society and has been supported by the general hospitals in Charlotte, North Carolina. The goals of the BRG are to assist health professionals and the general public in understanding and responding to complex moral issues in health care.

Projects on Hold

The following projects have fulfilled their initial goals. As of mid-1991, they were awaiting renewed funding and were relegated to inactive status.

Colorado Speaks Out on Health

Colorado Speaks Out on Health is the state's health decisions project. It completed its two-year educational program and study of public opinion on critical care issues in September 1988.

The Heartland Health Decisions Project

The Heartland Health Decisions Project was cosponsored as a nine-month pilot by the Heartland Health System, St. Joseph, Missouri, and the Midwest Bioethics Center, Kansas City, Missouri. Initiated in April 1989, it was designed as a communications network in which health policy makers and consumers in northwestern Missouri and northeastern Kansas could share views about critical health care issues.

Past Programs

Several small projects were initiated concurrently with the foundation-supported programs in the 1980s. They deserve mention because of their unique approach to organization and support.

The Goshen General Hospital
Ethics Committee

The Goshen (Indiana) General Hospital Ethics Committee initiated a project in 1982 entitled Just Caring. It was seen as an ideal opportunity to expand in a systematic way the discussion of medical–moral issues that already had been initiated in the community by the Goshen Hospital Ethics Committee as a means of gathering information to help the hospital formulate its own policies.

The project was aimed at the 140,000 people living in or around Elkhart County, of which Goshen is the county seat. The county's predominantly rural, small-town population reflects an interesting mix, including a disproportionate number of elderly and retired people, a large number of persons who face cyclical unemployment, a significant Amish population that pays for medical care in cash and usually shuns Medicare, and a large number of individuals of another religious group, the Faith Assembly, who refuse medical treatment on religious grounds.

Over a year's time, the project conducted 15 seminars that each were attended by 50 to 100 people. Nine separate task forces worked from the summer of 1986 through the winter of 1987 to organize the thoughts that emerged from the seminar discussions. A speaker's bureau, begun at the same time as the seminars, continues to send physicians, nurses, chaplains, and other representatives to community organizations to discuss ethical issues. The task force reports, as well as an issue agenda for the future, were published in a final report.[9] The project, though completed, remains an excellent example of a hospital-based health decision program.

Hawaii Health Care, Culture,
and Social Values Project

From 1985 to 1987, the Honolulu-based Institute for Religion and Social Change sponsored the Hawaii Health Care, Culture, and Social Values Project, which was particularly concerned with the ways in which bioethical issues are interpreted by various cultural and religious groups. The project's activities centered around workshops held in neighborhood and civic centers, various religious settings, union halls, and cultural centers.

Idaho "No Easy Choices" Project

A Prudential Foundation–supported initiative from 1985 to 1987, the Idaho "No Easy Choices" Project was sponsored by the Idaho Health Systems Agency. It placed volunteer project coordinators in each of the state's 44 counties to set up local meetings. A series of regional conferences later culminated in a statewide citizen's health care parliament attended by 72 delegates. Several recommendations from the parliament eventually were incorporated into state laws on the use of advance directives.

Iowa/Illinois Health Policy and Bioethics
in the Community Project

The Iowa/Illinois Health Policy and Bioethics in the Community Project, which spanned the Quad City region of the Iowa–Illinois border, was sponsored by the Iowa/Illinois Health Care Alliance. During its first year (1985), it focused on community discussion and education regarding resource allocation and access to health care. In 1986 (its last year), it turned its attention to issues of personal health decision making and patient autonomy.

Washington Health Choices

Based in Seattle, the Washington Health Choices project began in 1985 under the sponsorship of the Puget Sound Health Systems Agency. Starting with a leadership training conference attended by volunteers who later served as meeting organizers and discussion leaders, the project focused on allocation, access, and individual rights and responsibilities in making health care decisions. The project culminated in a statewide conference held in November 1986 at which delegates reviewed the conclusions of the local meetings and discussed strategies for addressing the concerns raised by their fellow citizens. A final report was prepared, and an executive summary of the report was distributed to more than 1,000 community leaders throughout the state.

American Health Decisions: A New Phase

In 1988, the community health decisions movement entered a new phase when representatives from the state projects met in Denver to lay the foundation for a national umbrella organization that would serve as a consortium of grassroots discussion networks among citizens committed to education and consensus development on ethical issues in health care. The organization, American Health Decisions, has since been incorporated as a nonprofit membership corporation. A primary goal of the AHD is to facilitate cooperation, collaboration, and mutual support among the member organizations.

The Health Decisions Process

Community health decisions (CHD) programs, as diverse as they seem, all follow a basic pattern for engaging the public: (1) development and distribution of a statement of purpose or mission that gives meaning and reason for public involvement and support, (2) development of a process for involving the public, and (3) design of a mechanism for ongoing public involvement in the program through dissemination of information and announcements of continued progress.

Premises and Principles

All of the CHD programs have a statement of purpose or mission and written objectives. In general, most share the premise that ethical issues relating to health care should be subject to wide public discussion. From this, two secondary premises are derived—one pertaining to personal decisions, the other to societal choices.

The premise underlying *personal decisions* acknowledges that patients and their families are often unprepared for the decisions they have to make in critical care settings, where the judgments and values of the provider can prevail. The American health care system generally lacks a mechanism for considering and incorporating the values of the patient or family into medical decisions.

The premise underlying *societal choices* also alludes to difficult choices, acknowledging that significant divergence exists between what is needed (or wanted) and the resources available. These choices are not clear and therefore result in hasty decisions or in nondecisions made either through default or because the options presented are not suitable. Almost as important as what we choose is how we arrive at that choice.

Because the public lacks knowledge and is isolated from the political process, health care decisions are based on the social values of those in power. Although social choice cannot be separated from the political process, U.S. systems of government and health care often fail to systematically develop a broad base of consensus for making decisions that are in the best interests of society.

Some community health decisions projects focus on guiding principles rather than premises. Arizona Health Decisions, for example, formulated the following principles, based on a community needs assessment and other research:[10]

1. Individual values are based on limited personal experiences with health care and bioethical issues.
2. People are eager to receive health care information that will enhance the quality of their lives, minimize suffering, and promote informed choices in health care use.
3. People want to be educated about bioethical issues so they can be empowered to make otherwise difficult health care choices.
4. There is a need for community resources to provide health care education and support for the individual decision-making process.
5. This community resource must be structurally and functionally independent of any existing health care provider or institution in order to avoid any conflict of interest and allow easy access by any person to unbiased information.
6. This community resource should facilitate the individual decision-making process by exploring alternatives rather than advocating one outcome over another.

7. This community resource could become a model for any community wanting to explore these issues in a community-based process.

The essence of many of these guiding principles is expressed in one form or another in nearly all of the other community health decisions projects. Table 2 provides a comparison of the topical areas addressed by the community health decisions projects and a summary of the processes used to (1) assess community values, (2) educate the community about ethical issues in health care, or (3) influence public policy.

Developing a Process for Community Involvement

Most of the successful projects have maintained their grassroots orientation by focusing on "bottom-up" activities. That is, the projects first elicit from individuals and communities their thoughts, desires, needs, and values and then design programs and outcomes to address these matters.

The model most often used for such a bottom-up effort is the three-phase Oregon approach to community involvement. This consists of (1) small-group meetings, where trained volunteers inform citizens of the issues and identify their areas of concern, (2) "town-hall" meetings, where larger numbers of people discuss and refine the input of the small-group discussions, and (3) a "parliament," where representatives selected at the town-hall sessions try to reach a community consensus on the issues chosen and to formulate recommendations that are forwarded to policy makers or providers. Details of the overall process are provided by Crawshaw[11] and Conviser.[12]

Many CHD projects chose variations of the Oregon model by seeking public opinion and value clarification through the use of surveys and questionnaires at community meetings. Colorado Speaks Out on Health, for example, used volunteer facilitators to distribute a 31-question survey to more than 400 business, religious, civic, charitable, professional, and educational groups. The questionnaire was designed as a tool to spur discussion and thought, not as a formal polling mechanism by which statistically valid data could be obtained.

Some of the projects, because of insufficient staff, time, or money, abbreviated various components of the Oregon process. Vermont Health Decisions, for example, combined the small-group and town-hall phases. It sponsored a total of 125 community forums involving about 2,800 people throughout the state from November 1989 through June 1990. Participants were asked to complete a brief questionnaire following the discussion.

Other projects, particularly those with academic ties, offer "top-down" activities, in which the assumed needs of the community are met with instructional or educational programs designed not so much to elicit values as

Table 2. Topical Areas Addressed by Currently Active Community Health Decisions Programs

Topical Areas Addressed	AZ	CA	GA	MA	NC	NE	NJ	NM	NY	OH	OR	TN	VT	WV	WI
Individual patient care issues															
Patient rights/informed consent											X		X		
Patient decision making									X				X		
End-of-life decisions		X					X		X			X			
Advance directives/PDSA	X	X		X	X	X	X		X		X	X	X	X	X
Care of elderly		X					X							X	
Proxy laws				X					X						
Institutional care issues															
Institutional ethics committees					X										
Long-term care					X					X					
Nursing ethics					X			X							
Cost containment/reimbursement						X									
Social health care issues															
Access to health care		X				X	X	X		X					
Health values and priorities	X	X	X	X			X	X		X	X				
Rationing/resource allocation	X	X									X	X			
Health insurance		X						X							
Public/community education	X						X								
Community ethics committees	X														
Health promotion											X				
Business ethics														X	
Environmental ethics														X	

to promote awareness of ethical issues. Examples include the Tennessee Guild for Ethical Health Decisions, the West Virginia Business and Professional Ethics Project, and the North Carolina Bioethics Resource Group. For the most part, these projects involve conferences, workshops, and seminars that are aimed at community members, but have little planning input from the community and give little attention to assessing, surveying, recording, or reporting public opinion and values.

Reaching the Disenfranchised

One criticism of the health decisions movement has been that the process of engaging the community, conducting discussions, and soliciting community opinion and values has usually resulted in a biased sample of community members, because the disenfranchised (for example, the poor, the unemployed, the homeless, and the disabled) and ethnic minorities are left out of the process. In Oregon, for example, it proved more difficult to get broad citizen participation in the large metropolitan Portland area than in the state's rural areas and small towns, where populations are more homogeneous.[13]

At least two reasons are given to explain the lack of participation by ethnic minorities and the disenfranchised. One is the language barrier. Oregon, for example, has the fastest growing and largest settlement of Russian immigrants in the country, but the Oregon Health Decisions has not provided Russian-language outreach to this group.

The other reason has more to do with subtle, unintended, tacit forms of intimidation and constraint felt by the disenfranchised in the process of assembly. For example, basic community forums usually are conducted at meetings of civic organizations, through membership organizations, in business settings, or in the homes of prominent citizens—all settings that tend to exclude or intimidate the poor, ethnic minorities, the unemployed, and the homeless. Although the health decisions movement recognizes these shortcomings, few projects have attempted to seek out representatives of disenfranchised groups.

There are some exceptions. One is the Bioethics Network of Ohio, which structures its program in a unique way. Three functional groups have been organized:

- A core group of about 34 community leaders who are chosen by the black community, blue-collar workers, and neighborhood centers for their sensitivity to the issues at hand and for their ability to speak on behalf of their constituents
- A policy-making forum consisting of legislators and elected public officials from the metropolitan Cleveland area
- A community forum that moves from neighborhood to neighborhood to hear scheduled witnesses air their views on specific problems

Discussions raised at the core group meeting are reported to the policy-making group, which produces its own commentary and reports back to the core group. A contingent of the core group then attends the community forum, the proceedings of which are reported back to the policy-making group. According to the director of the Center for Biomedical Ethics at Case Western Reserve University, this round-robin scheduling provides a steady stream of information and feedback, as well as a sense of accountability among the three functional groups.

Another exceptional program is the Heartlands Health Decisions Project, which conducted a demographic analysis of the citizens who participated in the project. It found that although small-group community meetings were a reasonable strategy for encouraging the uninsured and underinsured to speak out, one portion of the questionnaire that was used proved too difficult for participants to understand. The project's final report called for greater attention to developing a questionnaire that is easy to read.

The Heartlands town hall approach proved to be ineffective in reaching various minorities and the disenfranchised. The 91 town hall meetings brought in a total of 1,373 people, which represents only about 1 percent of the targeted population in the six counties of northeastern Kansas and northwestern Missouri.

The director of the Midwest Bioethics Center suggests that each county should have a community network committee responsible for bringing representatives of minority populations and the disenfranchised to the town-hall meetings.

In the fall of 1991, the W. K. Kellogg Foundation granted American Health Decisions (AHD) $90,000 to explore how to gain greater participation of ethnic and economic minorities in the community health decisions process. According to the chairman of the AHD's board, the purpose of the grant is not to determine health needs and values of minority groups, but rather to determine what steps and procedures will ensure that health decisions organizations across the nation at least "ring the right bell" when seeking minority involvement.[14] Three states (Georgia, New Mexico, California) will serve as test sites for the grant during 1992.

Ongoing Involvement

Successful CHD programs know how to maintain public interest during lulls in project activity. Even organizations that are "on hold" remain viable because they have managed to find a means of effective communication. In contrast, projects that have struggled and died have not maintained effective communication with the citizens who originally participated in the process. The newsletter is the most frequently used communication tool; every active health decisions group has one.

Another approach for maintaining continued interest is through the use of memberships. Many current health decision programs are membership organizations, with

personal, institutional, and corporate categories and fees ranging from $15 to $5,000.

Project activities that require cooperation, comment, review, or approval by an outside body often need follow-up by staff. Oregon Health Decisions had an implementation committee follow through on high priority resolutions developed in the 1984 parliament. Committee pressure, along with intensive media efforts, resulted in the introduction of proposals into the 1987 legislative session that increased the number of Oregonians who have advance directives.

Oregon Health Decisions has kept the interests of its constituency in mind. Its second project, Oregon Health Priorities in the 1990s, reexamined the issues identified at the first parliament but used a more structured group process that focused on influencing health program budget priorities for the 1989–1990 legislative session. The resulting report from the second parliament, *Quality of Life in Allocating Health Care Resources,* contains a list of 15 principles for allocating health care services.[15]

For its third project, the OHD was asked to build consensus on community values through a series of statewide community gatherings that prioritized health services in response to a series of bills passed by the 1989–1990 legislature that were aimed at increasing basic health care coverage for the state's citizens.

Oregon Health Decisions is preparing for its fourth project, a statewide series of community meetings that will focus on the ethical issues in public policies influencing life-style choices that can prevent illness and promote health. The project will seek to clarify the major values that define or determine life-style choices that result in healthy lives, as well as choices that result in premature death and avoidable disabilities.[16]

Outcomes and Results

Eventually one has to ask, "Is the health decisions movement working?" Answers depend on how the question is framed. It is actually two questions:

- Are the projects meeting their anticipated or stated program goals?
- Are the projects resulting in changes desired by the communities involved in the projects?

By and large, evaluation of either program goals or changes in health care delivery is nonexistent. Most of the stated project goals do not lend themselves to quantitative evaluation. Even survey and questionnaire data collected at community meetings are reported with the caveat that the numbers do not represent statistical significance.

However, there is evidence that most program goals have been achieved and that participating individuals and communities are satisfied with the outcomes. Although enlightenment has not been measured, it has been expressed. On the other hand, there is no evidence that exposure to ethical issues, consciousness raising, group discussions, and educational pursuits undertaken by the health decisions programs has changed individual beliefs, attitudes, behavior, or critical thinking regarding ethical problems.

Expanded Focus

In general, the newer projects have taken on a broader scope of activities than the original projects had envisioned. These original projects that have survived have expanded their activities to encompass emerging areas of interest, such as advance directives and ethics committees. Those projects that ceased to exist generally had only a single focus and did not attempt to expand.

Most community health decision programs continue to assess or monitor public opinion on specific issues or clarify community values on more general topics. There has been a general shift away from rights-based personal choices involving patient care to justice-based societal choices involving allocation of resources.

Two reasons could account for this shift. One may be the general public's perception that personal-choice issues tied to patient autonomy and dignity are finally being recognized and handled in more appropriate ways, through changes in institutional policies, court decisions, and legislative actions. The other reason may be the public's recognition and fear of impending disaster for all of society if changes are not made in the way the health care system is organized and operated.

The shift of problem focus from individual to society, however, presents a more difficult challenge for the health decisions movement. Community surveys, heightened awareness, values clarification, and consensus-building exercises were excellent ways to help individuals overcome their limitations in dealing with ethical issues at the bedside. The same exercises, however, when applied to societal problems such as the allocation of scarce resources are ineffective because societal issues lack a sense of immediacy and, more importantly, they involve more complex social, political, and economic processes. Thus, discussions of societal options regarding the allocation of resources, access to health services, and the financing of care have remained polite, profound, and prolific, but have had little demonstrable impact.

Even in Oregon, where there seemed to be a direct link between the 1987 legislature's decision to stop paying for organ transplants (except for kidney and cornea transplants) for Medicaid clients and the decision of the OHD's first parliament that providing prenatal care was a higher priority than providing transplants, the implied cause-and-effect relationship is stretched a bit. It is conceivable that the legislators could have voted as they did

for any number of other reasons. One could argue, of course, that the collective wisdom gained through community discussions needs to be internalized through gradual changes in attitudes and beliefs before any overt changes in behavior, such as changing one's vote on a particular measure, can be observed.

Risks of Political Action

Some health decisions programs have purposely avoided moving from discourse to *direct* political activity. To engage in advocacy through the political process, they claim, would interfere with the "value-neutral" nature of the education they provide and would stymie the objectivity and candidness of their surveys, discussions, and consensus-building efforts. They also recognize that efforts to politicize their activities would undermine much of their coalition building and could thereby jeopardize their corporate and foundation funding.

As was stated in the 1991 plan of action developed by the newly formed Georgia Health Decisions (GHD):

> The purpose of the Georgia Health Decisions process is to build consensus, but we *will not* be a lobbying or advocacy group pushing for specific types of legislation. Instead, we will serve as a resource to policy-makers and political leaders who must reach the political judgments needed to convert our consensus on health care values into specific legislation and administrative actions. Therefore, during Phase IV our work will center on education and further analysis that can inform the political process. Examples may include: forums for policy-makers, additional citizen surveys on selected issues, evaluation and analysis of issues, and comparative data studies of how health care delivery systems have worked in other environments.

Although remaining value neutral and nonpolitical may have benefits for emerging grassroots organizations, does neutrality accomplish much in the long run? The GHD plan assumes that policy makers and political leaders will convert consensus on health care values into specific legislation and administrative actions. But what if they don't? Sooner or later, the public will become weary of going through the process of values identification and clarification if changes do not materialize. In the past, projects that restricted their activities to opinion gathering, consciousness raising, or consensus building, without attaching the outcome to some other agenda, eventually failed.

Seeking consensus for its own sake is self-indulgent. In not being tied to some larger purpose or mission, the values defined in the process lose their value to decision makers.

New Directions and Actions

A number of projects recently initiated by CHD groups are exciting and unique.

Education about the Patient Self-Determination Act

Many groups have initiated educational projects about the Patient Self-Determination Act. The most elaborate of these has been created by California Health Decisions (CHD). The program's goal is to help 1 million Californians complete a durable power of attorney for health care (DPAHC) by 1995, targeting senior citizens, employee groups, and health professionals.

The CHD has also received a grant to produce a new educational video program and accompanying materials on the DPAHC. Another grant will make it possible for the CHD to convene a group of health decisions representatives from around the country to standardize advance directives education.

The CHD has also been part of the California Consortium on Patient Self-Determination, which was established in February 1991 as a coalition of groups representing health care facilities and providers, consumers, and bioethics experts from across the state, as well as representatives of the California Department of Health Services. One of the consortium's goals is to develop written materials that satisfy the requirements of the Patient Self-Determination Act.

In 1991, together with the Hastings Center and the Public Agenda Foundation, the CHD organized the Health Care Priorities and Community Values Project. This three-year project will include 1,000 community meetings throughout California, the development of educational material, and a major media campaign. The project is seen as a framework for a national model aimed at involving citizens in societal choices and bringing community values to bear on complex policy questions.

Wisconsin was the first state to mount a major statewide community health decisions program without the support of a major foundation, according to John M. Stanley, Ph.D., director of the program in biomedical ethics at Lawrence University, Appleton, and one of the founding members of the WHD. This was accomplished by collaborating with Wisconsin Public Television in developing the state's first community education program on advance directives. The program was aired during the course of community meetings in order to facilitate discussion.[17]

Ethics Workshops and Debating Program

The New Jersey Citizens' Committee on Biomedical Ethics has created a unique ethics education course that is taught at a growing number of high schools around the state. Known as the Ethics Workshop and Debating Program, the course brings students into the clinical setting to witness the impact that medical technology is having on patient care and to debate the ethical implications of this technology.

According to the chairwoman of the committee, the course reaches a wide audience and gives schools new ways to improve students' basic skills while producing informed citizens. "We had been criticized for not getting the so-called hard-to-reach populations like minorities in urban areas," she said. "The schools are the one place where we can reach all populations."[18] The course is intended primarily to improve students' ability to reason, vigorously support their opinions, and analyze problems and a wide variety of possible solutions.

Community-Based Bioethics Committee

A major effort of Arizona Health Decisions is the implementation of its free-standing, volunteer, community-based bioethics committee, called the Health Decisions Community Council (HDCC). The council was established for West Yavapai County after two years of planning.

Like institutional ethics committees, the HDCC is not a decision-making group, but rather serves as an impartial resource to any consumer or provider experiencing bioethical dilemmas and requesting assistance. The goal was to create a safe, respectful environment in which individuals feel supported and informed in their decision-making process. Council members represent a variety of constituencies, including medical, nursing, social work, religious, allied health, and lay community.

The HDCC is reaching a wider audience than initially expected. It is being used for regular case review processes and for retrospective case review by local health agency staff.

The Vermont Ethics Network is exploring the feasibility of establishing a communitywide process of inquiry and reflection for those who must act under moral uncertainty. The organization is now looking to hospital ethics committees for expertise in expanding the concept into the community.

The Bioethics Resource Group has helped establish ethics committees in the acute care hospitals of Charlotte, North Carolina. It offers continuing education and networking opportunities for those committees.

Task Force on Health Care Proxy Laws

Massachusetts Health Decisions staffs a task force to help shed light on the rather vague 1991 state health care proxy law. The task force devised a statement of understanding about the law, particularly on how it would relate to the Patient Self-Determination Act. The MHD also produced a health care proxy form and accompanying question-and-answer "primer" on its use.

Donald F. Phillips

The Future of Grassroots Efforts

Ethics attempts to answer the question, "What shall I do?" Social ethics broadens that question to "What shall *we* do?" Politics is the struggle for power to determine government outcomes; it is the attempt to control what is done collectively. Ethics and politics often intersect, and the majority of the health decisions groups would probably maintain that ethics should help determine what we choose to do politically.

The community health decisions movement, with its persona of ethical interest, may view itself as apolitical, but it is nonetheless a political movement in that its primary overall purpose is to influence, either directly or indirectly, the body politic. As the various state and regional programs shift their concerns from issues of individual choice in medical care and toward societal options in public health, the movement will encounter more difficult tasks and problems—and more politics.

One challenge will be "to introduce into the conversation values and claims of a less individualistic, more communitarian character."[19] This will require community health decision programs to hear and register more voices from different places, people, and perspectives—to aggressively expand into geographical and cultural areas heretofore beyond reach. This will necessitate new, creative, and ambitious approaches to community education and leadership. Until this is achieved, the movement will remain focused on what middle-class citizens believe the poor should be given, instead of on what all of us owe to and should provide for one another.

If the community health decisions movement does achieve a more communitarian character, it will still face the problem of continued support. Sooner or later, each program will pursue an idea or action that will not be favored by one or more of its coalition members.

In our time, the simple question of, "What shall I/we do?" has become more difficult to answer to everyone's satisfaction. Part of the problem may be the lack of a Rosetta Stone by which the language of ethics can be introduced into the political process. As Alasdair MacIntyre wrote, "There seems to be no rational way of securing moral agreement in our culture."[20] In moral debates today, there is a "conceptual incommensurability of rival arguments. . . . Every one of the arguments is logically valid or can be easily expanded so as to be made so; the conclusions do indeed follow from the premises. But the rival premises are such that we possess no rational way of weighing claims of one against the other."[21]

Put more simply, neither deontological ethics, with its attempts to provide rules of actions such as the Ten Commandments or the laws of the United States, nor teleological ethics, with its emphasis on the goals of "the good" or "justice," are able in U.S. society to provide an agreed-upon set of rules or goals. Even the newly defined feminist ethics of caring, which provides a morality based on respectability and relationships, does not appear to motivate business and government leaders.

Appeals to ethics may be of some use when brought to bear on corruption and reforms in government. But in the end, it may not be a question of achieving ethical reasoning—which community health decision groups have as a goal—but rather whether the groups can amass the votes necessary to replace existing politicians with others who are committed to different goals or to change the minds of current officials.

Appeals to traditional ethics in respect to such problems of justice as hunger, homelessness, and health care seem ineffectual. Appeals to an ethic of compassion and caring may well be intellectually correct, but apparently this ethic is not shared widely enough by the population or by governing elites to force necessary actions.

This situation speaks to a need for a reformulated approach to political ethics or ethical politics. The communitarian ethic sought may well include a component of caring and compassion. Such an ethic has to be adopted and accepted by all sectors within our society. The grassroots movement, as the intermediary between the unempowered and the empowered, could be the transforming element needed to define, design, and promote this new ethic—should it decide to do so.

References

1. Jennings, B. Community health decisions: A grassroots movement in bioethics. *Hastings Center Report* 18(3):Supplement 1–16, June/July, 1988.
2. Jennings.
3. Crawshaw, R., et al. Oregon health decisions: An experiment with informed community consent. *JAMA* 254:3213–16, 1985.
4. Hines, B. L. *Oregon and American Health Decisions: A Guide for Community Action on Bioethical Issues.* Washington, DC: Office of Health Planning, U.S. Department of Health and Human Services, 1985.
5. Crawshaw.
6. Conviser, R. A history of Oregon health decisions. Unpublished report, 1991.
7. Crawshaw.
8. Garland, M. J., and Hasnain, R. Health care in common: Setting priorities in Oregon. *Hastings Center Report* 20(5):16–18, September/October, 1990.
9. Goshen General Hospital. *Just Caring: Justice, Health Care, and the Good Society.* Goshen, IN: Goshen General Hospital Medical Ethics Committee, 1988.
10. Gallegos, T., and Mrgurdic, K. The community bioethics experiment: social work and health care decisionmaking. In submission, 1991.
11. Crawshaw.
12. Conviser.
13. Conviser.

14. Crawshaw.
15. Oregon Health Decisions. *Quality of Life in Allocating Health Care Resources.* Portland: Oregon Health Decisions, 1988.
16. Conviser.
17. Stanley, J. M. Private correspondence, 1991.
18. Strong, M. Personal communication, 1991.
19. Jennings, B. Democracy and justice in health policy. *Hastings Center Report* 20(5):22–23, September/October, 1990.
20. MacIntyre, A. *After Virtue: A Study in Moral Theory.* South Bend, IN: University of Notre Dame Press, 1981, pp. 6–8.
21. McIntyre.

Resources: Health Decisions Programs

California Health Decisions
505 S. Main Street, Suite 400
Orange, CA 92668
714/647-4920

New Jersey Citizen's Committee
on Biomedical Ethics, Inc.
Oakes Outreach Center
120 Morris Avenue
Summitt, NJ 07901-3948
908/277-3858

Oregon Health Decisions
921 S.W. Washington, Suite 723
Portland, OR 97205
503/241-0744

Arizona Health Decisions
Box 4401
Prescott, AZ 86302
602/778-4850

Part VI

The Individual and Society: Seeking Fairness

If individual ethics dilemmas tend to hinge on autonomy, then social ethics dilemmas tend to hinge on fairness — on whether justice is served by what is, or is not, done. But when what is considered fair by one individual or community is considered victimization by another individual or community, fairness becomes a weapon rather than a laudable goal. Nonetheless, it seems clear that practices, procedures, and decisions that are seen as fair by most, if not all, of the parties involved are most likely to meet with success. This is true whether it is a "micro" situation, such as which patient receives an organ transplant, or a "macro" situation, such as the growing debate over the plight of Americans who have no health insurance.

In this section, the question of fairness is examined from a number of perspectives. Daniel Callahan, Ph.D., offers guidance on the proper role of the health care system in a good and just society — and suggests that the current situation is a long way from ideal. Judith P. Swazey, Ph.D., and Renée C. Fox, Ph.D., look at the use — and misuse — of organ transplantation and its role as a metaphor for the uneasy (if not impossible) relationship between aggressive use of high technology for individuals and fairness in the larger society. Jean L. Forster, Ph.D., argues that when it comes to preventive health care and public health, individual interests are subsumed by community interest because some individual needs can be met only by community action. Steven Miles, M.D., and Allison August examine fairness in legal decisions regarding the right to die and come to the troubling conclusion that the autonomy of male patients is honored and protected by the courts, whereas the autonomy of female patients is devalued. Finally, Emily Friedman raises the broadest issue of fairness in health care by asking whether society, as a whole, and providers, in particular, are ethically committed to the tens of millions of Americans who must beg for health care as charity — and what the answer tells us about the ethics of the health care system itself.

Chapter 24

Modernizing Mortality:
Medical Progress and the Good Society

Daniel Callahan, Ph.D.

This paper [also published in *The Hastings Center Report*, January–February 1990, pp. 28–32] is adapted, with permission, from *What Kind of Life?: The Limits of Medical Progress,* Simon & Schuster. Copyright ©1990 by Daniel Callahan.

Daniel Callahan, Ph.D., is director of The Hastings Center, Briarcliff Manor, New York.

I n Condorcet's history of human progress, published in 1795, he wrote the memorable words that to this day animate the enterprise of scientific medicine:

Would it be absurd then to suppose that this perfection of the human species might be capable of indefinite progress; that the day will come when death will be due only to extraordinary accidents or to the decay of the vital forces, and that ultimately, the average span between birth and decay will have no assignable value? Certainly man will not become immortal, but will not the interval between the first breath that he draws and the time when in the natural course of events, without disease or accident, he expires, increase indefinitely?[1]

While such optimism is rarely expressed so unguardedly any longer, the hopes that are held out by scientists for the conquest of disease, and the public commitment to medical advancement, show how deeply embedded is its power. Lewis Thomas once said that he expected most major diseases of the present to be as well understood as the infectious diseases of the past. The present Director General of the World Health Organization, Dr. Hiroshi Nakajima, has stated that "the right to a long life, which might theoretically be averaged at 100 years, is a basic human right of every individual."[2]

The complexity of our present situation is not that such prophecies and optimism have been proved false, thus abandoning us to our present bodily fates. Medical and scientific advances in fact continue to come at a fast pace, and each one seems to open the way for still another. We do not yet know how long average life expectancy might be, or whether we can rid ourselves of most of our present diseases and infirmities. Those who have predicted the failure of this or that scientific dream have probably been more wrong over time than those who predicted their success. I do not, then, want to offer a brief against the possibility of further medical progress, even Condorcet's "indefinite progress." He has yet to be proved false, even if we can debate whether every medical advance should be called progress.

That point, however, is neither the end of the story nor the whole story. Only now have we come to see with any clarity the individual and social results of desiring, and trying to pay for, that kind of progress. We have found our mortality wanting, and we have tried to modernize it. What have we learned?

At the least we know that this can be an extraordinarily expensive economic venture, consuming resources at a rapid and growing rate, in lock step with the progress we make. Save perhaps in the care of the dying, we have been less slow to notice, or concede, the high human costs of chasing that progress. There is the growing fear of aging and death in the company of modern medicine, perhaps best demonstrated by a rising call for active euthanasia and assisted suicide. There is the greater sense of risk and vulnerability that greater medical knowledge ironically instills in us. Despite all our talk about death with dignity, there is the growing inability to find a way of coming to grips with the reality of death, a reality now seemingly transformed into wrenching choice rather than a deliverance of fate. There is the anxiety occasioned by our capacity to transform our biological condition without a comparable skill to transform our social condition; we know how to extend average life expectancy, but not how to cope with the consequences of an aging society.

That was not supposed to happen. We were meant in our quest for unlimited progress to overcome obstacles, to transform our human fate. Yet, as Michael Ignatieff has observed:

> the modern world, for very good reasons, does not have a vernacular of fate. Cultures that live by the values of self-realization and self-mastery are not especially good at dying, at submitting to those experiences where freedom ends and biological fate begins. Why should they be? Their strong side is Promethean ambition: the defiance and transcendence of fate. . . . Their weak side is submitting to the inevitable.[3]

That is not all. In our allocation of health care resources we are in a double jeopardy. We have neither been able to overcome our biological fate nor wisely to manage the resources necessary to accommodate even such fate as we have mastered.

The Mirage of Health

René Dubos once wrote movingly of the "mirage of health." "Complete and lasting freedom from disease," he observed, "is but a dream remembered from imaginings of a Garden of Eden."[4] We have yet, however, to enfold within our modern thinking about health care the implications of that simple but profound truth. If we cannot conquer all disease, or avoid all accidents, or overcome aging and death—*not now, not ever*—what should that truth mean for the devising of a health care system?

We can begin responding to that question by changing our understanding of medical progress, especially that version which seeks "indefinite progress." If that is construed to mean meeting all individual need for cure and avoiding death, it is a hopeless and ultimately damaging quest. If it might, instead, be understood as an effort to determine how best to live within the boundaries of a finite body and finite resources, then our task becomes one of finding a good balance and equilibrium, and of aiming for the kind of progress that most promotes it.

How could a goal of this kind be made plausible? The obstacles are powerful. "What has happened in the modern world," Michael Walzer has noted, "is simply that disease itself, even when it is endemic rather than epidemic, has come to be seen as a plague. And since the plague can be dealt with, it *must* be dealt with. People will not endure what they no longer believe they have to endure."[5]

Yet we must persuade people—persuade those people who are *ourselves*—that we will have to endure illness and death, convince ourselves that we are wrong in thinking we no longer have to accept disease. We will have to be convinced that a single-minded ambition to overcome our mortality will generate individual misery and societal distortion, that it will create a society in which we would not want to live. We will have to be persuaded that our desire for progress, understandable enough, can be preserved, but only if pointed in a different direction, one designed to enrich and intensify our lives, not to enlarge and to conquer the endless frontiers of mortality.

Consider how we now conduct our present health crusade. We focus on individual medical needs and wants, on this misery or that. We devise graphs of death and illness, work up ever more ambitious biomedical research lists, and we then seek as much money as can be had—and no amount is too much—to meet those demands. One reason we continue to want indefinite progress is that we constantly upgrade our needs to keep one jump ahead of our achievements. The more we get, the more we want. We manage brilliantly to keep ourselves dissatisfied. As a consequence, we make health an obsession and then try to spend our way out of it, and the cure soon becomes its own kind of disease.

The result is clearly seen in the growing proportion of our gross national product (GNP) going to health. It muscles aside everything else. Consider one set of figures. Thirty years ago 6 percent of the GNP went to health and 6 percent to education. It is still 6 percent for education, but 11.3 percent for health. Is that because our children are so well educated we need spend no more, or because our health has been declining over the past 30 years, and thus we need to spend more? The opposite is true in both cases.

The corrective to an imbalance of this kind cannot come from within the domain of health and medicine, which has no intrinsic limits. It must come from a coherent perspective on the general welfare of the society as a whole. That perspective is the only shield against those unending lists of statistics that show how many work days are lost from illness, or how many diseases are yet to be cured, or how many individual medical needs are going unmet, or how many wondrous research possibilities there are. All of those claims and lists are true and accurate, yet they also distort reality, which needs a wider lens to be seen clearly.

The so far irresistible force of such claims must be met by one just as powerful. That can only be the force of understanding that the overall welfare of our social, educational, economic, and cultural institutions—and the happiness of the individuals who draw their sustenance from those institutions—must be well nourished if health is to have a meaningful context. For it is their flourishing which is the point of good health. If good health becomes an end in itself—and some 40 percent of Americans report it to be their highest goal in life—then its quest begins to craze and impoverish us. That is all we will have, and we cannot forever hang on to that anyway.

Health and the Good Society

What kind of medicine is best for a good society, and what kind of society is best for a good medicine? Let me attempt a brief answer to those two questions. That medicine is best for a good society that contributes to the health necessary to make the society function well, to achieve its appropriate ends. The measure of that achievement, I propose, should be two-fold: There must, first, be a sufficient level of general good health to assure the viability of a society's social, cultural, and political institutions. There must, second, be a willingness to guarantee its citizens a decent baseline of public health and individual caring, and then beyond that as much—and only as much—individualized cure of disease as is compatible with overall societal needs.

Let me now turn to the second question: What kind of society is best for a good medicine? That society is best for a good medicine that understands that a society has many needs and dimensions, of which health is only one and itself no more than a means to other ends. It will be a society that comprehends that, however insistent the individual desire to overcome illness and forestall death, that desire must at some point be resisted so that other human ends can be sought and nourished, those that together respond to the full range of individual and social possibilities. A society excessively bent on conquering illness and death is certain both to fail and to harm many other values and human goods in the process. Life is to be lived for the sake of living a life, not for the sake of avoiding a death.

How can we fashion a notion of progress that can encompass that perception? Given the misery of disease and the hope for cure, it will not be an easy task to shift our priorities to a different vision of medical progress. My own suggested ranking would be: first, to give the highest priority once again to that most ancient of all medical values, that of caring for those we cannot (for scientific or economic reasons) cure—no one should ever be abandoned; second, we should focus on those well-established principles and practices of public health and primary care medicine that are most conducive to our common good at the least cost—good nutrition, disease prevention, immunization, antibiotics, primary care, and emergency medicine; and third (and last) we should pursue in a way that does not strain our general resources those advanced forms of high technology medicine that tend to benefit comparatively few individuals at comparatively high cost—organ transplantation, total parenteral nutrition (TPR), advanced intensive care services, and the like. I stress that these would be priorities only, not a rigid hierarchy. But a shift toward those priorities could lead to a dramatically different health care system in the future.

Is such a shift possible? I believe it is, but only if built upon a public discussion and debate of a kind heavily resisted in this country. It would require a consensus that many would consider dangerous. We will have to talk together and come to some agreement about what kind and level of health is sufficient for the good functioning of society. That goal will mean trying mutually to devise a picture of a coherent, well-proportioned society, one that finds a valid mix of health, education, defense, housing, welfare, culture, and recreation. We will no less have to talk together about the place of health in our individual lives. What is reasonable to aspire to, what health *ought* we to want (as distinguished from what we do want), what lack of health can we with help endure and learn to accept? We will have to talk about the kinds of demands it is reasonable to make upon our neighbor, our taxpaying fellow citizen, for care and for cure if we are unable to afford it ourselves. What do we owe each other, and what kind of a health care financing system are we willing to accept to make certain we discharge those obligations? We will have, in sum, to talk about the relationship between good health and the good self, between good health and the good society.

I would have it noted that those are basic moral issues, not the customary economic issues commonly used to talk about our health care crisis. They cannot be confronted adequately without a willingness to think together about human nature and human life, and to explore as a society the old and, for many, dangerously troubling ideas of the human good. Yet if the idea of a human good is troubling, a shock to the notion of pluralistic society that neither invokes nor shares a common view of the good, it is no less troubling to ignore it.

The need to allocate health care resources in relation to many other societal needs, and to ration curative medicine within the sphere of health care, requires some degree of satisfying consensus, some common notion of where we should be going. A consensus simply to limit health care is not enough. That can be done brutally, by the force of political coercion. A humane consensus to limit health care requires a meaningful rationale, a way of looking at society and individual life as a whole, that makes some sense to those who will have to accept the limits.

The more we can agree on the kind of society we want, and the sensible place of health care within it, the more likely we are to accept those limits. They will be our own self-imposed limits, a part of some full vision of the good of people and society. It will not be the young imposing limits on the old, or the rich upon the poor, or management on workers. We will be imposing limits upon ourselves, as a common action for the common good.

We will no less need to think about our own individual lives. We will in the future, for instance, have to pay an increasingly large share of our health care costs out of our own pockets. Almost all of the various health care proposals now being discussed have that as their message, either explicitly or implicitly. We will have to make choices about the kind of coverage we want, what we are willing to help pay for and what we are willing to forgo. Even a good program of guaranteed universal care for the indigent will not obviate those choices for everyone else. How much of what kind of health care can we afford? How much *ought* we be willing to afford? To ask that last question will be to ask how much we should value freedom from the threat of illness, from the danger of death. It will make us ask what kind of a life we want to live, and how the quest for health should fit into that life.

We can of course ask such questions wholly in private, but we would be much better advised to talk about them together, to hear what others have to say and how others have chosen to live. We will need each other's help.

How much risk of poor or impaired health should young parents run? Do the elderly have an obligation to avoid burdening their children with health or long-term care costs? That question will almost certainly once again surface as the elderly are forced to pay out-of-pocket a larger share of their health care costs, already now greater than when Medicare was passed in 1965 (18% now versus 15% then). Or is it the other way around, that children have an added obligation to take up the financial burdens of parental care—but, if so, to what extent and in what way? To think about questions of that kind will require our mutual help and enlightenment. They are all questions about the human good. We can pretend, or insist, that they are out of place in a free, pluralistic society that allows each individual to invent or discover his or her own human good. But that is a form of self-deception. They are real questions, and the kind we cannot well answer entirely on our own. Nor are they necessarily proof against the discovery of a consensus, a common way of looking at things, which we will find helpful and satisfactory, even if not perfect.

Private Good and Public Good

We have generally failed, both experts and lay people, to understand the way in which changing ideas of health bring with them changing ideas of our way of life; and how, in turn, changes in our way of life work back into alterations of our notions of health. To understand that is already to recognize that the supposed private sphere of our individual notions of health and happiness is deeply influenced by the society in which we live. It provides us with our images, stories, and paradigms. To grasp the way our public and private ideas of health work on and with each other is thus vital. It is undeniably a puzzle of uncertain dimensions, but at the core of the problem that faces us.

If, for instance, we believe that we should strive to eradicate all preventable pain and suffering, even at great cost to other goods and values, we will have no alternative but to give the highest priority to health care. If, moreover, we also believe that health and a sense of well-being are private and uniquely personal matters, then we are likely as a society to resist any common judgment about their meaning and value. We will favor policies of maximum individual choice. Yet it is precisely policies based on those values that are collapsing, both too expensive to implement and too little productive of individual satisfaction.

What can it mean, say, to use the language of "tradeoffs" as a way of resolving struggles about the provision of health care? Lacking any common ideas of individual good save that of self-determination and self-definition, it is a recipe for the play of power and interests, winner take all, not of reflection upon what might be best for people. What can it mean to talk about freedom of choice if that freedom becomes in the arena of allocation a war of all against all, each seeking maximum benefits maximally defined? That is a prescription for the ruination of all. What can it mean to seek "indefinite progress" in health if the cost of seeking it is to impoverish the rest of our lives? What is actually best for people?

Yet can we talk about "what is best for people," with all the overtones of moral judgment and substantive consensus that a phrase like that conveys? My response is: how can we not, finally, come to talk about that? Will we not in any event be talking about it implicitly, even if we try to stifle it? We already think that, in some sense, health is important. That is already one facet of a view of the human good; a general stance has been taken.

Now the task is to discover how, and in what way, health is important. There is no wholly neutral standpoint from which to do so. Since we must, moreover, come to some common political judgment about the allocation of health care resources, we will have to find a way to put together in some coherent fashion our various views on health and human life. We cannot solve our problem otherwise, except meanly and poorly, and we cannot avoid tacit and concealed answers to questions about the human good no matter what kind of solution we adopt.

Nor need we despair in advance of getting somewhere. We have much of value with which we can work, in our experience as well as our traditions. We have had at least fifty years of experience with high-technology medicine and we should have learned something by now. The most important insight is the most simple: medicine is just like everything else in the world. It can bring good and it can bring harm, often at the same time. It bewitches us as much as it benefits us. In the company of technology, we have had the experience in the United States of seeing how the demand for health care increases the more of it we get, but also how other cultures respond variously to that demand, and how different kinds of health care systems can be devised to cope with it.

We have had the experience of discovering, if we look, that the connection between health and happiness remains both important and yet indeterminate; there is no perfect symmetry. More research, of the right kind, could well improve that symmetry, but simply throwing one new device or drug after another at illness is not necessarily the way to go about it.

We are at an important historical juncture, our aspirations for indefinite progress at war with our limited resources and our experience of the mixed blessings of progress even when we can afford it. Our hope that we could avoid a genuinely serious crisis in health care costs through cost containment or other tactics has come to all too little. We can assume we have just not well learned how to make sensible tradeoffs and put proper incentives in place. Cost containment has not failed; it has just never been properly tried. We can, that is, convince ourselves that the problems we have encountered in the project of modernizing mortality, in seeking indefinite progress, in hoping for more life and better life, are just managerial and organizational in nature. There is nothing wrong with the goals. We just need to seek them more efficiently.

A Flawed Project?

Or we can understand those problems as evidence that there is something flawed about the project itself, about its very ends and purposes. Instead of assuming that more ingenuity and better cost-containment incentives will let us proceed apace, we might wonder whether our failures in efficiency bespeak a deeper lack of understanding of our own nature and limitations. We might wonder whether our lack of success in meeting individual health needs (always being redefined), or our repeated failure even to define what a "decent minimum" of health care would encompass, is just chance or, perhaps, the beginning of insight into the complexities and paradoxes of

the quest. We might wonder whether our ultimate problems with health care are not moral rather than practical, more about our chosen ends than our managerial means.

We have for many years now just drifted along, creating a health care system that not only costs too much for what it delivers, but fails also to deliver what it could for millions of people. It has led us to spend too much on health in comparison with other social needs, too much on the old in comparison with the young, too much on the acutely ill in comparison with the chronically ill, too much on curing in comparison with caring, too much on expensive individual health needs in comparison with less expensive societal health needs, and too much on extending the length of life rather than enhancing the quality of life.

Those are perhaps contentious convictions, but I think positions of that kind—however they may differ in detail and emphasis—will begin to emerge if we open up the moral questions in a full way. Once we have done so, we will find that they must be grappled with as moral questions. They cannot be adequately confronted if translated into more tractable political or economic problems. The relative priority we should accord the young and the old in the health care system, of length of life versus quality of life, of cure or care, for example, are deeply moral issues. They need answers on their merits, however awkward politically. This will happen only if we refuse to allow ourselves to be any longer comforted by those who would evade such questions to pursue, as if it is the true and full answer, a new try at efficiency, at "cutting the fat."

The faith in economic salvation from our problems should be put aside, along with the myth that a still larger research investment will allow us to turn some corner on costly care, or that a more informed, cost-conscious patient will make the decisive difference, or that technology assessment will do the trick. They are all ways of evading not just the hard choices, but the hard questions, and all the more seductive because some of them are truly needed and respond to part of the problem; they will just not be enough. It is as if the optimism of the scientific enterprise of medicine has infected the way we think about the social enterprise of medicine, that if we can make limitless scientific progress, we must therefore be able to make comparable progress in coping with its individual, economic, and political problems and costs. That is a profound mistake, but one whose power animates each new cost-containment and efficiency scheme.

What will it take to convince ourselves otherwise? Still greater deterioration in our system? One more failed cost-containment plan? One more stab at improved competition? And when they fail, will we continue to berate ourselves that we have not tried hard enough? Or blame the doctors for charging too much, the juries for awarding too heavy malpractice damages,

Daniel Callahan, Ph.D.

or the medical manufacturers for their cupidity? Will we, that is, round up the usual suspects? They are suspects, surely enough — and they must be dealt with — but it is a profound mistake to identify them as the ultimate problem. That problem is our aspiration for unlimited medical progress, which leads us to want more than we can get or can afford. Even if we can better manage our deranged health care system, we will be left with that far more profound issue. We need a change in our perspective, and of a penetrating kind.

The change cannot only be in our health care system, in its mechanisms, institutions, and practices. It must no less be a change in our values and goals, our ideas of good health and the good life. This change must, moreover, come from the inside, from ourselves, those selves that must wrestle with the fact that we are both patients or would-be patients, hurting and needy, alone with our individual needs, and yet also members of local communities, families, and a larger society, whose collective well-being gives our individuality a place and an enhanced meaning.

A health care system that took its point of departure from our need as individuals to be cared for, that promised never to abandon us, would bring us back into continuity with the richest and deepest traditions of medicine. A system that focused its vision of progress and research efforts on enhancing the quality of life rather than of holding off death, or on means of preventing illness and reducing the debilities of old age rather than on high technology cures, or on enhancing the general level of public health rather than the special curative needs of individuals, would be a more rounded and coherent system.

A health care system which understood that it was meant to be part of, and to serve the needs of, a broader social and political system, would be one less prone to think only of its own needs, or to forget that health is only a means to the living of a life, not its goal. A system that guaranteed a minimally decent level of health care for all, in turn asking each of us to rein in our private demands, would be a decent and manageable one. That is not an impossible ideal.

References

1. Antoine-Nicolas de Condorcet, *Sketch for a Historical Picture of the Progress of the Human Mind,* June Berraclough, trans. (New York: Library of Ideas, 1955), 200.
2. Lewis Thomas, "On the Science and Technology of Medicine," *Daedalus* (Winter 1977), 46; and Hiroshi Nakajima, "Address to the All-Union Conference on Physicians," WHO Press, Press Release WHO/37 (19 October 1988).
3. Michael Ignatieff, "Modern Dying," *The New Republic,* 26 December 1988, 28–33.
4. René Dubos, *Mirage of Health: Utopias, Progress, and Biological Change* (New York: Harper Colophon Books, 1979), 2.
5. Michael Walzer, *Spheres of Justice: A Defense of Pluralism and Equality* (New York: Basic Books, 1983), 8.

We Shall Overcome, Somehow:
Organ Replacement and the Meanings
of Medical Progress

Judith P. Swazey, Ph.D., and Renée C. Fox, Ph.D.

Judith P. Swazey, Ph.D., is president of The Acadia Institute, Bar Harbor, Maine. Renée C. Fox, Ph.D., is Annenberg Professor of the Social Sciences, University of Pennsylvania, Philadelphia.

This brief essay sets forth some of our increasingly troubled and critical reactions to the kinds of expansion that have taken place in organ replacement during the 1980s and early 1990s and the medical and cultural fervor by which that expansion has been driven.[1] The number, variety, and combinations of solid organs and other body parts being transplanted, along with the array of extracorporeal and implanted devices being routinely used, tested, or designed, have brought our society closer to the once-futuristic world of "rebuilt people."[2] As classically portrayed in science fiction, it is a world in which human beings are more and more composed of transplanted parts of one another, of other species, and of "man-machine unions" that "prosthetize" humans and humanize manmade organs.[3] It is the "spare parts" pragmatism, the vision of the "replaceable body" based on convictions about the possibility and desirability of limitless medical progress, and the escalating evangelistic ardor about the life-saving goodness of repairing and remaking people in this fashion that we have found particularly disturbing.

Our sociological and moral concerns have been deepened by the ways that we believe certain developments in organ replacement illuminate more general features of the nexus of health, medicine, and values in American society. Here, we are in accord with philosopher and bioethicist Daniel Callahan's convictions about the need for some fundamental value changes in our society with respect to the roles of health, illness, and medicine in our individual and collective lives.[4] Callahan is among those who are convinced that we need to openly and explicitly ration health care by establishing reasoned priorities for the medical goods and services we will provide. But any viable rationing effort, he contends, must be preceded by the arduous task of attempting to significantly alter the values that drive our so-called health care system.

Callahan, as do we and a number of other writers, sees three value changes as particularly essential to a recasting of what our society is seeking to accomplish through medicine and our provision of medical services. First, we must curb our aspirations for unlimited and infinite medical progress and in so doing relinquish our utopian belief in what the distinguished microbiologist René Dubos called the "mirage of health." "Complete and lasting freedom from disease," Dubos wrote 30 years ago, "is but a dream remembered from imaginings of a Garden of Eden designed for the welfare of man."[5] Second, we need to move away from the overweening emphasis that bioethics, in accord with America's value system, has given to individualism, autonomy, and rights[6] and place a greater emphasis on communitarian values, on public rather than personal health, and on the common good rather than the welfare of the individual. In this context, the value question becomes "how much health care is needed for the overall good or welfare of society?" Third, we need to place a greater value on the caring role of medicine and its practitioners, in contrast to the human and financial efforts we now devote to trying to cure all disease, prolong all lives, and overcome aging and death.

Health policy analyst Richard A. Rettig has portrayed the political dimensions of organ transplantation as constituting a "parable of our time."[7] This characterization, we would argue, applies not only to the matters that Rettig has analyzed, such as the financing of transplantation procedures, the certification of transplantation centers, and the management of organ procurement, but also to the deep-structured values undergirding and supporting our drive to avert death and, it is hoped, restore a measure of functional health through replacing failing vital organs with transplants or manmade surrogates.

Singly and jointly, we have spent many years studying the evolution of organ transplantation and the development and deployment of devices such as the artificial kidney and artificial heart, primarily through the medium of firsthand field research. There have been several aspects of these therapeutic innovations and their deployment that we have long found especially troubling. Prominent among them have been some components of the "we shall overcome" value system that is endemic in transplant physicians and artificial organ pioneers, and which infuses our societal perspectives on the meaning of medical progress and the goals of medical care. This ethos includes a classically American frontier outlook: heroic, pioneering, adventurous, optimistic, and determined. But it also involves a bellicose "death is the enemy" perspective, a rescue-oriented and often zealous determination to maintain life at any cost, and a relentless, hubris-ridden refusal to accept limits.

Another source of disquiet has been the disparity between social justice principles and practices concerning fairness and equity within the organ replacement arena. If a society is to engage in organ replacement endeavors, we believe there is a moral obligation to ensure equitable access to transplant waiting lists and to available organs for those accepted as prospective recipients, and, as has been attempted but imperfectly realized for dialysis, to vital artificial organs. Without such equity, for example, one observes again and again how specifically designated individuals have been privileged to become transplant candidates and then to obtain organs and funding by wielding special media, political, and economic resources they are in a position to command, including, during the Reagan years, the power of the presidency.[8]

Having closely tracked organ replacement endeavors from the 1950s to the present, we have recognized that our years in the field have made us more, rather than less,

emotionally and morally perturbable about many of their attributes and side effects. When, for example, we read about the various combinations and clusters of organs now being transplanted, the greater numbers of retransplants, estimates that up to 50,000 liver transplants a year may be needed in the United States to treat over 60 distinct diseases, and about the temporary use of diseased donor hearts to keep patients alive until a healthy donor heart can be found, we wonder, as does Callahan, "what kind of life" our values are driving us to seek, and whether our society can accept limits to medical progress.

We are not therapeutic nihilists, nor do we fail to appreciate the impressive medical, surgical, and technological progress that has been made with transplants and artificial organs during the past three decades. But we have come to feel that the missionarylike ardor about organ replacement that now exists, the overidealization of the quality and duration of life that can ensue, and the seemingly limitless attempts to procure and implant organs that are currently taking place have gotten out of hand. Reflecting on what she terms "the transplant odyssey," transplant nurse-specialist Patricia M. Park has written that "[w]hat is sometimes referred to as the 'miracle of transplantion' is just exactly that—sometimes. . . . For each case that can be made for the 'miracle of transplantation' though, a case can be made for the 'victims of transplanation' whose lives and hopes have been shattered by the experience. . . . Perhaps the most important issue in a critical examination of transplantation involves the need and criteria for responsible decisions about when to stop, when to say 'enough is enough' to the transplant process."[9]

In our view, the field of organ replacement currently epitomizes a very different and powerful tendency in American health care and in the value and belief system of our society's culture: our pervasive reluctance to accept the biological and human condition limits imposed by the aging process to which we are all subject and our ultimate mortality. It seems to us that much of the current organ replacement endeavor represents an obdurate, publicly theatricalized refusal to accept these limitations.

Paul Ramsey's *The Patient as Person*, published in 1970, has proved to be a prophetic analysis of our social and cultural problems in accepting limits on organ replacement and the care of dying patients. He wrote:

> If it is not possible for modern men, when the one "lone hope" is gone, to believe that this is not the end of hope, perhaps we might share the conviction of Socrates, who said, "Now it is time that we were going, I to die and you to live, but which of us has the happier prospect, is unknown to anyone but God." That outlook, too, might save men and doctors today from the triumphalist temptation to slash and suture our way to eternal life.[10]

We suspect that Ramsey would share our deepening reservations about the societal values underlying the growing intensity and expansion of the drive to sustain life and "rebuild people" through organ replacement. Our society seems to have accepted, in an unquestioning and even celebrated way, the merits of creating larger and larger numbers of what *New York Times* reporter Lawrence K. Altman graphically calls "patchwork people,"[11] whose quality of life often is dubious at best. "Our culture," Ramsey observed 20 years ago, "is already prepared for technocratizing the bodily life into a collection of parts in which consciousness somehow has residence for a time."[12]

Concomitantly, the determination to procure organs has become so powerful that at times there seems to be an almost predatory obliviousness to why and how most organs become available for transplantation. As health lawyer George Annas has observed, a "denial of reality" underlies the current policy of avidly promoting organ donation and transplantation, without publicly acknowledging the kinds of deaths—from causes such as vehicular accidents, homicides, and suicides—on which they are based.[13]

Since the first successful kidney transplants in the 1950s, one of transplantation's central value dimensions has involved defining the act of donating an organ as giving "a gift of life."[14] In recent years, however, the demand for organs has increasingly outstripped the supply, as, spurred by the advent of new more powerful immunosuppressive drugs such as cyclosporine and FK 506, burgeoning numbers of patients have been added to transplant waiting lists.[15] One of the "side effects" of strategies to procure more organs has been some significant alterations in the gift-exchange matrix of transplantation. In their desire to ameliorate the "shortfall" of transplantable organs and tissues, many members of the transplant community, along with some of the ethicists, lawyers, economists, and policy analysts closely involved with transplantation policies, seem to have systematically ignored or forgotten what has been learned about the meanings and dynamics of giving and receiving both live-donor and cadaver organs. The period from 1980 through the early 1990s, for example, saw renal transplanters expand their definition of eligible living donors to include persons who are "emotionally" as well as biologically related to prospective recipients, the inception of parent-to-child liver and lung transplants, and bone marrow transplants from infants conceived to serve as donors for their fatally ill siblings. These phenomena testify to an erosion, if not ending, of many of the informal taboos that previously restricted live donor transplants, and a marked reduction of the wariness with which most transplant teams approached these procedures, based on (1) their medical concerns about removing organs from healthy people and (2) their recognition of the ways that giving and receiving an organ can exacerbate problems in the relationships among donors, recipients, and their families.

The "supply-and-demand problem" associated with transplants also has catalyzed serious consideration of "rewarded gifting"—of ways in which donors or their families might be compensated in order to provide them with greater incentives to contribute organs. And, moving completely away from the gift-exchange framework, the conception of transplantable body parts as commodities gained considerable momentum in the free enterprise, market-oriented economic and political climate of the 1980s. Serious arguments began to be advanced for what some lawyers, economists, and policy analysts call the "commodification" and "marketification" of the "gift of life," inspiring various proposals to "solve" the transplant shortfall by developing licit ventures such as futures markets in "HBPs"—human body parts.[16]

For us, however, the most fundamental value question emerging from our long professional immersion in the world of "spare parts" medicine is whether, as poverty, homelessness, and lack of access to health care increase in our affluent country, it is justifiable for American society to be devoting so much of its intellectual energy and human and financial resources to the replacement of human organs. We realize that in terms of the ways our society provides, allocates, and expends resources within the "medical commons,"[17] the aggregate volume and costs of organ replacements are a relatively small portion of medical care activities and expenditures.[18] Nor, given the benefits that many patients may derive from transplants and artificial devices, do we advocate that all organ replacement endeavors should—or conceivably would—cease. But we have grown increasingly concerned that all the professional and public consideration given to transplants and pursuits such as a permanent artificial heart, and the societal value commitments that organ replacement epitomizes, are helping to divert attention and human and financial resources away from far more basic and widespread public and individual health care needs in our society.

Health policy analyst Emily Friedman has written, with passionate conviction, that a "silent, largely invisible epidemic [of] medical indigence" has become the most tragically serious health care problem in the United States; that "the noncoverage of the uninsured poor and their resultant lack of access [to health care] affect every American"; and that ignoring or accepting this situation puts us "all at risk," because "a society that forces its most vulnerable and needy members to beg for crumbs of care, or to go without care until they are dying, harms itself [and its moral fabric] even more than it harms the victims of its cruelty."[19] The predicament of these deprived and fragile members of our society has changed the ethical context of transplantation and artificial organs for us. Allowing American medicine and the society of which it is a part to become too caught up in repairing and rebuilding people through organ replacement, while health care continues to be defined as a private consumption rather than a social good and millions of people do not have adequate or even minimally decent care, speaks to a values framework and a vision of medical progress that we find medically and morally untenable.

Notes

1. This essay has been adapted from a forthcoming book by Fox, R., and Swazey, J. *Spare Parts: Organ Replacement in American Society.* New York City: Oxford University Press, 1992. See also Fox, R., and Swazey, J. *The Courage to Fail: A Social View of Organ Transplants and Dialysis.* 2nd ed. Chicago: University of Chicago Press, 1978. Swazey, J. The social context of medicine: Lessons from the artificial heart. *Second Opinion* 8:45–65, 1988. Swazey, J. P., Watkins, J. C., and Fox, R. C. Assessing the artificial heart: The clinical moratorium revisited. *International Journal of Technology Assessment in Health Care* 2(3):387–410, 1986.

2. Control of life. Pt. 3: Rebuilt people. *Life,* Sept. 24, 1965, pp. 66–84.

3. Asimov, I. The bicentennial man. In: I. Asimov. *The Bicentennial Man and Other Stories.* New York City: Ballantine, 1976, pp. 519–57.

4. This summary of Callahan's views is based on the following presentations and papers: Allocating health care resources: Can we change our way of life? Keynote speech, Vermont Health Decisions Conference, Rutland, VT, Sept. 27, 1990. Modernizing mortality: Medical progress and the good society. *Hastings Center Report* 20:28–32, Jan./Feb. 1990. Rationing medical progress: The way to affordable health care. *New England Journal of Medicine* 322:1810–13, June 21, 1990.

5. Dubos, R. *Mirage of Health: Utopias, Progress, and Biological Change.* New Brunswick, NJ: Rutgers University Press, 1987, p. 2.

6. Fox, R. C., and Swazey, J. P. Medical morality is not bioethics—Medical ethics in China and the United States. *Perspectives in Biology and Medicine* 27(3):336–60, Spring 1984.

7. Rettig, R. A. The politics of organ transplantation: A parable of our time. In: J. F. Blumstein and F. A. Sloan, editors. *Organ Transplantation Policy: Issues and Prospects.* Durham, NC: Duke University Press, 1989, pp. 191–228.

8. Childress, J. F. Some moral connections between organ procurement and organ distribution. *Journal of Contemporary Health Law and Policy* 3:85–110, 1987. Childress, J. F. Ethical criteria for procuring and distributing organs for transplantation. In: Blumstein and Sloan, pp. 87–113. Iglehart, J. K. Transplantation: the problem of limited resources.

9. Park, P. The transplant odyssey. *Second Opinion* 12:27,30, Nov. 1989.

10. Ramsey, P. *The Patient as Person: Explorations in Medical Ethics.* New Haven, CT: Yale University Press, 1970, p. 238.

11. Altman, L. With new boldness, surgeons create patchwork patients. *The New York Times,* Dec. 12, 1989, pp. C1, C14.

12. Ramsey, p. 193.

13. Annas, G. Feeling good about recycled hearts. *Second Opinion* 12:33–39, Nov. 1989.

14. Fox and Swazey, *The Courage to Fail,* chap. 1.

15. According to data collected by the United Network for Organ Sharing (UNOS), organs were procured from a total of 5,797 cadaveric and living donors in 1989 and from 6,145 such donors in 1990. During those same two years, the number of people on waiting lists for heart, heart–lung, kidney, liver, lung, and pancreas transplants totaled, respectively, 19,173 and 22,008. UNOS data also show that between 1987 and 1990, the number of people on waiting lists for these six most frequently performed solid organ transplants increased by over 61 percent, from 13,396 to 22,008. There also was a marked increase in the total number of these six transplant procedures performed between 1987 and 1990 from 11,992 to 15,164, plus over 500,000 tissue transplants in 1990. (Cate, F. H., and S. S. Laudicina. Transplantation white paper: Current statistical information about transplantation in America. The Annenberg Washington Program in Communication Policy Studies of Northwestern University and the United Network for Organ Sharing, pp. 2, 4, 6.)

16. Hansmann, H. The economics and ethics of markets for organs. In: Blumstein and Sloan, pp. 57–85. Several other papers in this volume also discuss the pros and cons of a market economy for transplantable organs and other body parts.

17. Hiatt, H. Protecting the medical commons: Who is responsible? *New England Journal of Medicine* 293:235–41, July 31, 1975.

18. To date, as Cate and Laudicina point out in the Annenberg–UNOS white paper, "available data on transplant costs is incomplete and far from perfect." Initial figures from the first national study on the costs of solid organ transplantation in 1988 indicate that lung and liver transplant operations are the most expensive single procedures, and kidney transplants the least costly, averaging hospital charges of $240,000, $235,000, and $51,000, respectively. However, these figures significantly understate the actual costs of transplantation, because they do not include items such as organ procurement charges, physician fees, and posthospital expenses such as immunosuppressive drugs. Cate and Laudicina, pp. 9, 14–15.

19. Friedman, E. The torturer's horse (Commentary/Caring for the Poor). *JAMA* 261:1481–82, Mar. 10, 1989.

New England Journal of Medicine 309:123–28, July 14, 1983.

A Communitarian Ethical Model for Public Health Interventions: An Alternative to Individual Behavior Change Strategies

Jean L. Forster, Ph.D.

Reprinted, with permission, from *Journal of Public Health Policy* 3(2):150–63, June 1982.

Jean L. Forster, Ph.D., is assistant professor in the School of Public Health at the University of Minnesota in Minneapolis.

Introduction

The problem of premature death, defined for the purposes of statistical comparison as death before the age of sixty-five, is one which presents a serious threat to Americans. An analysis by Vaupel indicates, by comparison to other countries, how significant the problem is. The United States ranks twenty-sixth among all nations in survival rates *to* age sixty-five, behind Bulgaria, Puerto Rico, and Hong Kong.[1] At the same time, Vaupel points out that the life expectancy for Americans *at* age sixty-five is just behind that of Sweden, which has the highest life expectancy in the world. This disparity makes the point clearly that the problem is truly one of premature death. Another way to state the problem dramatically, as Vaupel has done, is to indicate that the risk of premature death in the United States is 25%; one of four Americans dies before reaching age sixty-five.[1] Presented in this way, early death becomes a problem equal to or greater in magnitude than any we as a society or as individuals face.

However, one doesn't die of early death, but rather of a number of more definitive causes like heart disease, cancer, stroke, or accidents—causes which admit a more precise analysis in terms of prevention. One striking similarity about most of the leading causes of death for all ages is the presence of behavioral risk factors. Individual behaviors, oftentimes everyday habits and choices, directly or indirectly contribute to the ultimate cause of death. These include diet, smoking, alcohol and other drugs, lack of exercise, driving behavior, etc.[2]

In the past several years, these behavioral factors which contribute to chronic disease and premature death have been the focus of a call to redirect our health priorities. A document from the Ministry of National Health and Welfare of Canada, published in 1974, first made explicit this new direction.[3] Lalonde made the case that self-imposed risks and the environment are the main influences on the health of every age group of Canadians. He went on to indict individuals even for environmental problems, writing that "if the government is a mirror of the people's will, then the people must accept the blame for any sickness arising from the environment."[3]

To Lalonde and other policy makers, it seems to follow logically that if individual behavior is the cause of health problems, individual change must be the solution. In a similar vein, Knowles wrote in 1977, "The next major advances in the health of the American people will be determined by what the individual is willing to do for himself."[4] Since then both government agencies and private

Jean L. Forster, Ph.D.

organizations have followed suit in calling for an increase in individual responsibility for health and health care.[2,5] The assumptions of those who advocate a policy shift in this direction are that the cause of the health problem is faulty behavior, that the behavior in question is voluntary, and that the responsibility for change is the individual's. The focus is upon intervention at the time of use, for example of automobiles or alcohol, and so requires continual, active participation of the individual to avoid risks such as alcohol abuse or unsafe driving. Countermeasures to these individual behaviors typically include education/rehabilitation and/or punishment or disincentive. Interventions are based upon sophisticated analyses of the attitudes, beliefs, and other characteristics which distinguish those who display the behavior from those who don't. Though this individualistic way of analyzing health has been expressed publicly by health policy makers only recently, the assumptions have been part of the health care system and indeed the American ethos for a very long time. The assumptions are based upon the classical liberal belief in the individual's right to choose on the basis of his or her own best interests.

The public health tradition, as distinct from the rest of the health care system, has offered a different analysis of the problem and a different orientation to intervention. The mandate of public health has been prevention, and the arena of public health practice has been the community. The strategy of public health, beginning with sanitation and infectious diseases more than a hundred years ago, has been to analyze problems in terms of host, agent, and environment. The present-day success of this strategy, even with complex problems of chronic disease, injuries, and industrial hazards, is based upon the recognition that host, agent, and environment are each necessary but not alone sufficient components of health problems, and characteristics of the host alone do not determine illness. The entire community is assumed to be vulnerable and in need of protection. Therefore collective interventions are proposed which are mandatory, universal, and passive, to minimize the frequency of exposure and the amount of personal effort of those to be protected.[6] Prevention strategies on the community level utilize analysis of causative factors to determine the means available for reducing death and disability.[7]

The significant advances in health in the past century have been largely a consequence of public health interventions, and these advances are in turn a consequence of the change in policy and practice orientation from the individual to the community.[8] However, the change in orientation has not been without struggle. P. Barry has documented the difficulty in making the paradigmatic transition. She shows that health policy is at least a decade behind the theoretical reconceptualization and experimental verification of the effectiveness of the community approach to various health problems.[9]

In large part the struggle for acceptance of collective strategies toward modern health problems, despite their effectiveness, has been ideological and ethical in nature. The preemptory status of individual freedom and responsibility in all areas of our lives has caused even those who would be most likely to benefit directly from collective strategies to resist them in some cases (e.g., motorcycle riders' resistance to mandatory helmet laws).

The purpose of this paper is to show that the ethic of individual interest is insufficient to support efforts to solve our most pressing health problems. Using the example of passive auto restraints as a preventive measure against traffic injuries, I will argue that individual behavior-change strategies based on this ethic lead to unwelcome health outcomes and ethical problems, and that a communitarian context is required to justify and to achieve the goals of public health.

Nature of the Problem

Preventable injury is the third highest cause of deaths and disability in the United States, and traffic injuries account for over half of these deaths.[10] Fifty-three thousand people die in the United States annually as a result of traffic injury, of whom the great majority are under the age of sixty-five. The average traffic death results in a loss of twenty years of working life. An additional 750,000 people annually suffer serious injuries on the highway.[11] The odds are that one of three persons in the United States will experience serious injury from a traffic collision during their lifetime. Clearly, traffic injury constitutes a health problem of the highest magnitude.

A number of policy alternatives offer the potential to reduce the rate of auto collisions and/or the severity of the consequences of the impact. These alternatives include improving the design of the automobiles, improving the design of highways, improving the driving behavior of automobile users, and improving the accessibility of emergency medical services. However, research has shown that increasing the use of seat belts would have the greatest effect, at the lowest cost, of all measures that could be taken to improve highway safety.[12] Data from accident reports show that universal use of lap and shoulder belts could reduce fatalities by 40 to 80% (depending upon the size of the automobile) and reduce the overall frequency of injury by 20%.[13,14] Research done in Sweden by Volvo, for example, shows no fatalities in 28,000 collisions at speeds up to sixty miles per hour when lap and shoulder belts were used, as opposed to fatalities at speeds as low as twelve miles per hour when automobile users were unrestrained.[13]

Three policies are currently followed in various states and countries regarding the use of seat belts. The alternatives are: (1) persuasive strategies aimed at promoting voluntary use; (2) a coercive strategy which legally mandates use of belts which the user must actively employ; (3) a coercive strategy aimed at point of manufacture which requires passive restraints, either passive seat belts or airbags. This last strategy is not dependent for effectiveness upon individual decision, and the device is in place once and forever. No country or state currently requires use of passive restraint (the third strategy), although prior to the current Administration's review, a passive restraint standard would have been in effect for automobiles manufactured in the United States after 1983. Eighteen countries and several Canadian provinces currently require by law the use of safety belts (the second strategy). Great Britain and the United States are the only industrial nations which depend upon voluntary use of restraints (the first strategy) to protect automobile users.[10]

The United States does, however, require that manufacturers install seat belts as standard equipment. This regulation dates to the 1964 model year, when lap belts were required, and was updated in 1968 to specify lap and shoulder belts.[15] Strategies used to encourage use of seat belts, which are now paid for by, and available to virtually every automobile user, have been primarily education/persuasion and buzzer/light warning systems. In 1973 a continuous buzzer/light standard was put into place, and in 1974, an ignition interlock system was standard equipment on all autos sold in the United States.[15] However, an act of Congress in January 1975 removed this standard (and ended our only attempt to mandate use), and reduced the buzzer/light warning requirement to four to eight seconds following ignition.[15]

Since 1964, when seat belts became standard equipment in the United States, continuous media campaigns have urged their use. Efforts by both the auto industry and the National Safety Council to modify non-use behavior have used themes such as physician endorsement, personal and family responsibility, fear of disfigurement or disability, and exaggeration of personal risk to promote their use.[16] This almost twenty-year-long campaign represents the expenditure of millions of dollars, but despite this enormous outlay, only about 10% of auto front-seat occupants wear safety belts.[13] This figure is apparently impervious to change via the methods used to promote voluntary compliance. Numerous controlled studies which have measured the effects of media campaigns have shown no increase in seat belt use, even when the messages were designed by the best advertising experts, were based on market research, and subsequently won advertising industry awards.[12,16,17,18] The four-to-eight-second buzzer/light warning standard has been proven ineffective as well in promoting seat belt use.[19]

Even more surprising, in light of the failure of persuasive techniques to change behavior, are the levels of knowledge and attitude of the public concerning seat belts. Surveys have shown that 90% of the public express positive attitudes toward seat belts and the great majority know that seat belt use decreases injuries from collision.[12,13,20] In fact, over 50% of non-users in one survey actually favor compulsory seat belt use.[12] The factor which contributes most significantly to non-use is simply habit.[12,13,20] No personality characteristic, demographic variable, or experience significantly distinguishes user from non-user except whether the habit of use was developed. Despite popular belief, only a small percent of the public actively opposes seat belt use; most non-users simply do not believe that the risk of traffic injury to themselves (on the order of one in 100,000 trips) is high enough to worry about, with good reason. We routinely tolerate much higher personal risks in our everyday activities.

The Communitarian Ethic

In the face of the incredibly high but preventable toll of traffic injuries and the lack of any evidence that our current strategy to promote seat belt use is capable of reducing this toll, ethical argument in favor of compulsory seat belt use seems almost superfluous. Yet it is precisely a deeply entrenched ethical value which preempts our concern for reducing premature death on a policy level. Adherence to the ethic of individual freedom and responsibility forces us to define this problem in individual terms. Because the individual can choose to use seat belts, he or she must be permitted to choose, and is responsible for the outcome of the choice.

Arguments can be made for collective, coercive intervention more consistent with the public health tradition on several grounds. The utilitarian might easily make the case that in fact the burden of the outcome of individual choice in this and other cases is not even borne mostly by the individual. Consequently, where coercive strategies are suggested, it is usually on the grounds of the high economic costs of traffic injuries to society in terms of use of the health care system, increased insurance costs, and loss of productive years of work.[5] This argument is rejected here because it pits the individual and groups of individuals against society in a way even more obvious than the ethic of individual freedom, and therefore contributes to the same problems outlined below.

The communitarian justification for collective, coercive interventions, in this case mandatory passive restraint systems, is based upon the idea of community as a social value in itself, as developed by Wolff and expanded upon by Price.[21,22] Wolff describes a set of values which depend for their achievement and enjoyment upon a reciprocal awareness. That is, these values depend upon the context of mutually conscious effort, and so can neither be acquired nor enjoyed privately. He defines community as the state of affairs which promotes these values. Wolff has identified three functions of community: affective values which involve mutual awareness of shared culture and traditions; productive community which describes the enjoyment of the collective nature of work; and rational community, which is the process of collective deliberation upon social goals and choices.[21]

Wolff is careful to distinguish his notion of community from that of the social pluralists who are most often identified with the communitarian tradition. The concept of community advanced by the social pluralists is the outcome of the "attempt to impose collectivist sociology on individualist liberal political philosophy."[21] Social pluralism sees society as an aggregate of particularistic groups of communities, rather than as itself a human community. Identification with these smaller groups allows the individual to survive the destructive insecurity and alienation which result from the liberal political philosophy as it seeks to free the individual from the constraints of premodern community. At the same time, identification with a group whose interests parallel one's own allows the advancement of one group's interests against the interests of other groups. Group behavior becomes an extension of self-seeking individual behavior in the liberal political arena. The result is communitarian ideals which seek to preserve status and privilege, to emphasize differences, and to protect the status quo socially and economically.[21]

Thus the national policy agenda is set and resolved by the competitive interplay of special-interest groups. The assumption is that any interest of significance will, by definition, be able to make its concerns heard, and to influence the outcome of the political process. Furthermore, the outcome of the competitive interplay among these "countervailing forces" is assumed to represent a consensual decision maximizing the interests of all.[23,24]

However, as Wolff points out, a significant category of goods is excluded from the public agenda by this interest-oriented competitive process. These are goods which are not in the specific interest of any one group, but are in the general interest of all as a community, and so have no advocate in the competition among specific interests.[19] For this reason, problems of the environment, of the economy, and of the cities resist solution; any viable solution encounters considerable opposition from one or more powerful interest groups.[25] This political process is also one reason for the lack of national commitment to the public's health.

The idea of community articulated by Wolff, in contrast, emphasizes commonality and inclusiveness, cooperation, solidarity, and community as an end in itself, rather than as an instrument for achieving individual ends. It is the community of Wolff, and not that of the social pluralists, that I wish to show is consistent with the goals of public health.

While Wolff's notion of community seems limited to face-to-face groups and experiences, Price argues for the application of the same communitarian ideals to the policy arena on behalf of society-as-community, in tension with the pluralist concept of community.[22] He points out that it is quite possible to identify with collectivities and their purposes as well as with one's immediate associates, and that the achievement of collective purposes in a society as large as ours requires this identification. Price also traces the historic expression of these communitarian values in the United States, a history which emphasizes that the liberal individual values have not always been paramount, as some would have us believe.

Though the community Wolff describes is voluntaristic in nature, Price argues that voluntarism is not an essential component of the communitarian ethic. The literature on the common good supports the contention that communitarian values might require government coercion. The common good, as carefully defined by Douglass, seems fully congruent with Wolff's description of community values.[26] The benefits of the common good according to Douglass are universal, not reducible to private advantage, and dependent upon reciprocity. Normally, he says, the common good and the individual good coincide, but in a conflict, the common good takes precedence.

B. Barry develops further the role of the government in securing these values.[27] He makes the point explicitly that such values will not be advanced except by the state. While he says that these values are not necessarily superior to individual interests, they deserve an equal consideration. The community as a whole can act only through the state to obtain goods whose value can be enjoyed only in the context of the community.

Arneson has also noted that coercion by government is not incompatible with community, and in fact may facilitate its expression.[28] Coercion may be required to insure that all contribute a fair share to the provision of the common good, and that none succumb to the temptation to be the "free rider." Thus coercion may actually enhance community values by lifting the weight of suspicion that others might choose not to participate under a voluntary system.

It is important to recognize that social or distributive justice is a *sine qua non* of the communitarian ethic. The achievement of community is absolutely predicated upon a fair distribution of the benefits and burdens of society.[29] However, social justice does not guarantee the same set of goods that are protected by communitarian values. Social justice refers to goods which are still individualistic in nature, and which contribute to the private enjoyment of the individual. Communitarian values go beyond to protect the goods which people seek and enjoy in community with others. To the extent that health is denied to groups of people based on class or other characteristics of the group, it can be considered a distributive value. But health, as shall be argued in the next

Communitarian Values and Reduction in Premature Death

The goal of preventing premature death is best justified and accomplished by appealing to communitarian values. A communitarian ethic is a precondition to both solving the problem of premature death and to appreciating the outcome. As has been documented above, collective means—deliberate action on behalf of the entire community—are required to reduce the toll of preventable deaths from causes like highway injury. This enormous problem cannot be solved without collective measures because individual interest is not a sufficient motivation for behavior change in cases such as this where the risk to the individual is so low. In addition, the goal of reducing preventable deaths can be understood, and the outcome enjoyed, only in a communitarian context. It is only because we recognize such values as interdependence and mutual responsibility that a collective goal such as reducing highway injury makes sense and becomes important. As will be argued below, it is only in this context, too, that we can recognize the cost of an ethic of individual freedom.

The conflict between communitarian values and the prevailing prevention strategies, which focus ineffectively on voluntary behavior change rather than collective, coercive means, can be intuitively understood by use of an analogy made by Beauchamp.[30] He compares our tolerance of the high cost of early death to a story by Shirley Jackson called "The Lottery." She writes of a town where once a year everyone traditionally draws lots. The single loser is then stoned to death by the winners—the rest of the townspeople. The benefits believed to be gained by satisfying the tradition cause each person to participate, knowing that chances are very low that he or she will be the loser. However, the chances are close to 100% that a relative, neighbor, or other community member will be killed.

This analogy illustrates the horrifying result when individual choice is pitted against the social value of minimizing early death. An individual can choose not to use seat belts and argue against their imposition with a high degree of confidence that he or she will not be a loser, since the chances of death from highway injury are roughly one in 100,000 trips. However, it is an absolute surety that 53,000 people will die from traffic injuries per year, a large majority of them as a direct cost of the individual freedom to choose whether to use restraints.

The fact of the loss of this many members of the community exacts an enormous cost, not only in economic terms, but in terms of the complex fabric of interdependencies and reciprocal relationships. Each of these deaths represents a small tear in the fabric, affecting all of us to the extent that we are connected to each other, even distantly and as strangers.

An even greater cost than the actual fact of the deaths is the violence done to communitarian values by the existence of the "lottery" that pits our individual interests against certain death for some members of our community. As individuals we are forced to be indifferent to the preventable death of members of our community, because we have no way to express our concern for others individually. In the instance of auto safety restraints we cannot express our sense of obligation to others by our individual choice. Our decision to buckle up, despite our confusion on the issue, is never an effective expression of our responsibility for each other. This forced indifference for the well-being of the community diminishes the communitarian values of solidarity, altruism, and cooperation. We can develop and express these values only through a collective decision which connects limitations on our freedom to drive without restraints with our unknown neighbor's well-being.

Connecting limitations on our personal freedom to a communitarian ethic provides an alternative view of coercive public health measures. These measures have often been defined and resisted by the public as paternalistic intrusions by those who claim to act in the individual's best interests. However, when placed in the context of a communitarian ethic and seen as a collective response to a problem of the community, coercive measures provide opportunities for expression of our concern for the well-being of the whole community.

Indeed the case of highway injury illustrates Titmuss' point that the ways in which society organizes and structures social institutions can encourage or discourage the innate concern for the good of the whole in people.[31] Furthermore, it is truly, as Titmuss says, the responsibility of the state to eliminate the situations, such as the prevailing response to highway injury and other premature death, where people are unable to express these intuitive moral values.

Auto restraints and other cases of coercive public health interventions fit another characteristic of Titmuss' conception of the social gift, because the beneficiaries are most likely to be strangers, and not even specific strangers. For the lives saved are statistical lives—the ultimate "universal stranger" of Titmuss.[31] This characteristic also highlights the nature of the freedom from premature death as a common good. Though people may ordinarily conceive of protection from traffic injury as a private value, if weighed in a private calculation the need for protection is not apparent since the individual risk is so low. However, protection is in reality a need which can be seen only in collective terms, and a good measured and enjoyed only in the collective context. We cannot know if we have benefited individually from passive restraints, but we *can* appreciate the communal benefit of reduction in the number of highway injuries.

The communitarian critique of interventions to change individual behavior such as seat belt use does not rest upon the ineffectiveness of that intervention. Even if collective and individual strategies were equally effective, individual strategies would offend communitarian values because focus on the individual produces and reinforces isolation and alienation by assigning fault. While assignment of fault often contributes to the ineffectiveness of individual strategies by focusing on inappropriate or meaningless variables of a health problem, it also decreases our perception of personal susceptibility by defining artificial differences between ourselves and those who experience health problems like auto injuries. Ryan, in *Blaming the Victim*, points out that we see these problems as isolated and unexpected events, resulting from the defective behavior of rare individuals.[32] Thus assigning fault removes our moral responsibility to alter arrangements from which the majority derive benefit in order to solve social problems, because the problem has been taken out of the social context and placed in the individual who is suffering from the problem. Therefore we are told that traffic injuries are caused by faulty behavior, that they are preventable by individual use of seat belts, and so we have no collective responsibility for those who choose not to use them.

Collective measures like passive restraints to reduce premature death are characteristic of a renewal and re-application of the traditional mandate of public health which has been used in the past mostly to control infectious disease. Beauchamp has clearly articulated how the "new public health" is compatible and consistent with the communitarian ethic.[29,33] The focus of this postmodern public health is on controlling hazards rather than changing behavior, on prevention through control of market activities and other social structures which expose people to hazards, and on collective responsibility as opposed to self-interest. This focus is simply an extension of the ideas of Virchow, Pettenkofer, Biggs, and other founders of the public health movement. These people recognized that public health is a matter of community concern, that public health problems are linked to social and economic situations, and that structural mechanisms are required to control these problems.[34,35]

Beauchamp has also pointed out that the social norms which currently influence individual risk-taking behavior (such as alcohol use and driving behavior) are in effect protective of the community rather than of the individual. These norms prescribe limits to behavior which are often more stringent than maximum safe levels for individuals, and so reflect a concern for the effects of the behavior on the community. Beauchamp argues that our legal norms ought to at least reflect the social norms influencing risk-taking behavior.[36]

Limits on the Communitarian Ethic

Though prevention of premature death is an important social value it is not the only one. Critics of the collective perspective cite the danger that this ethic could be extended indefinitely to restrictions on personal freedom.[37,38] Some limits are required, and Beauchamp has discussed the general rules for their development.[39] The broad terms of these limits should be to respect the rights of privacy, autonomy, and individual freedom within reasonable limits; to weigh the goals of public health against other claims for social investment like education and elimination of poverty; to choose the least socially disruptive course which brings results; and to concentrate efforts on problems which are most severe.

The case for passive restraints is admittedly more obvious than for other collective strategies like control of alcohol and tobacco, which would bring considerable reduction in premature death, because the value attached to the use of these substances in our society is currently higher. Clearly the communitarian ethic cannot be applied against these hazards without regard for this value. Each problem requires careful analysis to determine what values are at stake, how intensely they are regarded, and what ethical justification could be applied to various strategies to control them.

Conclusion

If the persistent and pressing social problems like premature death, of which traffic injury is a very large factor, are to be solved, we must recognize that our current strategies are ineffective. Even more, these strategies of individual behavior change diminish communitarian values held intuitively by a large number of people, and deny us the opportunity to act upon these values in order to express our concern for others. Appeals to self-interest and to social cost for prevention of health problems leading to premature death should be replaced by strategies which reinforce communitarian values and encourage people to recognize their mutual dependencies and shared concern for the well-being of the community.

Acknowledgments

I want to thank Patricia Barry, Dan Beauchamp, JoAnne Earp, Nancy Lamson, David Price, Carol Runyan, and Allan Steckler for participating in discussions which stimulated the development of these ideas and/or commenting on drafts of this paper.

References

1. Vaupel, J. "Early Death: An American Tragedy," *Law Contemp. Probs.* 40 (1976): 73–121.

2. Office of the Surgeon General. *Healthy People.* Washington: DHEW, 1979.

3. Lalonde, M. *A New Perspective on the Health of Canadians.* Ottawa: Government of Canada, 1974.

4. Knowles, J. "The Responsibility of the Individual," in Knowles, J., ed., *Doing Better and Feeling Worse.* New York: W. W. Norton, 1977, pp. 57–80.

5. National Center for Health Education. *NCHE News,* Summer 1980.

6. Baker, S. "Childhood Injuries: The Community Approach to Prevention," *J. Pub. Health Policy* 2 (1981): 235–46.

7. Haddon, W. "Advances in the Epidemiology of Injuries as a Basis for Public Policy," *Pub. Health Rep.* 95 (1980): 411–21.

8. McGavran, E. "The Community as the Patient of Public Health," *Texas State J. Med.* 54 (1958): 719–23.

9. Barry, P. "Individual vs. Community Orientation in the Prevention of Injuries," *Prev. Med.* 4(1975): 47–56.

10. Waller, P. *Risk Avoidance Behavior and Traffic Safety.* University of North Carolina, Chapel Hill: Highway Safety Research Center, 1979.

11. Waller, P., et al. *Safety Belts: Uncollected Dividends.* Washington: National Highway Traffic Safety Administration, 1977.

12. Fhaner, G., and M. Have. "Seat Belts: Factors Influencing Their Use," *Accid. Anal. and Prev.* 5 (1973): 27–43.

13. Cropley, A., C. Knapper, and R. Moore. "A Clinical/Quantitative Analysis of Public Opinions of Seat Belts," *Int. Rev. App. Psych.* 26 (1976): 43–49.

14. Campbell, B., B. O'Neill, and B. Tingley. *Comparative Injuries to Belted and Unbelted Drivers of Sub-compact, Compact, Intermediate, and Standard Cars.* University of North Carolina, Chapel Hill: Highway Safety Research Center, 1974.

15. Grimm, A. "Use of Restraint Systems: A Review of the Literature," *HSRI Research Review* 11 (1980): 11.

16. Robertson, L., et al. "A Controlled Study of the Effect of TV Messages on Safety Belt Use," *Am. J. Pub. Health* 64 (1974): 1071–80.

17. University of Southern California. *An Experiment in the Use of Broadcast Media in Highway Safety.* Springfield: NTIS, 1971.

18. Phillips, B. *Evaluation of Safety Belt Education Program for Employees.* Washington: National Highway Traffic Safety Administration, 1976.

19. *Effectiveness of Various Safety Belt Warning Systems.* Washington: National Highway Traffic Safety Administration, 1976.

20. Knapper, C., A. Cropley, and R. Moore. "Attitudinal Factors in the Nonuse of Seat Belts," *Accid. Anal. and Prev.* 8 (1976): 241–51.

21. Wolff, R. *The Poverty of Liberalism.* Boston: Beacon Press, 1968, pp. 122–95.

22. Price, D. *Quest for Community.* Bloomington: Indiana University Foundation, 1977.

23. Berger, P., and R. Neuhaus. *To Empower People: The Role of Mediating Structures in Public Policy.* Washington: American Enterprise Institute for Public Policy Research, 1977.

24. Braybrooke, D., and C. Lindblom. *A Strategy of Decision.* New York: Free Press of Glencoe, 1963.

25. Thurow, L. *The Zero-Sum Society.* New York: Penguin Books, 1980.

26. Douglass, B. "The Common Good and the Public Interest," *Pol. Theory* 8 (1980): 103–17.

27. Barry, B. *Political Argument.* New York: Humanities Press, 1965, pp. 207–36.

28. Arneson, R. "Prospects for Community in a Market Economy," *Pol. Theory* 9 (1981): 207–27.

29. Beauchamp, D. "Public Health as Social Justice," *Inquiry* 13 (1977): 3–14.

30. Beauchamp, D. "Bloodsports," *Christian Century* 94 (1977): 237–38.

31. Titmuss, R. *The Gift Relationship.* New York: Pantheon Books, 1971, pp. 209–46.

32. Ryan, W. *Blaming the Victim.* New York: Pantheon Books, 1971.

33. Beauchamp, D. "Public Health and Individual Liberty," *Ann. Rev. Pub. Health* 1 (1980): 121–36.

34. Rosen, G. *From Medical Police to Social Medicine: Essays on the History of Health Care.* New York: Science History Publications, 1974.

35. Winslow, C. "The Contribution of Hermann Biggs to Public Health," *Am. Rev. Tuber.* 20 (1928): 1–15.

36. Beauchamp, D. Private communication.

37. Veatch, R. "Voluntary Risk to Health: the Ethical Issues," *J. Amer. Med. Assoc.* 243 (1980): 50–55.

38. Kass, L. "Regarding the End of Medicine and the Pursuit of Health," *The Public Interest* 40 (1975): 11–42.

39. Beauchamp, D. *Beyond Alcoholism.* Philadelphia: Temple University Press, 1980, pp. 152–82.

Chapter 27

Courts, Gender, and "The Right to Die"

Steven H. Miles, M.D., and Allison August

Reprinted, with permission, from *Law, Medicine, and Health Care* 18(1–2):85–95, Spring/Summer 1990.

Steven H. Miles, M.D., and Allison August are on the staff of the Extended Care Department at Hennepin County Medical Center, Minneapolis.

Public policy with regard to decisions to forgo life-sustaining medical care has dramatically changed over 15 years. Courts, legislatures, and professional bodies recognize a patient's right to refuse treatment despite civic or medical values that favor prolonging life. The United States Supreme Court has taken up this issue on an appeal of Missouri's Supreme Court decision ordering tube feeding for comatose Nancy Cruzan over her family's objections. The right to refuse life-sustaining treatment exemplifies a changing accommodation between controversial personal choices and the values our society holds collectively. As with other civil rights issues to come before the Court, the courts embody the very cultural canon they critique and redefine.

While the relevance of the American tenet of individualism to the "right to die" (properly, the "right to refuse life-sustaining treatment") is well recognized, the role of our culture's view of gender in these decisions is not appreciated.[1] A "right-to-die" case arises when a family member or, less often, a health care provider, asks a court to consider the legality of forgoing life-sustaining treatment. The final state appellate court rulings ordered continuation of life-prolonging care in two of 14 cases about profoundly ill, previously competent women who had not authored living wills. No such order was made in eight

similar cases involving men.[2] This difference is the result of an even more asymmetric gender-patterned reasoning within the cases.

This paper examines the different words and concepts that courts use in writing about men and women to imprint cultural views of gender onto final opinions. Judicial reasoning about profoundly ill, incompetent men accepts evidence of men's treatment preferences to define the standing of personal autonomy in decisions about life-sustaining treatment. Judicial reasoning about women defines the role of caregivers in making treatment decisions after either rejecting or failing to consider evidence of women's preferences with regard to life-sustaining treatment. This gender-patterned reasoning belies a premise of a universal, purportedly gender-neutral, right to refuse treatment. As the Massachusetts Supreme Court put it, "principles of equality and respect for individuals require the conclusion that a choice exists . . . [w]e recognize a general right in all persons to refuse medical treatment . . . [which] must extend to the case of an incompetent, as well as a competent patient, because the value of human dignity extends to both" (Saikewicz, MA, 1977). Though this premise endows men and women with an equal range of treatment options, exactly which treatment decision respects this "right" is problematic for particular comatose, demented, or retarded persons who cannot speak on their own behalf. It is both in the judicial conclusion that a patient's preference can be "constructed" from evidence of his or her values and in the empowerment of a third party when it cannot, that gender patterned reasoning arises.

We examine the gender pattern in all appellate-level, civil, state "right-to-die" cases involving incompetent, adult patients.[3] Our analysis is more akin to social criticism or semantic analysis than to conventional law review.[4] We examine judicial reasoning for three types of right to die cases, those involving: (1) previously competent persons who have not left written directives (e.g. living wills) for their care, (2) previously competent persons who have left written directives, and (3) persons who have never been competent. We close with a brief discussion of why gender-patterned reasoning might occur, its implications for other areas of judicial involvement in controversial personal choices, and of the possibility of reform to address this phenomenon.

Newly Incompetent Persons without Written Advance Directives

Most incompetent persons who are dependent on life-support were once competent but did not leave written directives (like living wills) for their care. The 22 decisions from 14 states addressing such situations are the bulk of state appellate level right-to-die decisions. Eight, from six states, concern men; 14, from 11 states, concern women. (See Table 1.)

Constructing a Treatment Preference: A Manly Way

In six of the eight cases involving men without advance directives, appellate courts constructed the patient's own preference for medical care from the memories and insights of family and friends. This "constructed preference" decisively supported the termination of life-sustaining treatment.

The case of Brother Fox (NY, 1981) was the first ruling about a previously competent man. New York's highest court allowed a respirator to be removed from an 83 year old Catholic brother at the request of the director of his Society, Father Eichner. In a ruling steeped in a "hyper-masculine" and uniquely entitled language of "Brother" and "Father," the court found "clear and convincing" evidence that "Brother Fox made the decision for himself." This conclusion was based on a formal Catholic discussion, three years before Mr. Fox became comatose, of the decision to remove a respirator from Ms. Quinlan (NJ, 1976). Mr. Fox agreed that the comatose Ms. Quinlan's respirator was extraordinary and

Table 1. Previously Competent Patients Without Living Wills

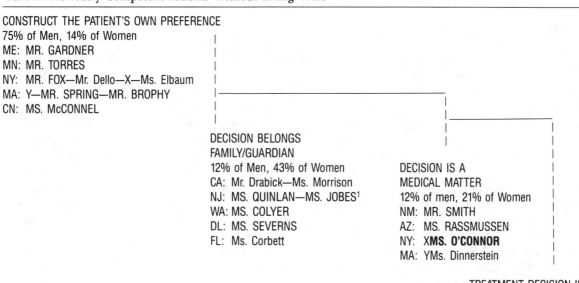

CONSTRUCT THE PATIENT'S OWN PREFERENCE
75% of Men, 14% of Women
ME: MR. GARDNER
MN: MR. TORRES
NY: MR. FOX—Mr. Dello—X—Ms. Elbaum
MA: Y—MR. SPRING—MR. BROPHY
CN: MS. McCONNEL

DECISION BELONGS
FAMILY/GUARDIAN
12% of Men, 43% of Women
CA: Mr. Drabick—Ms. Morrison
NJ: MS. QUINLAN—MS. JOBES[1]
WA: MS. COLYER
DL: MS. SEVERNS
FL: Ms. Corbett

DECISION IS A
MEDICAL MATTER
12% of men, 21% of Women
NM: MR. SMITH
AZ: MS. RASSMUSSEN
NY: X**MS. O'CONNOR**
MA: Y**Ms. Dinnerstein**

TREATMENT DECISION IS
MADE BY AN INSTITUTION
0% of Men, 21% of Women
MO: **MS. CRUZAN**
IL: **MS. LONGEWAY**
NJ: MS. CONROY

UPPER CASE: States Highest Court (Lower Case are State Appellate (but not highest) Court decisions

"—" shows sequential order of cases within a single state court system, superscripted letters show shifted rationales within the sequence. Cases not linked by hyphens are the only appellate level case for this class of persons in the state.

BOLD designates a decision ordering continued use of life support.

said that "he would not want any of this extraordinary business" done for him under similar circumstances. He repeated this view a few months before becoming comatose. [N.B. These offset abstracts are written by the author to illustrate points made in text.]

In 1987, A New York appellate court discovered "clear and convincing" evidence of the preference of a 33 year old exercise physiologist who became comatose after minor surgery. Mr. Delio was found to have made many statements about not wanting to receive life-support in the event of a coma to his wife, friends, and family in discussions about his father's recent illness and about cases in the media. He also made his wife promise not to keep him alive in such a situation.

The Maine Supreme Court (Gardner, 1987) found "clear and convincing" evidence of the preference to stop tube feeding of a 23 year old man who was comatose after falling from a pick-up truck. Two years before the accident, he told his girlfriend that "he would want to die" rather than be kept like the residents of the nursing home where the girlfriend worked. He made similar remarks to his mother, brother, and a friend before the accident. The court said that it did "not find it necessary to go beyond Gardner's own personal decision;" the "pre-accident decision by Gardner himself fully supports the relief granted. . . . Gardner is simply exercising his right to control the course of medical care."

The Minnesota Supreme Court (1984) ruled that a trial court properly constructed a man's preference for removal of a respirator. Mr. Torres was a 57 year old unmarried man who was comatose as a result of an accident with a hospital's restraining device. No one recalled remarks about life support although a close cousin testified that "he believed that [Mr. Torres] would want to have the respirator removed," a sentiment echoed by another male friend who cited Mr. Torres' unwillingness to wear a pacemaker.

In Spring (1980), the Massachusetts Supreme Court relied on the testimony of family to reach the "critical" conclusion that the demented man would choose to refuse dialysis. Mr. Spring had said nothing of his views of treatment.

In its Brophy decision (1986), the same court addressed a wife's suit to stop tube feedings for a comatose middle-aged paramedic-fireman. The Court concluded that "Brophy's judgment would be to decline the provision of food and water and to terminate his life." This conclusion was based on the wife's recollection that Mr. Brophy had said of Karen Quinlan ten years earlier, "I don't ever want to be on a life support system. No way do I want

to live like that; that is not living." He had made a similar comment about a man he had rescued who died after several months of therapy and about another event in the community. The court also noted a half-serious jest about a medical order of bed rest that Mr. Brophy made shortly before losing consciousness: "If I can't sit up to kiss one of my beautiful daughters, I may as well be six feet under."

In the two other cases involving men, a doctor and a brother were made responsible for deciding what should be done. The New Mexico Supreme court ruled that a guardian could not, without a living will, speak for comatose Mr. Smith's "right to die" (Smith, 1983). It said that these were "doctor[']s . . . medical decisions . . . as appropriate under current medical practice." A California court insisted that courts should not use constructed preference because a comatose man's "noncognitive state prevents him from choosing anything" and therefore the idea that his "right to choose" survives incompetence is "a legal fiction at best" (Drabick, 1988). Information about Mr. Drabick's values that was brought to court by his live-in partner and brothers was to be used to inform "the physician and family members or other persons who are making decisions for the patient" so that they can make a good faith decision about how to serve the patient's interests.

In striking contrast to the routine use of constructed treatment preferences for men, only two of the 14 appellate level cases addressing previously competent women without living wills take this approach. (See Table 1.)

In Elbaum (NY, 1989), an appellate court found "clear and convincing" evidence of a woman's desire not to be maintained on life-support. Ms. Elbaum had made her husband, sister, and son promise that they would try to remove life-support in such circumstances. She reportedly told her husband, "Murray, . . . I am telling you and I want you to tell me that you will not do anything to sustain my life in the event I am a vegetable." Similarly, in McConnell (CN, 1989), the court, relied on the testimony of a husband, two daughters and a son to conclude that a comatose 57 year old woman would not want tube feedings.[5]

We now examine why courts decline to construct the preferences of a large majority of previously competent women who do not leave written advance directives for their care.

Women: Values without Weight
Appellate court rulings show four major differences in how courts speak of previously competent women's or

men's moral preferences. The first difference is the courts' view that a man's opinions are rational and a woman's remarks are unreflective, emotional, or immature. Second, women's moral agency in relation to medical decisions is often not recognized. Third, courts apply evidentiary standards differently to evidence about men's and women's preferences. Fourth, life-support dependent men are seen as subjected to medical assault; women are seen as vulnerable to medical neglect. Not all of these differences are present in any one case. Each difference (e.g. language describing a woman's reasoning as immature) is present in at least three cases of the gender to which it is attributed and none of the cases of the opposite gender.

First, the judicial acceptance of constructed treatment preferences for incompetent men is associated with a ruling that a man's remarks reflects a mature, rational choice. Mr. Brophy reached a "judgment;" 23 year old Mr. Gardner was "very serious" when he told his friend he "would definitely want to die if he was ever in a vegetable state." The 33 year old Daniel Delio (whose Ph.D in exercise physiology, the court calls a "doctor of philosophy") expressed a "deeply held," "solemn, intelligent determination." Decisions affirming a man's choice allude to philosophical moralism. Much was made of Brother Fox's formal discussions of Catholic moral principles. Though it was not asserted that Mr. Brophy or Mr. Gardner had heard of it, John Stuart Mill's essay, *On Liberty,* was cited in affirming the construction of their decisions. Such extra-legal philosophical gloss is not present in the cases involving women.

Women's remarks, by contrast, are viewed as unreflective or emotional. Cases which reject a construction of a woman's treatment preference most clearly show this phenomenon.[6]

Ms. Quinlan (NJ, 1976), like Mr. Gardner, was a young adult who became comatose after an accident. Her father, with her mother's support, asked for legal permission to remove a respirator. Her statements to friends and family about not wanting to be kept alive on machines were rejected as a "remote and impersonal" emotional "distaste" or "wish," not as a rational conclusion. Later, in Conroy (NJ, 1985), the same court apologized for failing to accept evidence about Ms. Quinlan's views.

The seriousness of this apology, given this same court's rejection of a constructed preference for the comatose Ms. Jobes (NJ, 1987), is open to question. A close woman friend (who was a nurse) recalled that the 30 year old Ms. Jobes repeatedly said that if she [Jobes] were ever crippled like two profoundly ill persons that the friend was caring for, that she should not want to be kept alive. Ms. Jobes' husband and another friend cited similar conversations

about the case of Karen Quinlan. A cousin said that Ms. Jobes discussed, asked for, and acknowledged receiving a living will which was never found. The court ruled that these statements were "remote, general, spontaneous and . . . casual." Though impressed by their consistency, the court said that they were not "so clear, direct, and weighty and convincing as to enable the factfinder to come to a clear conviction, without hesitancy of the truth" of Ms. Jobes' treatment preference.

The Missouri Supreme Court (1988) characterized Ms. Cruzan's remarks about not wanting to be maintained if she could not be in a "halfway normal" condition as "informally expressed reactions," adding that it is "definitionally impossible" for such remarks to be equated with an informed refusal. New York's O'Connor decision (1988) fully illustrates the condescending view of women's "emotionalism."[7]

Ms. O'Connor was an elderly retired hospital administrator who was profoundly disabled after a series of strokes. The court was informed of many conversations with her daughters and coworkers occasioned by her hospital work, the illnesses of loved ones, and her own illnesses, in which the patient said that life support should not be used to prevent nature from taking its course if things could not get better. The court concluded that "although her expressions were repeated over a number of years, there is nothing other than speculation . . . that her expressions were more than immediate reaction to the unsettling experience of seeing or hearing of another unnecessarily prolonged death. Her comments that she would never want to lose her dignity before she passed away, that nature should be permitted to take its course, that it is 'monstrous' to use life-support machinery — are in fact no different than many of us might make after witnessing an agonizing death."

By contrast, men's emotions convey passionate conviction rather than a disordered mind. Thus, Mr. Delio (same age as Ms. Jobes) was described as "extremely distraught" over life-support for his dying father and Mr. Brophy was depicted throwing away a medal because the rescued person died on life-support, without these instances being taken as demonstrating immature reasoning. Two women may have acquired "rational" status by working in health care settings.[8] Courts accepted constructed preferences to stop life-support for Ms. McConnell (CN, 1989) and Ms. Peter [who also had an advance directive] (NJ, 1987).

A jargon of childlikeness is used to discount the maturity of persons when a preference is not constructed.

Only women are described as being in "fetal" postures (Quinlan, NJ, 1976; Conroy, NJ, 1985; Rasmussen, AZ, 1986) or an "infantile state" (Colyer, WA, 1983).[9] The court obliquely characterizes the serious conversations of the 31 year old Ms. Jobes as "off hand remark[s] . . . made by a person when young." Five previously competent persons are referred to by their first names (Ms. Quinlan, Ms. Colyer, Mr. Delio [NY, 1987], Mr. Drabick [CA, 1988], Ms. Cruzan [MO, 1988]). Only Mr. Delio has a treatment preference constructed. The legal familial relationship of "parens patriae" is only asserted in relation to women (Quinlan, Conroy, [below]; Cruzan, [see below]; Longeway, [IL, 1989]). The Massachusetts Supreme court rejected this legal-parentalism in the case of Mr. Brophy, as it sought to move "away from a *paternalistic* [emphasis added] view of what is 'best' for a patient toward a reaffirmation [of] . . . what decision will comport with the will of the patient" (MA, 1986).

Second, some courts simply do not recognize women's views. Ms. Dinnerstein's (MA, 1978) values are not even mentioned as the decision to forgo resuscitation is assigned to the doctor and consenting family. The court noted that Ms. Corbett (FL, 1986) had not written a living will without making any other comment on her own values.[10] In Conroy (1985), the nephew of a profoundly demented elderly woman proposed that her lifelong avoidance of doctors and medical care was evidence that she would not want to be sustained by a feeding tube in a nursing home. The New Jersey Supreme Court said that a patient's refusal of treatment might be deduced from a "consistent pattern of conduct with respect to prior decisions about his (sic) own medical care" but declined to illustrate this test with Ms. Conroy's life.[11]

Third, there are differences in the way probative standards are used vis a vis information about men's and women's values. Courts constructed Ms. Elbaum's (NY, 1989) and Ms. McConnell's (CN, 1988) treatment preferences because of very specific remarks they made about medical treatment. The six decisions accepting the proposed preferences of men incorporated evidence ranging from specific discussions (Fox, NY, 1981), to general discussions remote from the time and possibility of illness (Brophy, MA, 1986; Gardner, ME, 1987),[12] to constructions simply based on the man's character (Spring, MA, 1980; Torres, MN, 1986). With women, the "clear and convincing" standard is used to weigh evidence which is then often rejected as emotional, immature, remote, or nonspecific. Against the objection that evidence of Mr. Torres' views fell "far short of the evidentiary standards that ought to be met for a life and death issue," the Court said that a trial court had wide latitude according to its "sound discretion." No such latitude is afforded previously competent women.

Finally, men are depicted as subject to a medical assault; women are depicted as vulnerable to medical neglect. Mr. Delio "suffers the continued indignities and dehumanization created by his . . . helplessness." Mr. Torres "may well have wished to avoid the . . . ultimate horror . . . of being maintained in a limbo" (MN, 1986). Mr. Brophy is "in a condition which he would consider to be degrading" and is tube fed "baby food" (MA, 1986). Mr. Gardner's "utter helplessness" means that he suffers "the submission of the most private bodily functions to the attention of others," which the court suggests might be a "battery" (ME, 1987).[13]

By contrast, a woman's vulnerability summons aid. In New Jersey, the vulnerability of Ms. Quinlan (1976), Ms. Conroy (1985), and Ms. Jobes (1987) is the premise of an elaborate regulatory apparatus, because "an incompetent, like a minor child, is a ward of the state and the state's *parens patriae* power supports the authority of its courts" (Conroy). In Longeway (IL, 1989), the possibility that "greed may taint the [family's] judgment . . . to the point of fatal attraction" rationalizes the need for court approval of every decision to forgo nourishment. Ms. O'Connor (NY, 1988) and Ms. Cruzan (MO, 1988) are grouped with other patients who need "shelter" or would be at "grave risk" if courts accepted casual statements about not wanting life support.[14]

Who Makes Decisions for Women?

We now examine who is empowered to make treatment decisions on a woman's behalf when her preference is not constructed. Courts take several paths (see Table 1). Decision-making for six of 14 women (compared to one of eight men) is remanded to the family.[15] In three cases, the treatment choice is seen as a medical conclusion. In three other cases, courts reserved to themselves or a government agency the final decision as to proper medical care.

Three families were told to decide as they believe the woman would have done. After rejecting a construction of Ms. Quinlan's preference, the New Jersey Supreme court praised her father's moral character, and concluded that he should "render his best judgement . . . as to whether she would exercise" her right to refuse treatment. Likewise, the same court praised the "warm, close, and loving family" of the comatose Ms. Jobes as "best qualified to determine the medical decisions she would make" (NJ, 1987). Similarly, the Supreme Court of Washington said that "the unanimity of opinions expressed by Bertha's closest kin together with absence of any ill motives, . . . satisfied [the court] that Bertha's guardian [husband] was exercising his best judgment as to Bertha's personal choice when he requested removal of the life support system" (Colyer, 1983).

Appellate courts empowered three women's families to use their own judgment (rather than imagining the patient's preference) as to life-support.[16] In a narrow ruling, not mentioning how to discern Ms. Severns' own preference, the court simply said that her husband/

guardian, could "vicariously" assert Mrs. Severns constitutional right (DL, 1980). Ms. Severns, comatose after a car accident, had been a member of the Euthanasia Council of Delaware, and had said "that she did not want to be kept alive as a vegetable or by extraordinary means." Mr. Corbett was similarly empowered to act on behalf of his 75 year old comatose wife to remove a nasogastric tube by which she was being kept alive (FL, 1986). In Morrison, a daughter-conservator sued to remove a feeding tube from a comatose 90 year old woman. While a trial court felt that the patient "would probably concur" in the decision, the appellate court, relying on Drabick (CA, 1988), said that the daughter had made a decision in "good faith" because of the poor prognosis.

Courts ruled that treatment decisions for three women were primarily medical judgments.[17] Ms. Rasmussen's family would not speak on her behalf so the Arizona Supreme Court affirmed the judgment of a physician who in light of her "condition and prognosis" had ordered that resuscitation and hospitalization be withheld (AZ, 1986). In Dinnerstein (MA, 1978), the family (a physician-son and daughter) agreed with the physician to withhold resuscitation from a woman with advanced dementia and vascular disease (see above). The court found this decision to be "peculiarly within the competence of the medical profession as to what measures are appropriate to ease the imminent passing of an irreversibly terminally ill patient in light of the patient's history and condition and the wishes of her family."[18] The O'Connor decision is one of three ordering life support over the family's objections (see discussion of Storar and Cruzan).

In O'Connor, a hospital sued to place a feeding tube in a demented, bed bound, non-communicative woman after the patient's daughters refused to consent, saying that the patient would not want it. The daughters had closely cared for their mother throughout the course of her illness. The court rejected Ms. O'Connor's own statements as emotional. Then, it presented her as vulnerable. Then, in a manner reminiscent of how courts reject constructed treatment preferences for women patients, it rejected the "highest and most loving" motives [n.b. not reasoning] of the daughters, referring to these middle aged nurses exclusively by their first names, "Helen" and "Joan" (a form of appellation used to no other family of incompetent persons.) Then, it deferred to the physician's judgment in favor of treatment.

Finally, three state Supreme Courts, each considering women with close family who requested discontinuation of life-sustaining treatment, ruled that final decisions to forgo treatment should be made by the court or another official body (Conroy, NJ, 1985; Longeway, IL, 1989; Cruzan, MO, 1988).

The Missouri Supreme Court ordered tube feedings for a young woman rendered comatose by a car accident over the objections of family who, with the tacit support of the physicians, had gone to court to ascertain the legality of stopping tube feedings (Cruzan, 1988). Emphasizing Ms. Cruzan's vulnerability, the court rejected the constructed preference and the views of the "loving" parents with which Ms. Cruzan was "blessed." In expropriating the role of family, the court said that the "power to exercise third party choice arises from the state's authority, not the rights of the ward. The guardian is a delegatee of the state's *parens patriae* power."

Similarly the vulnerability of Ms. Longeway to ill-intentioned family members or the vulnerability of Ms. Conroy to abuses in the nursing home industry justified court or state ombudsman review of similar decisions.

To summarize, judicial reasoning about profoundly ill, incompetent men defines the standing of personal autonomy; judicial reasoning about women delineates the role of caregivers in these treatment decisions. A patient's treatment preference is constructed within the court ruling for 75 percent (6 of 8) of men and 14 percent (2 of 14) of women. This pattern is not the result of a few states. Of the 11 states with one or more cases of a *single* gender, nine show the gender pattern; only Connecticut (McConnell, 1989) and New Mexico (Smith, 1983) diverge. Three states (CA, MA, NY) address patients of both sexes. In California, the precedent making a brother responsible for medical decisions for Mr. Drabick (1988) was followed in empowering a proxy for Ms. Morrison (1988). In Massachusetts, where the first "right to die" case constructed a preference for a congenitally retarded man (Saikewicz, 1977), Ms. Dinnerstein's court (1978) did not mention her values, and the next two cases constructed preferences for previously competent men (Spring, 1980; Brophy, 1986). In New York, two courts constructed treatment preferences for men (Fox, 1981; Delio, 1987) before one rejected and one accepted constructions for women (O'Connor, 1988; Elbaum, 1989).[19] The gender pattern is seen over the entire 14 year history of these decisions.[20] It is unchanged by age or by whether or not the patient was comatose, or is supported by tube feedings as opposed to other technologies. It is not the result of chance.[21] We cannot examine the influence of a patient's race or social class. The judge's sex is rarely identified, though a large majority are men.

There are several reasons why courts are less likely to construct treatment preferences for women than for men. First, information about women's preferences or values may be less often brought to these courts[22] and is less vigorously sought as a way to resolve the treatment issue. Second, even when evidence of preferences is available, it is tested more rigorously against a "clear and convincing" standard. Third, courts tend to view women as dependent on medical care whereas men are portrayed as assaulted by it. When a woman's own preference is not constructed by the court, responsibility for decision-making is assigned to familial, professional, or societal caregivers. The one case in which a treatment decision for a man was assigned to a medical professional led to new legislation empowering family to speak on patients' behalf (Smith, NM, 1983). It is only when the treatment decisions are expropriated to professional or governmental caregivers that the court rejects the petition to discontinue life-sustaining treatment. We now briefly consider the role of gender in cases where a previously competent patient left written "right to die" directives and in cases of persons who were never competent.

Patients with Written Treatment Preferences

Few patients leave living wills or durable powers of attorney to guide their health care in anticipation of being incompetent and on life-support. Three cases examining the intent of such instruments have been resolved at the appellate level. Without comment, the Illinois Supreme Court vacated an appellate court ruling accepting the witnessed, handwritten living will of a competent woman who had undergone multiple surgeries for an advanced brain cancer (Prange, 1988). Two other appellate courts accepted similar documents in constructing a patient's preferences. A higher burden of proof was placed on bearers of the woman's directive than on the man's family.[23]

> The Florida Supreme Court accepted a six year old Living Will written by a terminally ill, comatose, and respirator-dependent man as evidence of the family's "good faith" judgment in constructing his preference to forgo life support (Landy, 1984).
> The New Jersey Supreme Court applied a more stringent standard before accepting 65 year old Ms. Peter's legal designation of the man with whom she lived to make health care decisions on her behalf (1987). The court said that the advance directive for health care must of itself or in concert with other evidence, provide "clear and convincing" evidence of the patient's desire to refuse treatment. The Court concluded that the legal document, with the testimony of the proxy and nine friends, provided the necessary "clear and convincing" evidence that Ms. Peter would choose to discontinue the nasogastric tube that was sustaining her.

Decisons about Persons Who Were Never Competent

Adults who were never competent have not stated views upon which treatment preferences can be constructed. In such cases, a court can either create the fiction of a morally choosing person or delegate decision-making to an agent who speaks for the patient's interests. The five decisions from three states are too few to permit generalization but are reminiscent of the findings seen in previously competent persons.

The most fanciful construction of a profoundly retarded person's preference was for a man (Saikewicz, MA, 1977). A guardian asked to withhold painful chemotherapy and transfusions which would only briefly extend Mr. Saikewicz's life. Reading from within Mr. Saikewicz's mind, the Massachusetts Supreme Court found that unlike most persons who would choose treatment, Mr. Saikewicz "would experience fear without understanding from which other patients draw strength." Thus, chemotherapy could be withheld because of "a regard for his actual interests and preferences." This precedent was used by an appellate court in that state for a never-competent woman (Hier, 1984).

The Washington Supreme Court built from its 1983 precedent of a previously competent woman for whom it said that family should decide (Colyer). It empowered guardians for a man and a woman to use their best judgment for never competent persons without contriving a preference (Hamline, 1984; Grant, 1987).

New York's highest court (Storar, 1981) infantilized an adult retarded man dying of cancer to disempower a mother (who had previously been appointed legal guardian to consent to radiation therapy) who wished to stop treatment. This case presages the case of Ms. O'Connor (NY, 1988) in which the same court removed a patient from intimately involved woman-family caregivers to require life-sustaining treatment. In Storar, a mother wanted her 52 year old son to receive hospice care rather than blood transfusions which were painful to him. While "understand[ing] and respect[ing] . . . [her] despair," the court cited Storar's mental age of 18 months to resolve the case as a matter of a parent's legal obligation to provide medical care to children. A dissenting judge noted that the mother "over his [Mr. Storar's] lifetime had come to know and sense his want and need and . . . had provided more love and affection for John than any other person or institution." He questioned why the medical providers had standing at all.

Discussion

Gender profoundly affects judicial analysis of right-to-die cases. Judicial reasoning about men stresses the role of personal autonomy in these controversial decisions. Judicial reasoning about women examines the role of caregivers. How does the purportedly gender-neutral legal framework for these decisions admit gender-patterned reasoning? What reforms might be possible? What is the relevance of this gender pattern to the other issues?

American jurisprudence and medical ethics posit the autonomous individual as an ideal moral agent whose rights are properly respected at least for decisions about the individual's personal life. This "rights-centered" ethic holds that a personal moral identity is created by affirming general moral rules which in the event of that person's subsequent incompetence are used by others who try to reason as the patient would. "Rights-centered" moral reasoning has been contrasted to "communal" or care-centered moral reasoning.[24] In this view, moral identity is expressed by how one lives in a complex, interdependent web of relationships rather than by individuation. Because "communal" moral reasoning entails a complex dialogue with others whose views and interests are a dialectical part of one's own values, persons with a communal style of reasoning employ a circumstantial moral casuistry in preference to using generalized rules.[25] Proponents hold that communal reasoning more adequately addresses interpersonal ethics in matters such as raising children, being a citizen, caring for profoundly disabled loved ones, or being ill in a grieving family.[26]

Gilligan and Lyon exemplify scholars who have associated the "rights" perspective with men; the "communal" with women.[27] If gender association of "rights" and "communal" modes of moral reasoning is a pervasive phenomenon, this fact challenges the premise that a gender-free public evaluation of a controversial personal choice will occur in a society which has a "rights-centered" legal system. An empowered "rights-centered" perspective will view an incompetent person's history of "communal" moral reasoning as inarticulate or immature in its failure to assert generalizable moral imperatives.[28] In the face of a presumption favoring treatment and a poorly articulated view of the authority of intimate communities of caregivers, communal reasoning renders women vulnerable to having controversial decisions about their care expropriated to professional or civic decision-makers. This expropriation will be augmented to the degree that society, in addition to being "rights" centered, subordinates women to empowered male doctors or judges. A semantic analysis of trial texts would be needed to fully assess the degree to which women's moral identities are not salient to their families, are inadequately presented to the court, or are discounted after being introduced. We believe that all of these mechanisms are probably operative.

This background clarifies the need for and possibilities of jurisprudential reform of gender patterned reasoning. Gender is fundamental to views of sexual difference in our culture; judges cannot be free of gender-associations.[29] A jurisprudential reform of gender-patterned reasoning in right-to-die cases would enable either "rights centered" or "communal" moral reasoning to determine the way to address and interpret the moral duties with regard to the care of a life-support dependent incompetent person.

Men and women might benefit from such a reform. We have seen how a woman's moral identity is more likely to be discounted as treatment decisions are assigned to family or in some cases, expropriated to politicized ideals of caregiving once the anchor of personal or family-centered decision-making is lost.[30] Theoretically, men are vulnerable to having life-sustaining care terminated too readily because of the credence courts give to the most trivial expression of a right not to be assaulted by medical care. This abuse does not occur because, to date, right-to-die cases are initiated when men's families bear their preferences to courts, thus asserting the families' concurrence with the view that the treatment is not wanted or is not serving the patient's interests. Judicial reform would preserve the safeguard for vulnerable men while preventing the expropriation of decisions about women from intimate caregivers.

Such reform is possible. Courts could forgo the attempt to construct a person's treatment preferences in the court and simply empower intimate caregivers to make decisions on behalf of an incompetent loved one, as was done in the Drabick ruling.[31] Intimate caregivers seem most likely to embody, promote, and interpret the patient's mode of moral thought. Such caregivers, using either "rights-centered" or "communal" moral reasoning for their loved one, would be most familiar with relevant medical or social circumstances. On the one hand, they would be less inclined to inflate casual remarks about "not wanting to be maintained in a vegetable state" to profound moral assertions. On the other, they would be less inclined to depersonalize the patient to serve politicized views of the duties owed our most vulnerable citizens. A court could more easily assess the present suitability of proxies than it could determine the patient's hypothetical preference. This framework is entirely compatible with the concept of durable powers of attorney for health care. There is no compelling evidence that worthy social purposes are advanced by expropriating these decisions from intimate caregivers to cumbersome judicial or executive branch bureaucracies. It is disingenuous to symbolically protect these vulnerable persons by court ordered life-support which most people and their caregivers do not want. It is unreasonable to believe that bureaucratic reasoning will yield better judgments than intimate caregivers in tragic circumstances. Indeed, the arbitrariness of gender patterned reasoning and its effect on the outcomes of these cases amply illustrates the vicissitudes of institutional reasoning.

Such gender patterned reasoning may be relevant to the debate about legal medical abortions, as well. The question of whether restrictions on abortion essentially devalue women's moral judgments or are a life-affirming policy which only incidently intrudes on women is hugely complicated by the fact that women become pregnant and men do not. The controversies over abortion and end-of-life medical care are both about medical treatments. Both test the social scope allowed to personal choice in matters of ultimate cultural value. Both rest on many of the same legal and political arguments. Roe v. Wade is often cited in support of autonomy with regard to decisions about life-sustaining treatment. "Pro-life" laws figured prominently in Attorney General Webster's arguments to the Missouri Supreme Court and its decision ordering life-support for Nancy Cruzan over the objections of her family and a construction of Ms. Cruzan's views. We find that women are disadvantaged in having their moral agency taken less seriously than that of men when a controversial medical decision is evaluated by a court. If this is generally true, the gender pattern in the "right-to-die" cases is more than a peephole on a troubling, but small, set of court decisions. The gender pattern is a lens which can magnify our understanding of the interaction of gender and jurisprudence.

References

This paper is made possible by the Henry J. Kaiser Family Foundation which supports Dr. Miles as a faculty scholar in General Internal Medicine. We are grateful to Mary Becker, Lisa Disch, Howard Eglit, Elizabeth Helsinger, Kathryn Hunter, John Lantos, Rebekah Levin, Joanne Lynn, Leora Auslander, John Paris, Karen Rothenberg, Carol Stocking, the Workshop on Feminist Theory at the University of Chicago, and the Center for Advanced Feminist Studies at the University of Minnesota for critiques of drafts of this paper and to the Society for the Right to Die for assistance in obtaining legal documents.

1. Gender is the social understanding of sexual difference, not simply social roles or biological differences. This conceptual framework often contrasts qualities such as strong and weak, public and private, rational and expressive, or material and spiritual. These qualities, encoded as masculine or feminine, are the basis of rules that interpret the experience and delineate the possibilities for women and men. J. Scott, "On Language Gender, and Working Class History," *International Labor and Working Class History,* 31 (Spring 1987):3–7.

2. The two women were Elbaum (NY, 1989) and McConnell (CN, 1989). The other twelve women were Colyer (WA, 1983), Conroy (NJ, 1985), Corbett (FL, 1986), Cruzan (MO, 1988), Dinnerstein (MA, 1978), Jobes (NJ, 1987), Longeway (IL, 1989), Morrison (CA, 1988), O'Connor (NY, 1988), Quinlan (NJ, 1976), Rasmussen (AZ, 1986), and Severns (DL, 1980). The eight men were Brophy (MA, 1986), Drabick (CA, 1988), Delio (NY, 1987), Fox (NY, 1981), Gardner (ME, 1987), Spring (MA, 1980), Smith (NM, 1983) and Torres (MN, 1984). (See note 3 for full citations of all cases.)

3. We discuss all patient cases addressed by state appellate level courts considering a petition to forgo life-sustaining treatment. When a case was heard at several appellate levels, only the final ruling is used. In focusing on civil cases, we do not discuss the Barber decision dismissing murder charges against physicians who removed life-support from a permanently comatose man with the written consent of his wife and eight children (Barber v Superior Ct. 147 Cal. App. 3d 1006,195 Cal. Reptr. 484 [1983]). We do not discuss regulatory or licensing actions. Trial court rulings that are not heard by appellate courts are often not recorded and are thus incompletely sampled; we use such rulings only as illustrative footnotes. Two federal district court rulings involving incompetent adults are discussed in footnotes as with other trial court rulings. Jurisprudence about children substantially differs from that pertaining to adults and is not discussed. Throughout the paper cases are referred to by the patient's name, year, and state.

Previously Competent Persons without Written Advance Directives: *In re Brophy,* 497 N.E.2d 626 (Mass., 1986); *In re Colyer,* 660 P.2d 738 (Wash., 1983); *In re Conroy,* 486 A.2d 1209 (N.J., 1985); *Corbett v. D'Alessandro,* 487 So.2d 368 (Fla. App. 2d., 1986); *Cruzan v. Harmon v. McCanse,* 760 S. W. 2d 408 (MO.banc, 1988); *In re Delio,* 129 AD2d 1 (N.Y. Sup. Ct. 1986); *In re Dinnerstein,* 380 N.E.2d 134 (Mass., 1978); *In re Drabick,* 245 Cal. Rptr. 840 (Cal. App 6 Dist., 1988); *Elbaum v. Grace Plaza,* AD2d, 2503E, (N.Y. Sup Ct. App. 1989); *Fox* (See Storar); *In re Joseph v. Gardner,* 534 A.2d 947 (Me. 1987); *In re Jobes,* 529 A.2d 434 (N.J., 1987); *In re Longeway,* Docket 67318, Ag. 24, (Il. Supr. Ct.) Nov 13,1989; *McConnell v. Beverly Enterprises,* 553 Atl. Rptr, 2d 596 (CN, 1989); *In re Morrison,* 253 Cal Rptr, 530(1988); *In re O'Connor,* 531 N.E. 2d. 607 (N.Y., 1988); *In re Quinlan,* 355 A. 2d 647(1976); *Rasmussen v. Fleming,* 741 P.2d 674 (Ariz., 1987); *Smith v. Fort,* No. 14,768 (N.M. 1983); *Severns v. Wilmington Medical Center,* 421 A. 2d 1334 (Del. 1980); *In re Spring,* 405 N.E.2d 115 (1980); *In re Torres,* 357 N.W.2d 332 (Minn. 1986).

Persons with Written Advance Directives: *John F. Kennedy Memorial Hospital v. Bludworth,* 452 So. 2d 921 (FLA. 1984) [hereinafter called *Landy*]; *In re Peter,* 529 A.2d 419 (N.J., 1987); *In re Prange* (1988) 121 Ill. 2d 570.

Never Competent Persons: *In re Grant,* 747 P.2d 445 (Wash., 1987); *In re Hamlin,* 687 P.2d 1372 (Wash., 1984); *In re Hier,* 464 N.E.2d 959 (Mass., 1984); *Superintendent of Belchertown State School v. Saikewicz* 373 Mass. 728, 370 N.E.2d 417 (1976); *In re Storar,* N.Y. 420 N.E.2d 64, (1981) [hereinafter also called *Fox*].

State Trial Courts: *In re Bayer,* No. 4131 (N.D. Burleigh County Ct./Feb 5,11,1987; *Lydia E. Hall Hospital v. Cinque,* 116 Misc.2d 477,455 N.Y.S. 2d 706 (N.Y.Sup.Ct. 1982); *Evans v. Bellevue Hospital* No. 16536/87, (N.Y. Sup. Ct. July 27, 1987) [hereafter called *Wirth*]; *In re Julie Evans,* No. E82-2173 (OR Douglas County Ct., Dec. 13, 1982); *Foody v. Manchester Memorial Hospital,* 40 Conn. Supp. 127,482 A.2d 713 (1984); *Hazelton v. Powhattan Nursing Home,* No. (Chancery) 68287 6 Va. Cir., 414 (1986); *Leach v. Akron General Medical Center,* 68 Ohio Misc. 1,426 N.E.2d 809 (1980); *In re Saunders,* 129 Misc.2d 45,492 N.Y.S.2d 510 (N.Y. Sup. Ct. 1985); *Severns v. Wilmington Medical Center,* 425

A.2d 156 (Del.Ch.1980); *In re Visbeck,* 210 N.J. Super. 527, 510 A.2d 125 (Ch.Div.1986); *Vogel v. Forman,* 134 Misc.2d 395, 512 N.Y.S.2d 622 (N.Y.Sup.Ct. 1986); *In re Weinstein,* 136 Misc.2d 931, 519 N.Y.S.2d 511 (N.Y.Sup.Ct.1987); *Workmans Circle Home v. Fink,* 135 Misc 2d.270 (N.Y., 1987)[hereafter called *Siegel*].

    Federal Trial Courts: *Gray v. Romeo,* Civ A. No. 87-0573B (U.S. Dist Ct., Rhode Is., 1988); *Newman v. Beaumont* EP-86-CA-276 (U.S. Dist Ct., West Texas, 1985).

4. A rationale for this type of critique may be found in R. A. Posner, "The Decline of Law as an Autonomous Discipline." *Harvard Law Review* 1987; 100:761–780.

5. Several trial courts have constructed women's preferences. Gray (Fed, 1988) constructed a preference from the conduct of Ms. Gray's lifestyle (see note 10). In Leach (OH, 1980), a comatose woman with Lou Gehrig's disease was found to have a "clear and convincing" preference to forgo treatment after a court heard of numerous conversations with 17 family members and friends going up to two days before her cardiac arrest that she did not want to be placed on life support systems and maintained in a vegetative state. In Bayer, a North Dakota trial court (1987) accepted a construction of a woman's preference. See also Hazelton, note 16.

6. See also discussion of Newman (Fed, 1988), note 14.

7. In Elbaum (NY, 1989) an appellate court overturned a lower Court which had rejected numerous statements by Ms. Elbaum as "emotional" and not contemplative.

8. The appellate decisions address two men and four women health care workers: Mr. Brophy (paramedic), Mr. Delio (exercise physiologist), Ms. McConnell (nurse), Ms. O'Connor (hospital administrator), Ms. Peter (hospital secretary), and Ms. Rasmussen (chiropractor). Excepting Ms. Rasmussen whose family was not involved in the litigation, all of the families of these persons used the patient's familiarity with health care to buttress the proposal that the patient would not want life-support.

9. The 52-year old Mr. Storar is described and legally treated as an infant, not as a man.

10. In Julie Evans (OR, 1982), a trial court authorized removing a ventilator from a comatose woman on the concurrence of her husband, mother and physician without mentioning her wishes.

11. This test was applied to comatose Ms. Gray (Fed, 1988). Her husband and guardian convinced the court that her "thoughtful and deep" (based on her love of classical music and reading) personal life and the fact that she was "private," "shy," and "meticulous about her appearance" justified the belief that she would not want treatment.

12. A lower court had said that Gardner's remarks were of a "casual" and "general nature" even as they were incorporated into a treatment preference (ME, 1987).

13. In Gray (Fed, 1988), a judge accepted a constructed refusal for Ms. Gray who was characterized as being "required to submit" to medical care. The Missouri Supreme Court (1988) rejected the views of the American Academy of Neurology which described Ms. Cruzan as a "prisoner of medical technology" who should be freed.

14. A Federal trial court (Newman, 1985) referred to the vulnerability of a comatose woman as it rejected a construction of her preference based on a conversation with her husband.

15. The construction of man's treatment preference by the court configures his family as virtuous witnesses to his preferences rather than as surrogate decision-makers. For example, the court commended Ms. Brophy's long and agonizing research, reflection, prayer, and consultation that preceded her conclusion that her husband's "life is over" but it based the ruling on its construction of his views, not hers (MA, 1986). Similarly, Mr. Spring's close family was "best informed" and thus "reliable" as the court reached its "critical construction of the demented man's preference to stop dialysis" (MA, 1980). By contrast, as shown below, a woman's family's faithfulness, knowledge, and love justify making them responsible for decision about her care.

16. In Hazelton (1986), a Virginia trial court acknowledged that an incompetent woman dying of a brain tumor had clearly expressed a preference against the use of life-support. Nevertheless, it concluded that existing law did not mandate the novel construction of these views into a present preference. Under existing law, the spouse had the right to act on her behalf and was doing so in a manner consonant with her wishes. A trial court allowed the family to act in "good faith" to exercise Ms. Foody's right to refuse the respirator (see note 22).

17. New Mexico's Supreme Court similarly attempted to medicalize decisions about whether to terminate dialysis for a comatose, demented man whose family and physicians proposed that the patient would not have wanted the treatment. The resulting uproar led to new legislation (Smith, 1983).

18. Two trial courts have similarly ruled for women. In Evans (OR, 1982), a trial court authorized removing a respirator from a comatose terminally ill woman on the concurrence of her husband, mother and physician. In Weinstein (NY, 1987), a court affirmed a petition to stop treatment by a sister who strongly believed that the patient would not want surgery after it analyzed medical benefits and burdens.

19. See also New York's remarkable trial court readings of living wills in note 23.

20. The two 1989 decisions which first accepted constructed treatment preferences for women (McConnell, NY; Elbaum, NY) do not signal a change in that both had made specific comments. The other four most recent decisions rejected preference constructions for women and expropriated women from families in ways that have no analogue in cases about men (Cruzan, MO, 1988; Jobes, NJ, 1987; Longeway, IL, 1989; O'Conner, NY, 1988).

21. There is less than one chance in 200 that the ratio of two of 14 constructed treatment preferences for women is equivalent to the six of eight constructed preferences for men (Chi square # 8.12, df 1, p. ff.005).

22. In Foody (CN, 1984), the court found no evidence to construct the treatment preference of a 42-year-old woman with a 24-year course of multiple sclerosis culminating in coma. Ms. Foody had normal intellectual function during her long course of increasing disability. The court described her as "resigned to the acceptance of her affliction . . . and its inevitable consequences." Her parents testified, "she rarely cried and was known . . . to have only once verbalized a complaint, stating: 'I have eyes but cannot see, I have legs but cannot walk.' "

Similarly, in Visbeck (NJ, 1986), a "decent, thoughtful, caring son who is mindful of his obligation to what is best for his [90 year old] mother" was "not able to recall any expression of views by his mother on treatment issues."

23. There are three New York trial court decisions addressing advance directives. In Cinque, a trial court readily accepted a man's signed request to stop dialysis (NY, 1982). In Wirth, a court rejected a homosexual man's assignment of medical decision-making to a man whom he wished to interpret his living will (NY, 1987). The court said that doctors, not the patient's designated surrogate decision-maker, properly interpret the living will. This rejection of Mr. Wirth's own intent more closely resembles how courts handle women. In Saunders (NY, 1985), a trial court was asked to rule on the validity of living will for an emphysematous woman who was not on life-support but who wished to be assured of the document's validity. The court said that the document was an informed refusal of treatment that could be used in good faith by health care providers. Absent specific legislation, the document could not be seen as binding on health care providers.

24. See, e.g., C. Gilligan, *In a Different Voice.* Harvard University Press. Cambridge, 1982. C. Gilligan, "Adolescent Development Reconsidered." *New Directions for Child Development.,* ed. Damon, William No. 37, Fall, 1987. S. Sherry, "Civic Virtue and the Feminine Voice in Constitutional Adjudication." *Virginia Law Review* 72 (1986):543–616.

25. This distinction is made by modern Aristotelian ethicists who critique the conventional Kantian ethics. Examples include M. Nussbaum, *Fragility and Goodness,* Cambridge University Press, NY 1986; A. Jonsen, S. Toulmin, *The Abuse of Casuistry,* University of California Press, 1988; A. MacIntyre, *After Virtue,* University of Notre Dame Press, 1984; and N. Scheman, "Individualism and the Objects of Psychology," in *Discovering Reality: Feminists Perspectives on Epistemology, Metaphysics, Methodology, and Philosophy of Science.* Eds S. Harding and M. B. Hintika, 1983, D. Reidel Pub Co. p. 231. Sherry's review (id.) elegantly discusses this difference in terms of the tension between republican and rights based civic theories, Aristotelian ethics, and gender related moral psychology.

26. Gilligan (1987) p. 67; R. N. Bellah, R. Madsen, W. M. Sullivan, et al., *Habits of the Heart.* Univ. of Cal. Press, Berkeley, 1985.

27. Gilligan op. cit., p. 73. The reason for this correlation is disputed. Some believe that it is the result of negotiating and living collectively in a subordinate social position. Others suggest that it is innately related to sex differentiated experience of pregnancy, childbirth and breastfeeding (See J. C. Tronto, "Beyond Gender Difference to a Theory of Care," *Signs* 12 (Winter, 1987):644–663). R. West, "Jurisprudence and Gender," *Univ. Chicago Law Rev.* 55 (January, 1988): 1–72 also discusses this relationship in a rich theoretical work.

28. See Gilligan (1982); and also I. Marcus, P. J. Spiegelman, E. C. Dubois, et al., "Feminist Discourse, Moral Values and the Law—A Conversation" *Buffalo Law Review* 34 (1985):60. Tronto. op. cit., 131.

29. We do not believe the individual cases could be contested as sex discrimination without a pattern of egregious sex-differentiated handling of such cases by a single court.

30. This analysis is indebted to the conceptual analysis of harms in gender-patterned jurisprudence outlined by R. West, op. cit.

31. Rhoden profoundly criticizes constructed treatment preferences, which she calls a "subjective" test. She points out that they place such a heavy burden on family that they have the effect of disempowering family. N. K. Rhoden, "Litigating Life and Death," *Harvard Law Rev.* 102 (1988):375–404.

Marcus et al., op. cit. similarly explore the jurisprudential issues of inclusive solutions.

Chapter 28

The Torturer's Horse

Emily Friedman

Ms. Friedman is an independent health policy analyst.

When people have no coverage for health care costs and cannot afford to pay for care themselves, the inevitable happens. Health care becomes charity doled out sporadically by those providers who are moved to do so—and not all providers are so moved. However, the lack of access of the medically indigent is not absolute; they usually receive last-minute interventions in emergency departments and delivery rooms. Beyond that, pickings are slim; the eroding availability of nonemergency care in most urban public hospitals has erased even this haven of last resort. These institutions have been overwhelmed by the needs of critically ill and injured patients and pregnant women.

But I do not believe that payment problems are the only barriers that separate the uninsured poor from providers. The gulf that has opened between physicians and hospitals on one side, and vulnerable would-be patients on the other, has darker origins.

For one thing, medical indigence is a silent, largely invisible epidemic. The health status indicators of low-income Americans are poorer than those of their more advantaged fellow citizens,[1-5] but their mortality and morbidity are not newsworthy. Occasionally medical indigence roars into public consciousness, usually in the case of a needy young transplant candidate or a patient who has been "dumped" by a hospital. But for the most part,

it does not happen under the noses of those who provide health care or who formulate its policy.

Furthermore, the medically indigent traditionally have not been members of mainstream middle-class society and thus suffer from social and cultural bias. Indeed, I wonder if medical indigence has bred the outcast state of the uninsured, or whether their outcast state has produced their lack of insurance. If a chronically mentally ill, unbathed, untidy, homeless black man had lavish private insurance, would he be treated by any physician or hospital from whom he sought care? Or would their prejudices lead them to consign him elsewhere? This question remains hypothetical, because, conveniently, such "unattractive" nonmainstream individuals almost never have private coverage.

So, although there are corners where the middle-class provider meets the uninsured patient (the emergency department being the most common arena), most insured Americans do not knowingly associate with the uninsured. The low-income uninsured are not our problem; they are somebody else's problem. Medical indigence does not happen to "us"; it happens to "them." The standard (and inaccurate) image in the middle-class mind of the medically indigent is nonwhite welfare mothers (who in reality are eligible for Medicaid) or dope dealers who refuse to use their ill-gotten gains to pay for care (as it happens, dope dealers usually pay cash).

The poet W. H. Auden described this passing of haves and have-nots in the night in "Musee des Beaux Arts":

About suffering they were never wrong,
The Old Masters; how well they understood
Its human position; how it takes place

While someone else is eating or opening a window or
    just walking dully along . . .
They never forgot
That even the dreadful martyrdom must run its
course
Anyhow in a corner, some untidy spot
Where the dogs go on with their doggy life, and
    the torturer's horse
Scratches its innocent behind on a tree.

Most insured Americans are like the torturer's horse, minding their own business while somewhere, in another part of the forest, the uninsured poor suffer. Some of this is the product of ignorance, but some of it is the product of bigotry. The poor, the nonwhite, the homeless, the oddball, the mad, and (increasingly) the very elderly are simply not considered as valuable as the white, employed, middle-class stereotype of American privilege.

This "us and them" syndrome underlying medical indigence is far more serious than it might appear, for the noncoverage of the uninsured poor and their resultant lack of access affect every American. As long as these vulnerable people are subject to the whims and prejudices of payers, providers, and society, we are all at risk.

We are at risk of disease and injury, because untreated and undetected conditions can spread or produce secondary effects. The untreated mentally ill, for example, time and again bring destruction on themselves and others. How many people have been killed or injured by mentally ill assailants armed with guns? It also seems likely, from the epidemiologic history of the acquired immunodeficiency syndrome, that if the illness had first struck the heterosexual middle class, rather than those who are social outcasts to some degree, its threat would have been confronted earlier.

Today, other diseases may be patiently waiting for their chance. They will probably strike the uninsured, the unimmunized, and the untreated first, for, as Constance Conrad, MD,[6] has observed, "Morbidity and mortality are not randomly distributed." Socioeconomic and racial differences in infant mortality, cancer mortality, and other health indicators reinforce this observation.[1-5,7-8] But viruses and microbes are no observers of social barriers; they may come for the rest of us, in time.

We are also at risk of further hampering American productivity and competitiveness as the work force includes more and more uninsured workers. Such employees are more likely to miss work, to lose jobs, to spend time at home with sick family members, and to spread what ails them to fellow employees. A recent federal study found that 12.8% of those working full-time and 23% of those working part-time in early 1987 were uninsured.[9] Part-time work is among the fastest-growing US employment sectors. Private coverage of dependents of working Americans is also declining.[10]

Furthermore, 47.7% of the working uninsured are employed in settings with 25 or fewer workers.[9] The self-employed (23.1% of whom are uninsured[9]) and others seeking individual policies are eligible only for a few expensive plans, most of which require extensive testing of the candidate to ensure that he or she does not actually need the insurance. In this age of the small business, this seems a strange way to encourage entrepreneurialism in the world marketplace.

We are also at risk because those found to be "uninsurable" due to past or current health problems or test results often cannot obtain affordable coverage at all.[11] Many individuals who are sick or in danger of becoming so are forced to remain in their current jobs or places of residence, fearful that if they change their circumstances, they will not be able to obtain insurance.

We hear announcements of potential genetic and other tests for latent alcoholism, predisposition to cancer, or hypertension. Some insurers have proposed testing not only individual applicants, but also members of small groups of employees.[11] As individuals subject to these risks are identified and denied coverage, medical indigence will grow. Already, the number of Americans with private coverage of hospital costs is dropping at the rate of 1 million a year.[12]

We are at risk of forgetting a basic rule: most fabrics unravel at the edges first. In dismissing the medically indigent as though they belong to another species, we dismiss the fact that the barrier between us and them is movable—and that it is moving closer to the rest of us all the time.

We have jeopardized ourselves because we have insisted on incorporating "us and them" thinking into our health policy. We have embraced the fallacy of the words written on the wall of a building in southern Texas in an area spared from the fury of the 1988 hurricane: "GILBERT IS A WIMP." Hurricane Gilbert left nearly 300 people dead, destroyed an area of Mexico, spawned destructive tornadoes in San Antonio, Tex, and left 500 000 Jamaicans without a place to live. But the person who wrote on the wall looked only at his or her neighborhood and saw no further.

The solution is obvious, however complex the logistics of effecting it may seem. Either all Americans must have reasonable coverage for the cost of appropriate health care, or physicians, hospitals, and other providers must be reasonably reimbursed for most of the care they provide to the uninsured. The problem is far too large to be solved by voluntary provider charity alone, although such charity will always be important. I prefer coverage to provider reimbursement, because it gives the patient more options and erases the stigma of charity that will otherwise continue to plague the uninsured.[13] Some analysts have proposed extension of Medicaid and Medicare; others have proposed universal coverage; still others prefer an incremental approach, beginning with mandated employer-based coverage of working Americans.

The emerging policy debate will center on whether funding should be public, private, or a mix; what services should be covered; and whether funding should go to coverage or to provider payment. What we do not need at this point is further discussion of whether the problem is serious, whether the uninsured poor are sufficiently "deserving," or whether the nation can "afford" to cover them. A nation that can afford nearly 1 million cesarean sections, more than a quarter million coronary artery bypass grafts, and a 25% annual increase in cosmetic surgery can afford basic care for everyone. Besides, we are not saving money by swelling the ranks of the medically indigent; they represent an enormous cost that we all pay. Almost any solution would be cheaper than last-minute care for those in extremis, provided in costly hospital settings.

The medically indigent also represent the risk of moral rot at the heart of our society, born of a callousness about those whose suffering we cannot see and therefore do not acknowledge. Bruce Bronzan (D, Calif), a state legislator, addressing the issue of access and justice, spoke last year of a comedian he had seen who ended his act with a serious statement: "Not to be loved is sad—but not to love is truly tragic."

Similarly, Representative Bronzan said, a society that forces its most vulnerable and needy members to beg for crumbs of care, or to go without care until they are dying, harms itself even more than it harms the victims of this cruelty. As writer Ron Dorfman observed, in another context: "We can have strangers in our midst, or we can have neighbors."[14] Should we continue to treat the most fragile members of our society as strangers, we will not be acting like the torturer's horse; we will be the torturers.

References

1. Woolhandler S, Himmelstein DU. Reverse targeting of preventive care due to lack of health insurance. *JAMA.* 1988;259:2872–2874.

2. Satariano WA, Belle SH, Swanson GM. The severity of breast cancer at diagnosis: a comparison of age and extent of disease in black and white women. *Am J Public Health.* 1986;76:779–782.

3. Bassett MT, Krieger N. Social class and black-white differences in breast cancer survival. *Am J Public Health.* 1986;76:1400–1403.

4. Wissow LS, Gittelsohn AM, Szklo M, Starfield B, Mussman M. Poverty, race, and hospitalization for childhood asthma. *Am J Public Health.* 1988;78:777–782.

5. Wise PH, Kotelchuck M, Wilson ML, Mills MA. Racial and socioeconomic disparities in childhood mortality in Boston. *N Engl J Med.* 1985;313:360–366.

6. Conrad C. When science doesn't support what we know. Presented at the Annual Meeting of the American Public Health Association; October 1, 1986; Las Vegas, Nev.

7. Hughes D, Johnson K, Rosenbaum S, Simons J, Butler E. *The Health of America's Children.* Washington, DC: Children's Defense Fund; 1988:3–12.

8. American Cancer Society Subcommittee on Cancer in the Economically Disadvantaged. *Cancer in the Economically Disadvantaged.* New York, NY: American Cancer Society; 1986.

9. Short PF, Monheit A, Beauregard K. Uninsured Americans: a 1987 profile. Presented at the Annual Meeting of the American Public Health Association; November 16, 1988; Boston, Mass.

10. Schur CL, Taylor AK. Choice of health insurance and the two-worker household. Presented at the Annual Meeting of the American Public Health Association; November 16, 1988; Boston, Mass.

11. Friedman E. Are risk pools being oversold as a solution? *Hospitals.* 1988;62:100–104.

12. *Source Book of Health Insurance Data: 1988 Update.* Washington, DC: Health Insurance Association of America; 1988:2–3.

13. Blendon RJ, Aiken LH, Freeman HE, Kirkman-Liff BL, Murphy JW. Uncompensated care by hospitals or public insurance for the poor: does it make a difference? *N Engl J Med.* 1986;314:1160–1163.

14. Dorfman R. The news media and the new nativism. *Quill.* 1986;74:14–15.

Other Titles on *Ethics*